CONTRIBUTORS

Sheryl Sommer, PhD, RN, CNE
VP Nursing Education & Strategy

Janean Johnson, MSN, RN
Nursing Education Strategist

Sherry L. Roper, PhD, RN
Nursing Education Strategist

Karin Roberts, PhD, MSN, RN, CNE
Nursing Education Coordinator

Mendy G. McMichael, DNP, MSN, RN
Nursing Education Specialist and
Content Project Coordinator

Marsha S. Barlow, MSN, RN
Nursing Education Specialist

Judy Drumm, DSN, RN, CPN
Nursing Education Specialist

Mary Jane Janowski, RN, MA
Nursing Technical Writer

Norma Jean Henry, MSN/Ed, RN
Nursing Education Specialist

Audrey Knippa, MS, MPH, RN, CNE
Nursing Education Coordinator

Pamela Roland, MSN, RN
Nursing Education Specialist

EDITORIAL AND PUBLISHING

Derek Prater
Spring Lenox
Michelle Renner
Mandy Tallmadge
Kelly Von Lunen

CONSULTANTS

Tracey Bousquet, MSN, BSN, RN
Pam DeMoss, MSN, RN
Virginia E. Tufano, EdD, MSN, RN
Loraine White, RN, BSN, RN

Intellectual Property Notice

ATI Nursing is a division of Assessment Technologies Institute®, LLC

Important Notice to the Reader

User's Guide

Welcome to the Assessment Technologies Institute® PN Pharmacology Nursing Review Module Edition 6.0. The mission of ATI's Content Mastery Series® review modules is to provide user-friendly compendiums of nursing knowledge that will:

- Help you locate important information quickly.

- Assist in your learning efforts.

- Provide exercises for applying your nursing knowledge.

- Facilitate your entry into the nursing profession as a newly licensed PN.

Organization

This review module is organized into units covering pharmacological principles (Unit 1) and medications affecting the body systems and physiological processes (Units 2 to 12). Chapters within these units conform to one of two organizing principles for presenting the content:

- Nursing concepts

- Medications

Nursing concepts chapters begin with an overview describing the central concept and its relevance to nursing. Subordinate themes are covered in outline form to demonstrate relationships and present the information in a clear, succinct manner.

Medications chapters include an overview describing a disorder or group of disorders. Medications used to treat these disorders are grouped according to classification. A specific medication may be selected as a prototype or example of the characteristics of medications in this classification. These sections include information about how the medication works, its therapeutic uses, and routes of administration. Next, you will find information about how complications, contraindications, and medication and food interactions, as well as nursing interventions and client education to help prevent and/or manage these issues. Finally, the chapter includes information on nursing administration of the medication and evaluation of the medication's effectiveness.

Application Exercises

Questions are provided at the end of each chapter so you can practice applying your knowledge. The Application Exercises include NCLEX-style questions, such as multiple-choice and multiple-select items, and questions that ask you to apply your knowledge in other formats, such as by using an ATI Active Learning Template. After the Application Exercises, an answer key is provided, along with rationales for the answers.

NCLEX® Connections

To prepare for the NCLEX-PN, it is important for you to understand how the content in this review module is connected to the NCLEX-PN test plan. You can find information on the detailed test plan at the National Council of State Boards of Nursing's Web site: https://www.ncsbn.org/. When reviewing content in this review module, regularly ask yourself, "How does this content fit into the test plan, and what types of questions related to this content should I expect?"

To help you in this process, we've included NCLEX Connections at the beginning of each unit and with each question in the Application Exercises Answer Keys. The NCLEX Connections at the beginning of each unit will point out areas of the detailed test plan that relate to the content within that unit. The NCLEX Connections attached to the Application Exercises Answer Keys will demonstrate how each exercise fits within the detailed content outline.

These NCLEX Connections will help you understand how the detailed content outline is organized, starting with major client needs categories and subcategories and followed by related content areas and tasks. The major client needs categories are:

- Safe and Effective Care Environment
  - Coordinated Care
  - Safety and Infection Control
- Health Promotion and Maintenance
- Psychosocial Integrity
- Physiological Integrity
  - Basic Care and Comfort
  - Pharmacological Therapies
  - Reduction of Risk Potential
  - Physiological Adaptation

An NCLEX Connection might, for example, alert you that content within a unit is related to:

- Pharmacological and Parenteral Therapies
  - Adverse Effects/Contraindications/Side Effects/Interactions
    - Identify a contraindication to the administration of a medication to the client.

QSEN Competencies

As you use the review modules, you will note the integration of the Quality and Safety Education for Nurses (QSEN) competencies throughout the chapters. These competencies are integral components of the curriculum of many nursing programs in the United States and prepare you to provide safe, high-quality care as a newly licensed PN. Icons appear to draw your attention to the six QSEN competencies:

- Safety: The minimization of risk factors that could cause injury or harm while promoting quality care and maintaining a secure environment for clients, self, and others.
- Patient-Centered Care: The provision of caring and compassionate, culturally sensitive care that addresses clients' physiological, psychological, sociological, spiritual, and cultural needs, preferences, and values.

- Evidence-Based Practice: The use of current knowledge from research and other credible sources, on which to base clinical judgment and client care.
- Informatics: The use of information technology as a communication and information-gathering tool that supports clinical decision-making and scientifically based nursing practice.
- Quality Improvement: Care related and organizational processes that involve the development and implementation of a plan to improve health care services and better meet clients' needs.
- Teamwork and Collaboration: The delivery of client care in partnership with multidisciplinary members of the health care team to achieve continuity of care and positive client outcomes.

Icons

Icons are used throughout the review module to draw your attention to particular areas. Keep an eye out for these icons:

 This icon is used for NCLEX connections.

 This icon is used for content related to safety and is a QSEN competency. When you see this icon, take note of safety concerns or steps that nurses can take to ensure client safety and a safe environment.

 This icon is a QSEN competency that indicates the importance of a holistic approach to providing care.

 This icon, a QSEN competency, points out the integration of research into clinical practice.

 This icon is a QSEN competency and highlights the use of information technology to support nursing practice.

 This icon is used to focus on the QSEN competency of integrating planning processes to meet clients' needs.

 This icon highlights the QSEN competency of care delivery using an interprofessional approach.

 This icon indicates that a media supplement, such as a graphic, animation, or video, is available. If you have an electronic copy of the review module, this icon will appear alongside clickable links to media supplements. If you have a hardcopy version of the review module, visit www.atitesting. com for details on how to access these features.

Feedback

ATI welcomes feedback regarding this review module. Please provide comments to: comments@atitesting.com.

TABLE OF CONTENTS

UNIT 1   ## Pharmacological Principles

CHAPTERS

› Pharmacokinetics and Routes of Administration
› Safe Medication Administration and Error Reduction
› Dosage Calculation
› Intravenous Therapy
› Adverse Effects, Interactions, and Contraindications

NCLEX® CONNECTIONS

When reviewing the chapters in this unit, keep in mind the relevant sections of the NCLEX® outline, in particular:

Client Needs: Safety and Infection Control

› Relevant topics/tasks include:

» Accident/Error/Injury Prevention

› Identify client allergies and intervene as appropriate.

› Evaluate the appropriateness of a health care provider order for the client.

» Reporting of Incident/Event/Irregular Occurrence/Variance

› Identify situations requiring completion of incident/event/irregular occurrence/variance report (medication administration error, client fall).

› Acknowledge and document practice error.

Client Needs: Pharmacological Therapies

› Relevant topics/tasks include:

» Adverse Effects/Contraindications/Side Effects/ Interactions

› Identify a contraindication to the administration of prescribed or over-the-counter medication to the client.

» Dosage Calculation

› Perform calculations needed for medication administration.

» Medication Administration

› Follow the rights of medication administration.

› Collect required client data prior to medication administration.

› Calculate and monitor intravenous (IV) flow rate.

chapter 1

Overview

- Pharmacokinetics refers to how medications travel through the body. Medications undergo a variety of biochemical processes that result in absorption, distribution, metabolism, and excretion.

Phases of Pharmacokinetics

- Absorption is the transmission of medications from the location of administration (gastrointestinal [GI] tract, muscle, skin, or subcutaneous tissue) to the bloodstream. The most common routes of administration are enteral (through the GI tract) and parenteral (by injection). Each of these routes has a unique pattern of absorption.
  - The rate of medication absorption determines how soon the medication will take effect.
  - The amount of medication absorbed determines its intensity.
  - The route of administration affects the rate and amount of absorption.

ROUTE	BARRIERS TO ABSORPTION	ABSORPTION PATTERN
Oral	› Medications must pass through the layer of epithelial cells that line the GI tract.	› Varies greatly due to the following variables: » Stability and solubility of the medication » GI pH and emptying time » Presence of food in the stomach or intestines » Other medications currently being administered » Forms of medications (enteric-coated pills, liquids)
Sublingual/buccal	› Gastric pH can inactivate medication if swallowed before it dissolves.	› Absorbed quickly systemically through highly vascular mucous membrane
Other mucous membranes (e.g., rectal, vaginal)	› Presence of stool in rectum or infectious material in vagina limits tissue contact.	› Easily absorbed with both local and systemic effects
Inhalation via mouth or nose	› Inspiratory effort.	› Rapidly absorbed through alveolar capillary network
Intradermal/topical	› Epidermal cells closely packed.	› Absorption slow and gradual › Effects primarily local, but systemic as well, especially with lipid-soluble medications passing through subcutaneous fatty tissue

ROUTE	BARRIERS TO ABSORPTION	ABSORPTION PATTERN

Subcutaneous and intramuscular	› Capillary wall has large spaces between cells, so there is no significant barrier.	› Rate of absorption is determined by:
		» Solubility of the medication in water
		  › Highly soluble medications will be absorbed in 10 to 30 min.
		  › Poorly soluble medications will be absorbed more slowly.
		» Blood perfusion at the site of injection
		  › Sites with high blood perfusion (e.g., mucous membranes) have rapid absorption.
		  › Sites with low blood perfusion (e.g., skin) have slow absorption.

IV	› No barriers.	› Immediate – administered directly into blood › Complete – all of it reaches the blood

- Distribution is the transportation of medications to sites of action by bodily fluids. Distribution can be influenced by the ability to:
  - Travel to the site of action through the bloodstream. (Peripheral vascular or cardiac disease can delay medication distribution.)
  - Leave the bloodstream by traveling between the capillaries' cells.
    - Plasma protein binding: Medications compete for protein-binding sites within the bloodstream, primarily albumin. The ability of a medication to bind to a protein can affect how much of the medication will leave and travel to target tissues. Two medications can compete for the same binding sites, resulting in either toxicity or decreased bioavailability.
    - Barriers: Medications that are lipid-soluble or have a transport system can cross the blood-brain barrier or the placenta.
- Metabolism (biotransformation) changes medications into less active or inactive forms by the action of enzymes. This occurs primarily in the liver, but it also takes place in the kidneys, lungs, bowel, and blood.
  - Factors influencing the rate of medication metabolism
    - Age – Infants have limited medication-metabolizing capacity. The aging process also can influence medication metabolism, but it varies by individual. In general, hepatic medication metabolism tends to decline with age.
    - An increase in certain medication-metabolizing enzymes – This can metabolize a particular medication sooner, requiring an increase in dosage of that medication to maintain a therapeutic level. It also can cause an increase in the metabolism of other medications that are being used concurrently.
    - First-pass effect – Some oral medications are inactivated on their first pass through the liver and can require a higher dose to achieve a therapeutic effect, or must be given by a nonenteral route because of their high first-pass effect. These medications usually are given by alternate routes, such as sublingual or IV.

- Similar metabolic pathways – When two medications are metabolized by the same pathway, they can interfere with the metabolism of one or both of the medications. In this way, the rate of metabolism can decrease for one or both of the medications, leading to medication accumulation.
- Nutritional status – A malnourished client can be deficient in the factors that are necessary to produce specific medication-metabolizing enzymes, consequently impairing medication metabolism.

- Outcomes of metabolism
  - Increased renal excretion of medication
  - Inactivation of medications
  - Increased therapeutic effect
  - Activation of pro-medications (also called pro-drugs) into active forms
  - Decreased toxicity when active forms of medications are converted to inactive forms
  - Increased toxicity when inactive forms of medications are converted to active forms

- Excretion is the elimination of medications from the body, primarily through the kidneys. Elimination also takes place through the liver, lungs, bowel, and exocrine glands. Renal dysfunction can lead to an increase in duration and intensity of medication response, so BUN and creatinine levels should be monitored.

- Medication responses – Plasma medication levels can be regulated to control medication responses. Medication dosing attempts to maintain plasma levels between the minimum effective concentration (MEC) and the toxic concentration. A plasma medication level is in the therapeutic range when it is effective and not toxic. Therapeutic levels are well established for many medications; use these levels to monitor a client's response.

- Therapeutic index (TI) – Medications with a high TI have a wide safety margin. Therefore, there is no need for routine serum medication level monitoring. Medications with a low TI require close monitoring of serum medication levels. Monitor peak levels based on the route of administration. For example, an oral medication might have a peak of 1 to 3 hr after administration. If the medication is given IV, the peak time might occur within 10 min. (*Refer to a drug reference or pharmacist for specific medication peak times.*) For trough levels, blood is drawn immediately before the next medication dose regardless of the route of administration.

- Half-life (t½) refers to the period of time needed for the medication to be reduced by 50% in the body. Liver and kidney function can affect half-life. It usually takes four half-lives to achieve a steady state of serum concentration (medication intake = medication metabolism and excretion).

SHORT HALF-LIFE	LONG HALF-LIFE
› Medications leave the body quickly (4 to 8 hr).	› Medications leave the body more slowly (24+ hr). There is a greater risk for medication accumulation and toxicity.
› Short-dosing interval or minimum effective concentration (MEC) will drop between doses.	› Medications are given at longer intervals without loss of therapeutic effects.
	› Medications take a longer time to reach a steady state.

- Pharmacodynamics (mechanism of action) describes the interactions between medications and target cells, body systems, and organs to produce effects. These interactions result in functional changes that are the mechanism of action of the medication. Medications interact with cells in one of two ways.

  ○ An agonist is a medication that can mimic the receptor activity regulated by endogenous compounds. For example, morphine is classified as an agonist because it activates the receptors that produce analgesia, sedation, constipation, and other effects.

  ○ An antagonist is a medication that can block normal receptor activity regulated by endogenous compounds or receptor activity caused by other medications. For example, losartan (Cozaar), an angiotensin II receptor blocker, is classified as an antagonist. Losartan works by blocking angiotensin II receptors on blood vessels, which prevents vasoconstriction.

  ○ Partial agonists can act as an agonist/antagonist and have limited affinity to receptor sites. For example, nalbuphine acts as an antagonist at mu receptors and an agonist at kappa receptors, causing analgesia with minimal respiratory depression at low doses.

Routes of Administration

NURSING IMPLICATIONS BY ROUTE OF ADMINISTRATION
Oral or enteral (tablets, capsules, liquids, suspensions, elixirs)

› Contraindications for administration include vomiting, absence of gag reflex, difficulty swallowing, and decreased level of consciousness.	› In general, administer on an empty stomach (1 hr before meals, 2 hr after meals). However, some should be administered with food.
› Have client sitting upright, in Fowler's position, unless contraindicated, to facilitate swallowing.	› Follow manufacturer's directions for crushing, cutting, and diluting medication. A complete list can be found at the Institute for Safe Medication Practice's website (www.ismp.org).
› Administer irritating medication with small amounts of food.	
› Do not mix with large amounts of food or beverages in case the client is unable to consume the entire quantity.	› Enteric-coated or time-release medication must be swallowed whole to prevent faster absorption.
› Avoid administration with contraindicated foods or beverages such as grapefruit juice.	› Use liquid form of medication to facilitate swallowing whenever possible.

Sublingual (under the tongue) and buccal (between the cheek and the gum)	
› Instruct the client to keep the medication in place until it is absorbed.	› The client should not eat or drink while the tablet is in place.

Liquids, suspensions, elixirs	
› Follow directions for dilution and mixing.	› The base of the meniscus (lowest fluid line) is at the level of the desired dose.

Transdermal (medication stored in a skin patch and absorbed through the skin)	
› Instructions to client should include the following: » Apply patches as provided to ensure proper dosing. » Wash skin with soap and water, and dry thoroughly before applying new patch.	» Place patch on a hairless area of the skin, and rotate sites to prevent skin irritation. Verify removal of previous patch before applying new one.

NURSING IMPLICATIONS BY ROUTE OF ADMINISTRATION

Topical

› Apply with a glove, tongue blade, or cotton-tipped applicator.

› Never apply with a bare hand.

Instillation (drops, ointments, sprays; generally used for eyes, ears, and nose)

› Eyes
  » Use surgical aseptic technique when instilling medication.
  » Have the client sit upright or lie supine with the head tilted slightly and looking up at ceiling.
  » Rest dominant hand on the client's forehead, hold dropper above conjunctival sac approximately 1 to 2 cm, drop medication into center of sac, and have client close eye gently.
  » Apply gentle pressure with finger and a clean tissue on nasolacrimal duct for 30 to 60 seconds to prevent systemic absorption of medication.
› Ears
  » Use medical aseptic technique when administering medication.
  » Have the client sit upright or maintain side-lying position.

  » Straighten ear canal by pulling auricle upward and outward for adults, or down and back for children. Hold dropper 1 cm above ear canal, instill medication, and then gently apply pressure with finger to tragus of the ear.
› Nose
  » Use medical aseptic technique when administering medication.
  » Place client supine with head positioned to allow medication to enter appropriate nasal passage.
  » Use dominant hand to instill drops, supporting head with nondominant hand. Hold end of the dropper about 1.5 cm above nostril.
  » Instruct the client to breathe through mouth, stay in a supine position, and avoid blowing nose for 5 min after instillation.

Nasogastric and gastrostomy tubes

› Check for proper tube placement.
› Use syringe, and allow medication to flow in by gravity, or gently push plunger of syringe to promote flow.
› General guidelines
  » Do not give sublingual medications through the tube; give them under the tongue.
  » Do not crush specially prepared oral medications (extended/time-release, fluid-filled, enteric-coated).

  » Use liquid forms of medications.
  » Check compatibility of medications before mixing.
  » Do not mix medications with enteral feedings.
  » Administer medications one at a time.
› To prevent clogging, flush tubing before and after each medication with at least 15 mL warm sterile water. When administration of medications is complete, flush with at least 15 mL warm sterile water.

Suppositories

› Follow manufacturer's directions for storage.
› Wear gloves for procedure.
› Remove foil wrapper, and lubricate suppository if necessary.
› Rectal suppositories
  » Position client in left lateral position.
  » Insert just beyond internal sphincter.
  » Instruct client to retain medication 20 to 30 min for stimulation of defecation and 60 min for systemic absorption.

› Vaginal suppositories
  » Position client supine with knees bent, and feet flat on the bed and close to hips (modified lithotomy position).
  » Suppositories generally are inserted with an applicator.
  » Instruct the client to remain in position for a prescribed amount of time.

NURSING IMPLICATIONS BY ROUTE OF ADMINISTRATION

Inhalation (medications usually administered through metered-dose inhalers [MDI] or dry-powder inhalers [DPI])

› For an MDI, instruct the client to:
  » Remove cap from inhaler.
  » Shake inhaler five to six times.
  » Hold inhaler with mouthpiece at the bottom.
  » Hold inhaler with thumb near mouthpiece and index and middle fingers at top.
  » Hold inhaler approximately 2 to 4 cm (1 to 2 in) away from front of mouth.
  » Take a deep breath, and then exhale.
  » Tilt head back slightly, and press inhaler. While pressing inhaler, begin a slow, deep breath that should last for 3 to 5 seconds to facilitate delivery to the air passages.
  » Hold breath for 10 seconds to allow medication to deposit in airways.
  » Take inhaler out of mouth, and slowly exhale through pursed lips.
  » Resume normal breathing.

› A spacer can be used to keep medication in device longer, thereby increasing amount of medication delivered to the lungs and decreasing amount of the medication in the oropharynx. If a spacer is used, instruct the client to:
  » Remove covers from mouthpieces of inhaler and spacer.
  » Insert MDI into the end of the spacer.

  » Shake inhaler five to six times.
  » Exhale completely, and then close mouth around spacer mouthpiece. Continue as with an MDI.

› For a DPI, instruct the client to:
  » Avoid shaking device.
  » Take the cover off the mouthpiece.
  » Follow directions of manufacturer for preparing medication, such as turning wheel of inhaler.
  » Exhale completely.
  » Place mouthpiece between lips, and take a deep breath through mouth.
  » Hold breath for 5 to 10 seconds.
  » Take inhaler out of mouth, and slowly exhale through pursed lips.
  » Resume normal breathing.
  » If more than one puff is prescribed, wait length of time directed before administering second puff.
  » Remove canister, and rinse inhaler, cap, and spacer once a day with warm running water, and dry completely before using again.

Parenteral

› General considerations for parenteral medications
  » Vastus lateralis site is usually recommended for infants and children younger than 2 years of age.
  » After age 2, the ventrogluteal site can be used. It accommodates 2 to 5 mL of fluid in adults. The deltoid site has smaller muscle mass and can accommodate only up to 2 mL of fluid.
  » Use needle size and length appropriate for type of injection and client size. Syringe size should approximate volume of medication.

  » Use tuberculin syringe for solution volume less than 0.5 mL.
  » Rotate injection sites to enhance medication absorption, and document each site used.
  » Do not use injection sites that are edematous, inflamed, or have moles, birthmarks, or scars.
  » If caring for a client who has received IV medication, monitor for therapeutic and adverse effects.
  » Discard all sharps (broken ampules, bottles, needles) in designated containers. Containers should be leak- and puncture-proof.

NURSING IMPLICATIONS BY ROUTE OF ADMINISTRATION

Intradermal

› Usually used for tuberculin testing or checking for medication/allergy sensitivities.
› Can be used for some cancer immunotherapy.

› Use small amounts of solution (0.01 to 0.1 mL) in tuberculin syringe with fine-gauge needle (26- to 27-gauge) in lightly pigmented, thin-skinned, hairless sites (inner surface of mid-forearm or scapular area of back) at a 5° to 15° angle with bevel up.

Subcutaneous

› Appropriate for small doses of nonirritating, water-soluble medications and is commonly used for insulin and heparin.
› Sites are selected for adequate fat-pad size (abdomen, upper hips, lateral upper arms, thighs).

› Use 3/8- to 5/8-inch, 25- to 27-gauge needle, or insulin syringe of 28- to 31-gauge. Inject no more than 1.5 mL of solution. For average-size client, pinch up skin, and inject at 45° to 90° angle. For obese client, use 90° angle.

Intramuscular

› Appropriate for irritating medications, solutions in oils, and aqueous suspensions.
› Common sites include ventrogluteal, deltoid, and vastus lateralis (pediatric). Dorsogluteal site is not recommended due to its proximity to sciatic nerve.

› Use needle size 18 to 27 (usually 22- to 25-gauge), 1 to 1½ inches long, and inject at 90° angle. Volume injected is usually 1 to 3 mL. If greater amount is required, divide into two syringes and use two sites.

Z-Track

› Type of IM injection that prevents medication from leaking back into subcutaneous tissue.

› Often used for medications that cause visible and/or permanent skin stains, such as certain iron preparations.

IV

› Appropriate for administration of medications, fluid, and blood products.
› Vascular access devices can be for short-term use (catheters) or long-term use (infusion ports).

› If caring for a client who has received IV medications, monitor for therapeutic and adverse effects.

Epidural

› Appropriate for administration of opioid analgesia (morphine [Duramorph] or fentanyl) via infusion pumps.

› A catheter is advanced through a needle that is inserted into epidural space at the level of fourth or fifth vertebrae.

 View Video: Sites for Medication Administration

ROUTE	ADVANTAGES	DISADVANTAGES
Oral	› Safe, inexpensive, easy, and convenient.	› Highly variable absorption. › Inactivation can occur by GI tract or first-pass effect. › Client must be cooperative, conscious, and have an intact gag reflex. › Contraindications include nausea and vomiting.
Subcutaneous and IM	› For medications that are poorly absorbed or cannot be absorbed by the GI tract. › Appropriate for administering medications that are meant for slow absorption for extended period of time (depot preparations).	› IM injections are associated with higher cost. › IM injections are inconvenient for client due to need to remove clothing. They can be difficult for client or family to administer. › Pain with the risk for local tissue damage and nerve damage. › Risk for infection at the injection site.
IV	› Onset is rapid, and absorption into the blood is immediate, which provides immediate response. › Allows control over the precise amount of medication administered. › Allows for administration of large volumes of fluid. › Irritating medications can be administered with free-flowing IV fluid.	› Associated with an even higher cost. › More inconvenient due to the degree of technical skill required, and might not always be successful. Client's activity can be limited. › Immediate absorption of medication into blood can be potentially dangerous if wrong amount, or the wrong medication, is administered. › Increased risk for infection or embolism.

APPLICATION EXERCISES

1. A client is prescribed phenobarbital (Luminal) for a seizure disorder. The medication has a long half-life of 4 days. Based on this half-life, the medication most likely will be prescribed

    A. once a day.

    B. twice a day.

    C. three times a day.

    D. four times a day.

2. A nurse educator is reviewing medication dosages and factors that influence medication metabolism with a group of nurses. Medication dosages can need to be decreased for which of the following reasons? (Select all that apply.)

    _____ A. Increased renal excretion

    _____ B. Increased medication-metabolizing enzymes

    _____ C. Liver failure

    _____ D. Peripheral vascular disease

    _____ E. Concurrent use of medication metabolized by the same pathway

3. A nurse is preparing to administer eye drops to a client. Which of the following are appropriate nursing interventions related to this procedure? (Select all that apply.)

    _____ A. Using medical aseptic technique

    _____ B. Asking the client to look up at the ceiling

    _____ C. Having the client lie in a side-lying position

    _____ D. Dropping medication into the center of the client's conjunctival sac

    _____ E. Instructing the client to close the eye gently

4. A nurse is reinforcing discharge teaching with a client who has a new prescription for a transdermal medication. Which of the following statements by the client indicates understanding of the teaching?

    A. "I will clean the site with an alcohol swab prior to applying the patch."

    B. "I will rotate the application sites weekly."

    C. "I will apply the patch to an area of skin with no hair."

    D. "I will place the new patch on the site of the old patch."

5. A nurse is reviewing a client's health record and notes a new prescription by the provider to verify the trough level of the client's medication. Which of the following actions should the nurse take?

    A. Have a blood specimen obtained immediately prior to the next dose of medication.

    B. Verify that the client has received the medication for 24 hr before obtaining a blood specimen.

    C. Ask the client to provide a urine specimen after the next dose of medication.

    D. Begin administering the medication, and obtain a blood specimen.

6. A nurse is reviewing with a client a new prescription for a medication to take via metered-dose inhaler (MDI) with a spacer. What instructions should the nurse reinforce with the client? Use the ATI Active Learning Template: Medication to complete this item to include the following:

    A. Indications: Identify the medication absorption pattern and a barrier to absorption.

    B. Client Education: Describe the steps for using an MDI with a spacer.

APPLICATION EXERCISES KEY

1. A. **CORRECT:** Medications with long half-lives remain at their therapeutic levels between doses for long periods of time. This medication can be administered once a day.

   B. INCORRECT: Medications with long half-lives remain at their therapeutic levels between doses for long periods of time. It is unlikely this medication will be prescribed twice a day.

   C. INCORRECT: Medications with long half-lives remain at their therapeutic levels between doses for long periods of time. It is unlikely this medication will be prescribed three times a day.

   D. INCORRECT: Medications with long half-lives remain at their therapeutic levels between doses for long periods of time. It is unlikely this medication will be prescribed four times a day.

   (N) NCLEX® Connection: Pharmacological Therapies, Expected Actions/Outcomes

2. A. INCORRECT: Increased renal excretion can decrease concentration of the medication, requiring an increased dosage.

   B. INCORRECT: Increased medication-metabolizing enzymes can decrease the concentration of the medication. This can require increasing the dosage of the medication.

   C. **CORRECT:** Liver failure can decrease metabolism and thus increase the concentration of a medication. This can require decreasing the dosage of medication.

   D. INCORRECT: Peripheral vascular disease can impair distribution, thus requiring more of the medication.

   E. **CORRECT:** When two medications are metabolized in the same way, they can compete for metabolism, thereby increasing the concentration of one or both medications. This can require decreasing the dosage of one or both medications.

   (N) NCLEX® Connection: Pharmacological Therapies, Adverse Effects/Contraindications/ Side Effects/Interactions

3. A. INCORRECT: Surgical aseptic technique is used to administer eye drops.

   B. **CORRECT:** The client should look up at the ceiling to avoid the drop falling on the cornea and increasing intraocular pressure.

   C. INCORRECT: The client should sit or lie supine to facilitate proper administration of eye drops.

   D. **CORRECT:** The nurse should drop the medication into the center of the conjunctival sac to promote distribution.

   E. **CORRECT:** The client should close the eye gently to allow improved distribution of the medication.

   (N) NCLEX® Connection: Pharmacological Therapies, Medication Administration

4. A. **INCORRECT:** The skin should be washed with soap and water and dried thoroughly before applying a transdermal medication.

    B. **INCORRECT:** Application sites should be rotated on a daily basis to prevent skin irritation.

    C. **CORRECT:** Transdermal medication should be applied to a hairless area of skin to promote absorption of the medication.

    D. **INCORRECT:** Application sites should be rotated on a daily basis to prevent skin irritation.

    Ⓝ NCLEX® Connection: Pharmacological Therapies, Medication Administration

5. A. **CORRECT:** To verify trough levels of a medication, a blood specimen is obtained immediately before the next dose of medication.

    B. **INCORRECT:** Trough levels are based on the time the medication is administered, not how long a client has been receiving a medication.

    C. **INCORRECT:** Trough levels are based on monitoring serum medication levels, not urine levels.

    D. **INCORRECT:** Trough levels are obtained immediately prior to medication administration, not with or after medication administration.

    Ⓝ NCLEX® Connection: Pharmacological Therapies, Medication Administration

6. *Using the ATI Active Learning Template: Medication*

    A. Indications

    - Medication Absorption Pattern: Rapidly absorbed through the alveolar capillary network
    - Barrier to Absorption: Inadequate respiratory effort

    B. Client Education

    - Remove cap from mouthpieces of inhaler and end of the spacer.
    - Insert the MDI into the end of the spacer.
    - Shake the inhaler/spacer five or six times.
    - Exhale completely, and close the mouth around the spacer mouthpiece.
    - Hold the inhaler with the thumb near the mouthpiece and index and middle fingers at the top.
    - Tilt the head back slightly, and depress the inhaler. While depressing the inhaler, begin a slow deep breath that should last 3 to 5 seconds.
    - Hold breath for 10 seconds.
    - Remove the mouthpiece, and slowly exhale through pursed lips.
    - Resume normal breathing.

    Ⓝ NCLEX® Connection: Pharmacological Therapies, Medication Administration

chapter **2**

Overview

- The providers who are legally permitted to write prescriptions in the United States include physicians, advanced practice nurses, dentists, and physician assistants. These providers are responsible for:
  - Obtaining the client's medical history and physical examination.
  - Diagnosing.
  - Prescribing medications.
  - Monitoring the response to therapy.
  - Modifying medication prescriptions as necessary.

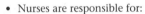

- Nurses are responsible for:
  - Having knowledge of federal, state (nurse practice act), and local laws, and health care facility policies that govern the prescribing, dispensing, and administration of medications.
  - Preparing, administering, and evaluating client responses to medications.
  - Developing and maintaining an up-to-date knowledge base of medications administered, including uses, mechanisms of action, routes of administration, safe dosage range, side effects, adverse responses, precautions, and contraindications.
  - Maintaining acceptable practice and skill competency.
  - Determining accuracy of medication prescriptions.
  - Reporting all medication errors.
  - Safeguarding and storing medications.

Medication Category and Classification

- Nomenclature
  - Chemical name is the name of the medication that specifies its chemical composition.
  - Generic name is the official or nonproprietary name that is given by the United States Adopted Names Council. Each medication has only one generic name.
  - Trade name is the brand or proprietary name given by the company that manufactures the medication. One medication can have multiple trade names.

- Prescription medications are administered under the supervision of providers. Some medications can be habit-forming or have potential harmful effects and require more stringent supervision.

  ○ Uncontrolled substances require monitoring by a provider, but do not pose a risk of abuse and/or addiction. Antibiotics are an example of uncontrolled prescription medications.

  ○ Controlled substances have a potential for abuse and dependence and are categorized into schedules. Heroin is a medication in Schedule I and has no medical use in the United States. Medications categorized in Schedules II through V have approved applications. Each level has a decreasing risk of abuse and dependence. For example, morphine (Duramorph) is a Schedule II medication that has a greater risk of abuse and dependence than phenobarbital (Luminal), which is a Schedule IV medication.

  ○ New medications in development undergo rigorous testing procedures established by the Food and Drug Administration (FDA) to determine both effectiveness and safety before approval. However, newly released drugs can have previously unreported adverse effects that, if observed, nurses can report online at www.fda.gov/medwatch.

KNOWLEDGE REQUIRED PRIOR TO MEDICATION ADMINISTRATION	
Medication category/class	› Medications are organized according to pharmacological action, therapeutic use, body system, chemical composition, and safe use during pregnancy. » For example, lisinopril (Zestril) is an angiotensin-converting enzyme inhibitor (pharmacological action) and an antihypertensive (therapeutic use).
Mechanism of action	› This is how the medication produces the desired therapeutic effect. » For example, glipizide (Glucotrol) is an oral hypoglycemic agent that lowers blood glucose levels primarily by stimulating pancreatic islet cells to release insulin.
Therapeutic effect	› This is the preferred and expected effect for which the medication is administered to a specific client. One medication can have more than one therapeutic effect. » For example, one client receives acetaminophen (Tylenol) to lower fever, whereas another client receives it to relieve pain.
Side effects	› These are usually expected and inevitable at a therapeutic dose. » For example, morphine given for pain relief usually results in constipation. Side effects are usually identified according to body system.
Adverse effects	› These are undesired, inadvertent, and unexpected dangerous effects of the medication. Adverse effects usually are identified according to body system. » For example, the antibiotic gentamicin can cause hearing impairment.
Toxic effects	› Medications can have specific risks and manifestations of toxicity. » For example, a client taking digoxin (Lanoxin) should be monitored closely for dysrhythmias, a sign of cardiotoxicity. Hypokalemia places this client at greater risk for digoxin toxicity.

KNOWLEDGE REQUIRED PRIOR TO MEDICATION ADMINISTRATION	
Medication interactions	› Medications can interact with each other, resulting in desired or undesired effects. » For example, a desired interaction results from giving the beta-blocker atenolol (Tenormin) concurrently with the calcium channel blocker nifedipine (Procardia) to prevent reflex tachycardia. » An example of an undesired interaction is prescribing omeprazole (Prilosec) is concurrently with phenytoin (Dilantin). This can increase the serum level of the anticonvulsant. › Obtain a complete medication history, and be knowledgeable of clinically significant interactions.
Precautions/ Contraindications	› A specific disease or condition can be a contraindication for a particular medication. » For example, tetracycline can stain developing teeth and should not be administered to children under 8 years of age. › Some medications should only be used cautiously. » For example, vancomycin (Vancocin) is excreted unchanged in the kidneys and requires caution in a client who has renal impairment.
Preparation, dosage, administration	› It is important to know any special considerations for preparation, recommended dosages, and how to administer the medication. » For example, morphine is available in several formulations. Oral doses of morphine are generally higher than parenteral doses due to extensive first-pass effect. Clients who have chronic, severe pain, as with cancer, generally are given oral doses of morphine.
Nursing implications	› Know how to monitor therapeutic effects, prevent and treat adverse effects, provide for comfort, and instruct client in the safe use of medications.

Medication Prescriptions

- Each facility has written policies related to medication prescriptions. Policies include which providers can write, receive, and transcribe medication prescriptions.

- Types of Medication Prescriptions
  - Routine/standing prescription
    - A routine/standing prescription identifies medications to give on a regular schedule. It can have a termination date. Without a specified termination date, the prescription will be in effect until the provider discontinues it or the client is discharged.
    - Certain medications such as opioids and antibiotics must be represcribed within a specified amount of time or will automatically be discontinued.
  - Single/one-time prescription
    - A single/one-time prescription specifies giving a medication once at a specified time or as soon as possible. For example, a one-time prescription instructs the nurse to administer warfarin (Coumadin) 5 mg PO at 1700.

- Stat prescription

  - A stat prescription specifies giving a medication only once, and immediately. For example, a stat prescription instructs the nurse to administer digoxin 0.125 mg IV bolus stat.

- PRN prescription

  - A PRN prescription stipulates at what dosage, what frequency, and under what conditions a medication can be given. The nurse uses clinical judgment to determine the client's need for the medication. For example, a PRN prescription instructs the nurse to administer morphine sulfate 2 mg intermittent IV bolus every 1 hr PRN for pain.

- Components of a Prescription

  - The client's name

  - Date and time of prescription

  - Name of medication (can be generic or trade, depending on policy)

  - Dosage of medication

  - Route of administration

  - Time and frequency of medication administration – exact times or number of times per day (dictated by facility policy or specific qualities of the medication)

  - Signature of prescribing provider

- Communicating Medication Prescriptions

  - Origination of medication prescriptions

    - Medication prescriptions are written in the client's health record by the provider or a nurse who takes a verbal or telephone prescription from a provider. If the nurse writes a medication prescription in the client's health record, facility policy specifies how much time the provider has in which to sign the prescription (usually 24 hr). Medication prescriptions are transcribed or entered electronically into the medication administration record (MAR) by a nurse or other provider.

  - Receiving a telephone prescription

    - If possible, have a second nurse listen on an extension.

    - Ensure that the prescription is complete and correct by reading back to the provider: the client's name, name of the medication, dosage, time of administration, frequency, and route.

    - Remind the provider that the prescription must be signed within the specified amount of time.

    - Enter the prescription in the client's health record.

- Medication Reconciliation

  - The Joint Commission requires policies and procedures for medication reconciliation. The nurse should compile a list of all current medications, with correct dosages and frequency. This list should be compared with new prescriptions and reconciled to resolve any discrepancies. This becomes the current list from which medications should be administered. This process should take place on admission, when transferring between units or facilities, and at discharge.

Data Collection Prior to Medication Therapy

- The following information should be obtained prior to the initiation of medication therapy, and updated as necessary.
  - ○ Health History
    - Age
    - Diagnosed health problems and current reason for seeking care
    - All medications currently being taken (prescription and nonprescription): name, dose, route, and frequency of each medication
    - Any adverse and side effects possibly related to medication therapy, as well as therapeutic effects
    - Use of herbal or natural products for medicinal purposes
    - Use of caffeine, tobacco, alcohol, and/or street drugs

    - Client's understanding of the purpose of the medications along with the client's beliefs, feelings, and concerns
    - All known medication and food allergies
  - ○ Physical Examination
    - A systemic physical examination provides a baseline for evaluating therapeutic effects of medication therapy and detecting possible side and adverse medication effects.

Six Rights of Safe Medication Administration

- Right Client
  - ○ Verify the client's identification each time a medication is given. The Joint Commission requires using two client identifiers when administering medications.
    - Acceptable identifiers include the client's name, an assigned identification number, telephone number, birth date, or another person-specific identifier.
    - Check identification bands for name, identification number, and/or photograph.
    - Check for allergies by asking the client, looking for an allergy bracelet, and reviewing the medication administration record.
    - Bar code scanners can be used to identify clients.
- Right Medication
  - ○ Correctly interpret the medication prescription (verify completeness and clarity).
    - Read the label three times: when selecting the container, removing the dose from container, and replacing the container.
    - Leave unit-dose medication in its package until administration.
    - With automated medication dispensing systems, the same checks are required and can be adapted.
- Right Dose
  - ○ Calculate the correct medication dose, and have a second qualified nurse check the calculations.
  - ○ Check a drug reference to ensure the dose is within the usual range.

- Right Time
  - Administer medication on time to maintain a consistent therapeutic blood level.
    - It is generally acceptable to administer the medication 30 min before or after the scheduled time. However, refer to the drug reference or institution policy for exceptions.
- Right Route
  - The most common routes of administration are oral, topical, subcutaneous, IM, and IV.
  - Select the correct preparation for the prescribed route (for example, otic versus ophthalmic topical ointment or drops).
  - Know how to administer medication safely and correctly.
- Right Documentation
  - Immediately record medication, dose, route, time, and any pertinent information, including the client's response to the medication.
  - For some medications, in particular those to alleviate pain, evaluate and document the client's response later, perhaps after 30 min.

 View Video: Safe Administration of Medications

Additional Considerations

- Data collection
  - Collect appropriate data before administering medication (for example, check apical heart rate before giving digitalis preparations). Identify physical and psychosocial factors that can affect medication response.

- Education
  - As part of informed consent, provide accurate information about the medication therapy and its implications (therapeutic response, side and adverse effects). To individualize the instructions, determine what the client already knows, needs to know, and wants to know about the medication.
- Evaluation
  - Determine the effectiveness of the medication based on the client's response, as well as the occurrence of side and adverse effects.
- Medication Refusal
  - Clients have the right to refuse to take a medication. Determine the reason for refusal, provide information regarding the risk of refusal, notify the appropriate health care personnel, and document refusal and actions taken.

Medication Error Prevention

- Common Medication Errors
  - Wrong medication or IV fluid
  - Incorrect dose or IV rate
  - Wrong client, route, or time

- ○ Administration of known allergic medication
- ○ Omission of dose
- ○ Incorrect discontinuation of medication or IV fluid
- • Use the nursing process to prevent medication errors
  - ○ Data Collection
    - ▪ Ensure knowledge of the medication to be administered. Use appropriate resources.
      - □ Providers, including nurses, physicians, and pharmacists
      - □ Poison control centers
      - □ Sales representatives from drug companies
      - □ Nursing pharmacology textbooks and drug handbooks
      - □ *Physicians' Desk Reference*
      - □ Newsletters including *The Medical Letter on Drugs and Therapeutics* (bimonthly)
      - □ Professional journals
      - □ Professional websites
    - ▪ Obtain information about the client's medical diagnoses and conditions related to medication administration, such as ability to swallow; allergies; and heart, liver, and kidney disorders.
      - □ Identify client allergies.
      - □ Obtain necessary preadministration data (heart rate, blood pressure).
      - □ Omit or delay doses as indicated by the client's condition.
    - ▪ Determine whether the medication prescription is complete – to include name of client, date and time, name of medication, dosage, route of administration, time, frequency, and signature of prescribing provider.
    - ▪ Interpret the medication prescription accurately.
      - □ The Institute for Safe Medication Practices is a nonprofit organization working to educate providers and consumers regarding safe medication practices. Tools have been developed to decrease the risk of medication errors. Go to www.ismp.org for a complete list.
        - ▸ Error-Prone Abbreviation List – abbreviations that have been associated with a high number of medication errors
        - ▸ Confused Medication Name List – soundalike and lookalike medication names
        - ▸ High-Alert Medication List – medications that, if given in error, have a high risk for resulting in significant harm
    - ▪ Question the provider if the prescription is unclear or seems inappropriate for the client's condition. Refuse to administer a medication if it is thought to be unsafe. Notify the charge nurse or supervisor.
    - ▪ Dosage changes are usually made gradually. Question the provider if abrupt and excessive changes in dosages are made.
  - ○ Planning
    - ▪ Identify client outcomes for medication administration.
    - ▪ Set priorities.

○ Implementation

- Avoid distractions during medication preparation (poor lighting, ringing phones). Interruptions can increase the risk of error.

- Check the labels for the medication name and concentration. Read labels carefully. Measure doses accurately, and double-check high-alert medications, such as insulin and heparin, with a colleague.

- Doses are usually one to two tablets, or one single-dose vial. Question multiple tablets or vials for a single dose.

- Follow the Six Rights of Medication Administration consistently. Take the MAR to the bedside.

- Do not administer medications that someone else prepared.

- Encourage clients to become part of the safety net, informing them about medications and the importance of proper identification before medications are administered. Omit or delay a dose if the client questions the size of a dose or appearance of a medication.

- Follow correct procedures for all routes of administration.

- Communicate clearly both verbally and in writing.

- Use verbal prescriptions only for emergencies, and follow facility protocol for telephone prescriptions.

- Omit or delay doses as indicated by the client's condition, and document and report appropriately.

- Follow all laws and regulations regarding controlled substances when preparing and administering medications. Keep controlled substances in a locked area. Discarding of an excess of a controlled substance should be witnessed by another licensed provider.

- Only leave medication at the bedside if allowed by facility policy (for example, topical medication).

○ Evaluation

- Evaluate client response to a medication, and document and report appropriately.

- Recognize side and adverse effects, and document and report appropriately.

- Report all errors, and implement corrective measures immediately.

  □ Complete an unusual occurrence report within the specified time frame, usually 24 hr. This report should include:

    ▸ The client's identification.

    ▸ The name and dose of the medication.

    ▸ The time and place of the incident.

    ▸ An accurate and objective account of the event.

    ▸ Who was notified.

    ▸ What actions were taken.

    ▸ The signature of the person completing the report.

  □ This report does not become a part of the client's permanent record, and the report should not be referenced in another part of the record.

APPLICATION EXERCISES

1. A nurse is preparing a client's medications. Which of the following are legal responsibilities of the nurse? (Select all that apply.)

_____ A. Maintaining skill competency

_____ B. Determining the dosage

_____ C. Monitoring for adverse effects

_____ D. Safeguarding medications

_____ E. Identifying the client's diagnosis

2. A nurse is reviewing a client's health record and notes a new prescription by the provider for lisinopril (Zestril) 10 mg PO every day. The nurse should recognize this as which of the following types of prescription?

A. Single prescription

B. Stat prescription

C. Routine prescription

D. PRN prescription

3. A nurse is reviewing a new prescription for ondansetron (Zofran) 4 mg PO PRN nausea and vomiting for a client who has hyperemesis gravidarum. The nurse should clarify which of the following parts of the prescription with the provider?

A. Name

B. Dosage

C. Route

D. Time

4. A newly hired nurse asks another nurse about how to accept a telephone prescription. Which of the following statements by the newly hired nurse indicates understanding of the discussion?

A. "A second nurse enters the prescription into the client's health record."

B. "Another nurse should listen to the phone call."

C. "The provider can clarify the prescription when he signs the health record."

D. "The 'read back' is omitted if this is a one-time prescription."

5. A nurse on a medical unit is collecting data from a client before administration of medications. Which of the following data should the nurse include? (Select all that apply.)

_____ A. Use of herbal teas

_____ B. Daily fluid intake

_____ C. Current health status

_____ D. Previous surgical history

_____ E. Food allergies

6. A nurse educator is reviewing prevention of medication errors with a group of newly hired nurses. What actions can nurses take based on the use of nursing process to prevent medication errors? Use the ATI Active Learning Template: Basic Concept to complete this item to include the following:

A. Nursing Interventions: Using the Underlying Principle of nursing process to prevent medication errors, describe:
   - Three data-collection actions.
   - One planning action.
   - Four implementation actions.
   - Three evaluation actions.

APPLICATION EXERCISES KEY

1. A. **CORRECT:** Maintaining skill competency and using appropriate administration technique are legal responsibilities of the nurse.

    B. INCORRECT: Determining medication dosage is the responsibility of the provider.

    C. **CORRECT:** A nurse is legally responsible for monitoring for side and adverse effects of medications.

    D. **CORRECT:** Safeguarding of medications, such as controlled substances, is a legal responsibility of the nurse.

    E. INCORRECT: A nurse should be aware of a client's diagnosis, but identifying a diagnosis is the role of the provider.

    Ⓝ NCLEX® Connection: Pharmacological Therapies, Medication Administration

2. A. INCORRECT: A single prescription is for a medication to be given once at a specified time or as soon as possible.

    B. INCORRECT: A stat prescription is for a medication only given once, and immediately.

    C. **CORRECT:** A routine prescription identifies a medication that is given on a regular schedule. This medication is administered every day until discontinued.

    D. INCORRECT: A PRN prescription specifies giving a medication only when a client needs it, for example, for pain relief.

    Ⓝ NCLEX® Connection: Pharmacological Therapies, Medication Administration

3. A. INCORRECT: The generic and trade name are included in the prescription.

    B. INCORRECT: The dosage of 4 mg is included in the prescription.

    C. INCORRECT: The route is identified as oral in the prescription.

    D. **CORRECT:** The time or frequency of medication administration is not included and should be clarified with the provider.

    Ⓝ NCLEX® Connection: Safety and Infection Control, Accident/Error/Injury Prevention

4. A. INCORRECT: The nurse who receives the telephone prescription should enter it into the client's health record to prevent errors in translation.

   B. **CORRECT:** A second nurse should listen to a telephone prescription to prevent errors in communication.

   C. INCORRECT: The nurse verifies that the prescription is complete and accurate at the time it is received by reading it back to the provider.

   D. INCORRECT: A telephone prescription includes reading back all types of medication prescriptions.

   Ⓝ NCLEX® Connection: Pharmacological Therapies, Medication Administration

5. A. **CORRECT:** Use of herbal products, which often contain caffeine, is important to determine prior to medication administration because caffeine can affect medication biotransformation.

   B. INCORRECT: Daily fluid intake is important, but it is not part of data collection prior to medication administration.

   C. **CORRECT:** Current health status should be reviewed because new prescriptions can cause alterations in current health status.

   D. INCORRECT: Surgical history is important, but it is not part of data collection prior to medication administration.

   E. **CORRECT:** Food allergies should be included in data collection prior to medication administration to identify any potential interactions.

   Ⓝ NCLEX® Connection: Pharmacological Therapies, Medication Administration

6. *Using the ATI Active Learning Template: Basic Concept*

A. Nursing Interventions
- Data Collection
  - Use appropriate resources to ensure adequate knowledge of the medication.
  - Have information about the client's diagnosis and conditions.
  - Verify the medication prescription is complete.
  - Interpret prescription accurately.
  - Clarify concerns regarding accuracy of the prescription and appropriate use for client.
  - Determine whether dosage changes are appropriate.
- Planning
  - Identify client outcomes for medication administration.
  - Determine priorities.
- Implementation
  - Avoid being distracted during medication preparation.
  - Verify labels for medication accuracy, dosages, alerts, and following facility protocol.
  - Question unusual quantities.
  - Follow the Six Rights of Medication Administration.
  - Do not give medications others prepare.
  - Encourage the client's participation in knowing about medications and their administration.
  - Follow correct procedure for administration.
  - Use verbal prescriptions only in an emergency, and follow telephone protocol per facility.
  - Follow laws and regulations regarding controlled substances.
  - Follow facility policy regarding medications allowed to remain at the bedside.
- Evaluation
  - Evaluate the client's response to medication, document, and report.
  - Recognize side and adverse effects, document, and report.
  - Report errors and implement corrective actions immediately.

Ⓝ NCLEX® Connection: Pharmacological Therapies, Medication Administration

chapter 3

Overview

- Basic medication dose conversion and calculation skills are essential for the provision of safe nursing care.
- Nurses are responsible for administering the correct amount of medication by calculating the appropriate amount of medication to give. Types of calculations include:
  - Solid oral medication
  - Liquid oral medication
  - Injectable medication
  - Correct dose based on the client's weight
  - IV infusion
- Nurses can use three different methods for dosage calculation. These are ratio and proportion, desired over have, and dimensional analysis.
- Standard conversion factors include:
  - 1 mg = 1,000 mcg
  - 1 g = 1,000 mg
  - 1 kg = 1,000 g
  - 1 oz = 30 mL
  - 1 L = 1,000 mL
  - 1 tsp = 5 mL
  - 1 tbsp = 15 mL
  - 1 tbsp = 3 tsp
  - 1 kg = 2.2 lb
  - 1 gr = 60 mg
- General Rounding Guidelines
  - Rounding up: If the number to the right is equal to or greater than 5, round up by adding 1 to the number on the left.
  - Rounding down: If the number to the right is less than 5, round down by dropping the number, leaving the number to the left as is.
  - For dosages less than 1.0, round to the nearest hundredth.
    - For example (rounding up): 0.746 mL = 0.75 mL. The calculated dose is 0.746 mL. Look at the number in the thousandths place (6). Six is greater than 5. To round to hundredths, add 1 to 4 in the hundredths place and drop the 6. The rounded dose is 0.75 mL.
    - Or (rounding down): 0.743 mL = 0.74 mL. The calculated dose is 0.743 mL. Look at the number in the thousandths place (3). Three is less than 5. To round to the hundredth, drop the 3 and leave the 4 as is. The rounded dose is 0.74 mL.

○ For dosages greater than 1.0, round to the nearest tenth.

- For example (rounding up): 1.38 = 1.4. The calculated dose is 1.38 mg. Look at the number in the hundredths place (8). Eight is greater than 5. To round to the tenth, add 1 to the 3 in the tenth place and drop the 8. The rounded dose is 1.4 mg.

- Or (rounding down): 1.34 mL = 1.3 mL. The calculated dose is 1.34 mL. Look at the number in the hundredths place (4). Four is less than 5. To round to the tenth, drop the 4 and leave the 3 as is. The rounded dose is 1.3 mL.

SOLID DOSAGE

Example: A nurse is preparing to administer phenytoin (Dilantin) 0.2 g PO every 8 hr. The amount available is phenytoin 100 mg/capsule. How many capsules should the nurse administer per dose? (Round the answer to the nearest whole number.)

Using Ratio and Proportion

STEP 1: *What is the unit of measurement to calculate?*
capsule

STEP 2: *What is the dose needed? Dose needed = Desired.*
0.2 g

STEP 3: *What is the dose available? Dose available = Have.*
100 mg

STEP 4: *Should the nurse convert the units of measurement?*
Yes (g ≠ mg)
Equivalents:
1 g = 1,000 mg (1 x 1,000)
0.2 g = 200 mg (0.2 x 1,000)

STEP 5: *What is the quantity of the dose available?*
1 capsule

STEP 6: *Set up an equation and solve for X.*

$$\frac{Have}{Quantity} = \frac{Desired}{X}$$

$$\frac{100\ mg}{1\ capsule} \times \frac{200\ mg}{X\ capsule(s)}$$

X = 2

STEP 7: *Round if necessary.*

STEP 8: *Reassess to determine whether the amount to give makes sense.*
If there are 100 mg capsules and the prescribed amount is 0.2 g (200 mg), it makes sense to give 2 capsules. The nurse should administer phenytoin 2 capsules PO every 8 hr.

Using Desired Over Have

STEP 1: *What is the unit of measurement to calculate?*
capsule

STEP 2: *What is the dose needed? Dose needed = Desired.*
0.2 g

STEP 3: *What is the dose available? Dose available = Have.*
100 mg

STEP 4: *Should the nurse convert the units of measurement?*
Yes (g ≠ mg)
Equivalents:
1 g = 1,000 mg (1 x 1,000)
0.2 g = 200 mg (0.2 x 1,000)

STEP 5: *What is the quantity of the dose available?*
1 capsule

STEP 6: *Set up an equation and solve for X.*

$$\frac{Desired \times Quantity}{Have} = X$$

$$\frac{200\ mg \times 1\ capsule}{100\ mg} = X\ capsule(s)$$

2 = X

STEP 7: *Round if necessary.*

STEP 8: *Reassess to determine whether the amount to give makes sense.*
If there are 100 mg capsules and the prescribed amount is 0.2 g (200 mg), it makes sense to give 2 capsules. The nurse should administer phenytoin 2 capsules PO every 8 hr.

Using Dimensional Analysis

STEP 1: *What is the unit of measurement to calculate?*
capsule

STEP 2: *What quantity of the dose is available?*
1 capsule

STEP 3: *What is the dose available? Dose available = Have.*
100 mg

STEP 4: *What is the dose needed? Dose needed = Desired.*
0.2 g

STEP 5: *Should the nurse convert the units of measurement?*
Yes (g ≠ mg)
1,000 mg = 1 g

STEP 6: *Set up an equation and solve for X.*

$$X = \frac{Quantity}{Have} \times \frac{Conversion\ (Have)}{Conversion\ (Desired)} \times \frac{Desired}{}$$

$$X\ capsule(s) = \frac{1\ capsule}{100\ mg} \times \frac{1,000\ mg}{1\ g} \times \frac{0.2\ g}{}$$

X = 2

STEP 7: *Round if necessary.*

STEP 8: *Reassess to determine whether the amount to give makes sense.*
If there are 100 mg capsules and the prescribed amount is 0.2 g (200 mg), it makes sense to give 2 capsules. The nurse should administer phenytoin 2 capsules PO every 8 hr.

LIQUID DOSAGE

Example: A nurse is preparing to administer erythromycin estolate 0.25 g PO every 6 hr. The amount available is erythromycin estolate oral suspension 250 mg/mL. How many mL should the nurse administer per dose? (Round the answer to the nearest whole number.)

Using Ratio and Proportion

STEP 1: *What is the unit of measurement to calculate?*
mL

STEP 2: *What is the dose needed? Dose needed = Desired.*
0.25 g

STEP 3: *What is the dose available? Dose available = Have.*
250 mg

STEP 4: *Should the nurse convert the units of measurement?*
Yes (g ≠ mg)
Equivalents:
1 g = 1,000 mg (1 x 1,000)
0.25 g = 250 mg (0.25 x 1,000)

STEP 5: *What is the quantity of the dose available?*
1 mL

STEP 6: *Set up an equation and solve for X.*

$$\frac{Have}{Quantity} = \frac{Desired}{X}$$

$$\frac{250\ mg}{1\ mL} = \frac{250\ mg}{X\ mL}$$

X = 1

STEP 7: *Round if necessary.*

STEP 8: *Reassess to determine whether the amount to give makes sense.*
If there are 250 mg/mL and the prescribed amount is 0.25 g (250 mg), it makes sense to administer 1 mL. The nurse should administer erythromycin estolate oral suspension 1 mL PO every 6 hr.

Using Desired Over Have

STEP 1: *What is the unit of measurement to calculate?*
mL

STEP 2: *What is the dose needed? Dose needed = Desired.*
0.25 g

STEP 3: *What is the dose available? Dose available = Have.*
250 mg

STEP 4: *Should the nurse convert the units of measurement?*
Yes (g ≠ mg)
Equivalents:
1 g = 1,000 mg (1 x 1,000)
0.25 g = 250 mg (0.25 x 1,000)

STEP 5: *What is the quantity of the dose available?*
1 mL

STEP 6: *Set up an equation and solve for X.*

$$\frac{Desired \times Quantity}{Have} = X$$

$$\frac{250 \ mg \times 1 \ mL}{250 \ mg} = X \ mL$$

1 = X

STEP 7: *Round if necessary.*

STEP 8: *Reassess to determine whether the amount to give makes sense.*
If there are 250 mg/mL and the prescribed amount is 0.25 g (250 mg), it makes sense to administer 1 mL. The nurse should administer erythromycin estolate oral suspension 1 mL PO every 6 hr.

Using Dimensional Analysis

STEP 1: *What is the unit of measurement to calculate?*
mL

STEP 2: *What quantity of the dose is available?*
1 mL

STEP 3: *What is the dose available? Dose available = Have.*
250 mg

STEP 4: *What is the dose needed? Dose needed = Desired.*
0.25 g

STEP 5: *Should the nurse convert the units of measurement?*
Yes (g ≠ mg)

$$\frac{1,000 \ mg}{1 \ g}$$

STEP 6: *Set up an equation and solve for X.*

$$X = \frac{Quantity}{Have} \times \frac{Conversion \ (Have)}{Conversion \ (Desired)} \times \frac{Desired}{}$$

$$X \ mL = \frac{1 \ mL}{250 \ mg} \times \frac{1,000 \ mg}{1 \ g} \times \frac{0.25 \ g}{}$$

X = 1

STEP 7: *Round if necessary.*

STEP 8: *Reassess to determine whether the amount administer makes sense.*
If there are 250 mg/mL and the prescribed amount is 0.25 g (250 mg), it makes sense to administer 1 mL. The nurse should administer erythromycin estolate oral suspension 1 mL PO every 6 hr.

INJECTABLE DOSAGE

Example: A nurse is preparing to administer heparin 8,000 units subcutaneously every 8 hr. The amount available is heparin injection 10,000 units/mL. How many mL should the nurse administer per dose? (Round the answer to the nearest tenth.)

Using Ratio and Proportion

STEP 1: *What is the unit of measurement to calculate?*
mL

STEP 2: *What is the dose needed? Dose needed = Desired.*
8,000 units

STEP 3: *What is the dose available? Dose available = Have.*
10,000 units

STEP 4: *Should the nurse convert the units of measurement?*
No

STEP 5: *What is the quantity of the dose available?*
1 mL

STEP 6: *Set up an equation and solve for X.*

$$\frac{\text{Have}}{\text{Quantity}} = \frac{\text{Desired}}{\text{X}}$$

$$\frac{10,000 \text{ units}}{1 \text{ mL}} = \frac{8,000 \text{ units}}{\text{X mL}}$$

X = 0.8

STEP 7: *Round if necessary.*

STEP 8: *Reassess to determine whether the amount to administer makes sense.*
If there are 10,000 units/mL and the prescribed amount is 8,000 units, it makes sense to administer 0.8 mL. The nurse should administer heparin injection 0.8 mL subcutaneously every 8 hr.

Using Desired Over Have

STEP 1: *What is the unit of measurement to calculate?*
mL

STEP 2: *What is the dose needed? Dose needed = Desired.*
8,000 units

STEP 3: *What is the dose available? Dose available = Have.*
10,000 units

STEP 4: *Should the nurse convert the units of measurement?*
No

STEP 5: *What is the quantity of the dose available?*
1 mL

STEP 6: *Set up an equation and solve for X.*

$$\frac{\text{Desired x Quantity}}{\text{Have}} = \text{X}$$

$$\frac{8,000 \text{ units x 1 mL}}{10,000 \text{ units}} = \text{X mL}$$

0.8 = X

STEF 7: *Round if necessary.*

STEP 8: *Reassess to determine whether the amount to administer makes sense.*
If there are 10,000 units/mL and the prescribed amount is 8,000 units, it makes sense to administer 0.8 mL. The nurse should administer heparin injection 0.8 mL subcutaneously every 8 hr.

Using Dimensional Analysis

STEP 1: *What is the unit of measurement to calculate?*
mL

STEP 2: *What quantity of the dose is available?*
1 mL

STEP 3: *What is the dose available? Dose available = Have.*
10,000 units

STEP 4: *What is the dose needed? Dose needed = Desired.*
8,000 units

STEP 5: *Should the nurse convert the units of measurement?*
No

STEP 6: *Set up an equation and solve for X.*

$$\text{X} = \frac{\text{Quantity}}{\text{Have}} \times \frac{\text{Conversion (Have)}}{\text{Conversion (Desired)}} \times \frac{\text{Desired}}{}$$

$$\text{X mL} = \frac{1 \text{ mL}}{10,000 \text{ units}} \times \frac{8,000 \text{ units}}{}$$

X = 0.8

STEP 7: *Round if necessary.*

STEP 8: *Reassess to determine whether the amount to administer makes sense.*
If there are 10,000 units/mL and the prescribed amount is 8,000 units, it makes sense to administer 0.8 mL. The nurse should administer heparin injection 0.8 mL subcutaneously every 8 hr.

DOSAGES BY WEIGHT

Example: A nurse is preparing to administer cefixime (Suprax) 8 mg/kg/day PO divided in equal doses every 12 hr to a toddler who weighs 22 lb. The amount available is cefixime suspension 100 mg/5 mL. How many mL should the nurse administer per dose? (Round the answer to the nearest whole number.)

Using Ratio and Proportion

STEP 1: *What is the unit of measurement to calculate?*
kg

STEP 2: *Set up an equation and solve for X.*

$$\frac{2.2\ lb}{1\ kg} = \frac{\text{Client weight in lb}}{X\ kg}$$

$$\frac{2.2\ lb}{1\ kg} = \frac{22\ lb}{X\ kg}$$

X = 10

STEP 3: *Round if necessary.*

STEP 4: *Reassess to determine whether the equivalent makes sense.*
If 1 kg = 2.2 lb, it makes sense that 22 lb = 10 kg.

STEP 5: *What is the unit of measurement to calculate?*
mg

STEP 6: *Set up an equation and solve for X.*
mg x kg/day = X
8 mg x 10 kg = 80 mg

STEP 7: *Round if necessary.*

STEP 8: *Reassess to determine whether the amount makes sense.*
If the prescribed amount is 8 mg/kg/day divided in equal doses every 12 hr and the toddler weighs 10 kg, it makes sense to give 80 mg/day, or 40 mg every 12 hr.

STEP 9: *What is the unit of measurement to calculate?*
mL

STEP 10: *What is the dose needed? Dose needed = Desired.*
40 mg

STEP 11: *What is the dose available? Dose available = Have.*
100 mg

STEP 12: *Should the nurse convert the units of measurement?*
No

STEP 13: *What is the quantity of the dose available?*
5 mL

STEP 14: *Set up an equation and solve for X.*

$$\frac{\text{Have}}{\text{Quantity}} = \frac{\text{Desired}}{X}$$

$$\frac{100\ mg}{5\ mL} = \frac{40\ mg}{X\ mL}$$

X = 2

STEP 15: *Round if necessary.*

STEP 16: *Reassess to determine whether the amount to give makes sense.*
If there are 100 mg/5 mL and the prescribed amount is 40 mg, it makes sense to give 2 mL. The nurse should administer cefixime suspension 2 mL PO every 12 hr.

Using Desired Over Have

STEP 1: *What is the unit of measurement to calculate?*
kg

STEP 2: *Set up an equation and solve for X.*

$$\frac{2.2\ \text{lb}}{1\ \text{kg}} = \frac{\text{Client weight in lb}}{X\ \text{kg}}$$

$$\frac{2.2\ \text{lb}}{1\ \text{kg}} = \frac{22\ \text{lb}}{X\ \text{kg}}$$

X = 10

STEP 3: *Round if necessary.*

STEP 4: *Reassess to determine whether the equivalent makes sense.*
If 1 kg = 2.2 lb, it makes sense that 22 lb = 10 kg.

STEP 5: *What is the unit of measurement to calculate?*
mg

STEP 6: *Set up an equation and solve for X.*
mg x kg/day = X
8 mg x 10 kg = 80 mg

STEP 7: *Round if necessary.*

STEP 8: *Reassess to determine whether the amount makes sense.*
If the prescribed amount is 8 mg/kg/day divided in equal doses every 12 hr and the toddler weighs 10 kg, it makes sense to give 80 mg/day, or 40 mg every 12 hr.

STEP 9: *What is the unit of measurement to calculate?*
mL

STEP 10: *What is the dose needed? Dose needed = Desired.*
40 mg

STEP 11: *What is the dose available? Dose available = Have.*
100 mg

STEP 12: *Should the nurse convert the units of measurement?*
No

STEP 13: *What is the quantity of the dose available?*
5 mL

STEP 14: *Set up an equation and solve for X.*

$$\frac{\text{Desired x Quantity}}{\text{Have}} = X$$

$$\frac{40\ \text{mg x 5 mL}}{100\ \text{mg}} = X\ \text{mL}$$

2 = X

STEP 15: *Round if necessary.*

STEP 16: *Reassess to determine whether the amount to give makes sense.*
If there are 100 mg/5 mL and the prescribed amount is 40 mg, it makes sense to give 2 mL. The nurse should administer cefixime suspension 2 mL PO every 12 hr.

Using Dimensional Analysis

STEP 1: *What is the unit of measurement to calculate?*
kg

STEP 2: *Set up an equation and solve for X.*

$$\frac{2.2 \text{ lb}}{1 \text{ kg}} = \frac{\text{Client weight in lb}}{X \text{ kg}}$$

$$\frac{2.2 \text{ lb}}{1 \text{ kg}} = \frac{22 \text{ lb}}{X \text{ kg}}$$

X = 10

STEP 3: *Round if necessary.*

STEP 4: *Reassess to determine whether the equivalent makes sense.*
If 1 kg = 2.2 lb, it makes sense that 22 lb = 10 kg.

STEP 5: *What is the unit of measurement to calculate?*
mg

STEP 6: *Set up an equation and solve for X.*
mg x kg/day = X
8 mg x 10 kg = 80 mg

STEP 7: *Round if necessary.*

STEP 8: *Reassess to determine whether the amount makes sense.*
If the prescribed amount is 8 mg/kg/day divided in equal doses every 12 hr and the toddler weighs 10 kg, it makes sense to give 80 mg/day, or 40 mg every 12 hr.

STEP 9: *What is the unit of measurement to calculate?*
mL

STEP 10: *What quantity of the dose is available?*
1 mL

STEP 11: *What is the dose available? Dose available = Have.*
100 mg

STEP 12: *What is the dose needed? Dose needed = Desired.*
40 mg

STEP 13: *Should the nurse convert the units of measurement?*
No

STEP 14: *Set up an equation and solve for X.*

$$X = \frac{\text{Quantity}}{\text{Have}} \times \frac{\text{Conversion (Have)}}{\text{Conversion (Desired)}} \times \frac{\text{Desired}}{}$$

$$X \text{ mL} = \frac{5 \text{ mL}}{100 \text{ mg}} \times \frac{40 \text{ mg}}{}$$

X = 2

STEP 15: *Round if necessary.*

STEP 16: *Reassess to determine whether the amount to give makes sense.*
If there are 100 mg/5 mL and the prescribed amount is 40 mg, it makes sense to give 2 mL. The nurse should administer cefixime suspension 2 mL PO every 12 hr.

IV FLOW RATES

- Nurses calculate IV flow rates for large-volume continuous IV infusions and intermittent IV bolus infusions using electronic infusion pumps (mL/hr) and manual IV tubing (gtt/min).
- IV infusions using electronic infusion pumps
  - Infusion pumps control an accurate rate of fluid infusion. Infusion pumps are able to deliver a specified amount of fluid during a specified amount of time. For example, an infusion pump can deliver 150 mL in 1 hr or 50 mL in 15 min.

Example: A nurse is caring for a client who is receiving dextrose 5% in water (D_5W) 500 mL IV to infuse over 4 hr. The nurse should make sure the IV infusion pump delivers how many mL/hr? (Round the answer to the nearest whole number.)

Using Ratio and Proportion, Desired Over Have, and Dimensional Analysis

STEP 1: *What is the unit of measurement to calculate?*
mL/hr

STEP 2: *What is the volume needed? Volume needed = Volume.*
500 mL

STEP 3: *What is the total infusion time? Time available = Time.*
4 hr

STEP 4: *Should the nurse convert the units of measurement?*
No

STEP 5: *Set up an equation and solve for X.*

$$\frac{\text{Volume (mL)}}{\text{Time (hr)}} = X$$

$$\frac{500 \text{ mL}}{4 \text{ hr}} = X \text{ mL/hr}$$

$$125 = X$$

STEP 6: *Round if necessary.*

STEP 7: *Reassess to determine whether the IV flow rate makes sense.*
If the amount prescribed is 500 mL to infuse 4 hr, it makes sense to administer 125 mL/hr. The nurse should make sure the IV pump delivers D_5W 500 mL IV at 125 mL/hr.

Example: A nurse is is caring for a client who is receiving cefotaxime (Claforan) 1 g intermittent IV bolus. Available is cefotaxime 1 g in 100 mL of 0.9% sodium chloride (0.9% NaCl) to infuse over 45 min. The nurse should make sure the IV infusion pump delivers how many mL/hr? (Round the answer to the nearest whole number.) (Note that a PN might not administer the IV medication, but must know how to monitor the infusion and ensure the correct rate of infusion.)

Using Ratio and Proportion, Desired Over Have, and Dimensional Analysis

STEP 1: *What is the unit of measurement to calculate?*
mL/hr

STEP 2: *What is the volume needed? Volume needed = Volume.*
100 mL

STEP 3: *What is the total infusion time? Time available = Time.*
45 min

STEP 4: *Should the nurse convert the units of measurement?*
No (mL = mL)
Yes (min ≠ hr)

$$\frac{1 \text{ hr}}{60 \text{ min}} = \frac{X \text{ hr}}{45 \text{ min}}$$

X = 0.75

STEP 5: *Set up an equation and solve for X.*

$$\frac{\text{Volume (mL)}}{\text{Time (hr)}} = X$$

$$\frac{100 \text{ mL}}{0.75 \text{ hr}} = X \text{ mL/hr}$$

$$133.3333 = X$$

STEP 6: *Round if necessary.*
133.3333 = 133

STEP 7: *Reassess to determine whether the IV flow rate makes sense.*
If the amount prescribed is 100 mL to infuse over 45 min (0.75 hr), it makes sense to administer 133 mL/hr. The nurse should make sure the IV pump delivers cefotaxime 1 g in 100 mL of 0.9% NaCl IV at 133 mL/hr.

- Manual IV infusions
  - If an electronic infusion pump is not available, regulate the IV flow rate using the roller clamp on the IV tubing. When setting the flow rate, count the number of drops that fall into the drip chamber over the period of 1 min. Then calculate the flow rate using the drop factor on the manufacturer's package containing the administration set. The drop factor is the number of drops per milliliter of solution.

Example: A nurse is preparing to administer lactated Ringer's (LR) 1,500 mL IV to infuse over 10 hr. The drop factor of the manual IV tubing is 15 gtt/mL. The nurse should set the manual IV infusion to deliver how many gtt/min? (Round the answer to the nearest whole number.)

Using Ratio and Proportion and Desired Over Have

STEP 1: *What is the unit of measurement to calculate?*
gtt/min

STEP 2: *What is the volume needed?*
Volume needed = Volume.
1,500 mL

STEP 3: *What is the total infusion time? Time available = Time.*
10 hr

STEP 4: *Should the nurse convert the units of measurement?*
No (mL = mL)
Yes (hr ≠ min)

$$\frac{1\ hr}{60\ min} = \frac{10\ hr}{X\ min}$$

X = 600 min

STEP 5: *Set up an equation and solve for X.*

$$\frac{Volume\ (mL)}{Time\ (min)} \times Drop\ factor\ (gtt/mL) = X$$

$$\frac{1,500\ mL}{600\ min} \times 15\ gtt/mL = X\ gtt/min$$

37.5 = X

STEP 6: *Round if necessary.*
37.5 = 38

STEP 7: *Reassess to determine whether the IV flow rate makes sense.*
If the amount prescribed is 1,500 mL to infuse over 10 hr (600 min), it makes sense to administer 38 gtt/min. The nurse should set the manual IV infusion to deliver LR 1,500 mL IV at 38 gtt/min.

Using Dimensional Analysis

STEP 1: *What is the unit of measurement to calculate?*
gtt/min

STEP 2: *What is the quantity of the drop factor that is available?*
15 gtt/mL

STEP 3: *What is the total infusion time? Time available = Time.*
10 hr

STEP 4: *What is the volume needed? Volume needed = Volume.*
1,500 mL

STEP 5: *Should the nurse convert the units of measurement?*
No (mL = mL)
Yes (hr ≠ min)

$$\frac{1\ hr}{60\ min}$$

STEP 6: *Set up an equation and solve for X.*

$$X = \frac{Quantity}{1\ mL} \times \frac{Conversion\ (Have)}{Conversion\ (Desired)} \times \frac{Volume}{Time}$$

$$X\ gtt/min = \frac{15\ gtt}{1\ mL} \times \frac{1\ hr}{60\ min} \times \frac{1,500\ mL}{10\ hr}$$

X = 37.5

STEP 7: *Round if necessary.*
37.5 = 38

STEP 8: *Reassess to determine whether the IV flow rate makes sense.*
If the amount prescribed is 1,500 mL to infuse over 10 hr (600 min), it makes sense to administer 38 gtt/min. The nurse should set the manual IV infusion to deliver LR 1,500 mL IV at 38 gtt/min.

Example: A nurse is caring for a client who is receiving ranitidine (Zantac) 50 mg by intermittent IV bolus. Available is ranitidine 50 mg in 100 mL of 0.9% sodium chloride (0.9% NaCl) to infuse over 30 min. The drop factor of the manual IV tubing is 10 gtt/mL. The nurse should make sure the manual IV infusion delivers how many gtt/min? (Round the answer to the nearest whole number.)

(Note: A PN might not administer the IV medication, but must know how to monitor the infusion and ensure the correct rate of infusion.)

Using Ratio and Proportion and Desired Over Have

STEP 1: *What is the unit of measurement to calculate?*
gtt/min

STEP 2: *What is the volume needed? Volume needed = Volume.*
100 mL

STEP 3: *What is the total infusion time? Time available = Time.*
30 min

STEP 4: *Should the nurse convert the units of measurement?*
No

STEP 5: *Set up an equation and solve for X.*

$$\frac{\text{Volume (mL)}}{\text{Time (min)}} \times \text{Drop factor (gtt/mL)} = X$$

$$\frac{100 \text{ mL} \times 10 \text{ gtt/mL}}{30 \text{ min}} = X \text{ gtt/min}$$

33.3333 = 33

STEP 6: *Round if necessary.*
33.3333 = 33

STEP 7: *Reassess to determine whether the IV flow rate makes sense.*

If the amount prescribed is 50 mL to infuse over 30 min, it makes sense to administer 33 gtt/min. The nurse should make sure the manual IV infusion delivers ranitidine 50 mg in 100 mL of 0.9% NaCl IV at 33 gtt/min.

Using Dimensional Analysis

STEP 1: *What is the unit of measurement to calculate?*
gtt/min

STEP 2: *What is the quantity of the drop factor that is available?*
10 gtt/mL

STEP 3: *What is the total infusion time? Time available = Time.*
30 min

STEP 4: *What is the volume needed? Volume needed = Volume.*
100 mL

STEP 5: *Should the nurse convert the units of measurement?*
No

STEP 6: *Set up an equation and solve for X.*

$$X = \frac{\text{Quantity}}{1 \text{ mL}} \times \frac{\text{Conversion (Have)}}{\text{Conversion (Desired)}} \times \frac{\text{Volume}}{\text{Time}}$$

$$X \text{ gtt/min} = \frac{10 \text{ gtt}}{1 \text{ mL}} \times \frac{100 \text{ mL}}{30 \text{ min}}$$

X = 33.3333

STEP 7: *Round if necessary.*
33.3333 = 33

STEP 8: *Reassess to determine whether the IV flow rate makes sense.*

If the amount prescribed is 100 mL to infuse over 30 min, it makes sense to administer 33 gtt/min. The nurse should make sure the manual IV infusion delivers ranitidine 50 mg in 100 mL of 0.9% NaCl IV at 33 gtt/min.

APPLICATION EXERCISES

1. A nurse is caring for a client who is receiving cefotaxime (Claforan) 1 g by intermittent IV bolus. The amount available is cefotaxime 1 g in dextrose 5% in water (D_5W) 100 mL to infuse over 45 min. The drop factor shown on the package of IV tubing is 10 gtt/mL. The nurse should make sure the manual IV infusion delivers how many gtt/min? (Round the answer to the nearest whole number.)

2. A nurse is caring for a client who is receiving clindamycin (Cleocin) 200 mg by intermittent IV bolus. The amount available is clindamycin injection 200 mg in 100 mL 0.9% sodium chloride (0.9% NaCl) to infuse over 30 min. The nurse should make sure the IV pump delivers how many mL/hr? (Round the answer to the nearest whole number.)

3. A nurse is preparing to administer furosemide (Lasix) 80 mg PO daily. The amount available is furosemide oral solution 40 mg/5 mL. How many mL should the nurse administer? (Round the answer to the nearest whole number.)

4. A nurse is preparing to administer dextrose 5% in water (D_5W) 750 mL IV to infuse over 6 hr. The nurse should set the IV pump to deliver how many mL/hr? (Round the answer to the nearest whole number.)

5. A nurse is preparing to administer haloperidol (Haldol) 2 mg PO every 12 hr. The amount available is haloperidol 1 mg/tablet. How many tablets should the nurse administer? (Round the answer to the nearest whole number.)

6. A nurse is preparing to administer amoxicillin (Amoxil) 20 mg/kg/day PO divided in equal doses every 12 hr to a preschool child who weighs 44 lb. The amount available is amoxicillin suspension 250 mg/5 mL. How many mL should the nurse administer per dose? (Round the answer to the nearest whole number.)

7. A nurse is preparing to administer heparin 15,000 units subcutaneously every 12 hr. The amount available is heparin injection 20,000 units/mL. How many mL should the nurse administer per dose? (Round the answer to the nearest tenth.)

8. A nurse is preparing to administer acetaminophen (Tylenol) 650 mg PO every 6 hr PRN for pain. The amount available is acetaminophen liquid 500 mg/5 mL. How many mL should the nurse administer per dose? (Round the answer to the nearest tenth.)

APPLICATION EXERCISES KEY

1. **22** gtt/min

Using Ratio and Proportion and Desired Over Have

STEP 1: *What is the unit of measurement to calculate?*
gtt/min

STEP 2: *What is the volume needed? Volume needed = Volume.*
100 mL

STEP 3: *What is the total infusion time? Time available = Time.*
45 min

STEP 4: *Should the nurse convert the units of measurement?*
No

STEP 5: *Set up an equation and solve for X.*

$$\frac{Volume\ (mL)}{Time\ (min)} \times Drop\ factor\ (gtt/mL) = X$$

$$\frac{100\ mL \times 10\ gtt/mL}{45\ min} = X\ gtt/min$$

22.2222 = X

STEP 6: *Round if necessary.*
22.2222 = 22

STEP 7: *Reassess to determine whether the IV flow rate makes sense.*
If the amount prescribed is 100 mL to infuse over 45 min, it makes sense to administer 22 gtt/min. The nurse should make sure the manual IV infusion delivers cefotaxime 1 g in D_5W 100 mL IV at 22 gtt/min.

Using Dimensional Analysis

STEP 1: *What is the unit of measurement to calculate?*
gtt/min

STEP 2: *What is the quantity of the drop factor that is available?*
10 gtt/mL

STEP 3: *What is the total infusion time? Time available = Time.*
45 min

STEP 4: *What is the volume needed? Volume needed = Volume.*
100 mL

STEP 5: *Should the nurse convert the units of measurement?*
No

STEP 6: *Set up an equation and solve for X.*

$$X = \frac{Quantity}{1\ mL} \times \frac{Conversion\ (Have)}{Conversion\ (Desired)} \times \frac{Volume}{Time}$$

$$X\ gtt/min = \frac{10\ gtt}{1\ mL} \times \frac{100\ mL}{45\ min}$$

X = 22.2222

STEP 7: *Round if necessary.*
22.2222 = 22

STEP 8: *Reassess to determine whether the IV flow rate makes sense.*
If the amount prescribed is 100 mL to infuse over 45 min, it makes sense to administer 22 gtt/min. The nurse should make sure the manual IV infusion delivers cefotaxime 1 g in D_5W 100 mL IV at 22 gtt/min.

 NCLEX® Connection: Pharmacological Therapies, Dosage Calculation

2. **200** mL/hr

Using Ratio and Proportion, Desired Over Have, and Dimensional Analysis

STEP 1: *What is the unit of measurement to calculate?*
mL/hr

STEP 2: *What is the volume needed? Volume needed = Volume.*
100 mL

STEP 3: *What is the total infusion time? Time available = Time.*
30 min

STEP 4: *Should the nurse convert the units of measurement?*
No (mL = mL)
Yes (min ≠ hr)

$$\frac{1\,hr}{60\,min} = \frac{X\,hr}{30\,min}$$

X = 0.5

STEP 5: *Set up an equation and solve for X.*

$$\frac{Volume\,(mL)}{Time\,(hr)} = X$$

$$\frac{100\,mL}{0.5} = X\,mL/hr$$

200 = X

STEP 6: *Round if necessary*

STEP 7: *Reassess to determine whether the IV flow rate makes sense.*
If the amount prescribed is 100 mL to infuse over 30 min (0.5 hr), it makes sense to administer 200 mL/hr. The nurse should make sure the IV pump delivers clindamycin injection 200 mg in 100 mL 0.9% NaCl IV at 200 mL/hr.

 NCLEX® Connection: Pharmacological Therapies, Dosage Calculation

---

3. **10** mL

Using Ratio and Proportion

STEP 1: *What is the unit of measurement to calculate?*
mL

STEP 2: *What is the dose needed? Dose needed = Desired.*
80 mg

STEP 3: *What is the dose available? Dose available = Have.*
40 mg

STEP 4: *Should the nurse convert the units of measurement?*
No

STEP 5: *What is the quantity of the dose available?*
5 mL

STEP 6: *Set up an equation and solve for X.*

$$\frac{Have}{Quantity} = \frac{Desired}{X}$$

$$\frac{40\,mg}{5\,mL} = \frac{80\,mg}{X\,mL}$$

X = 10

STEP 7: *Round if necessary.*

STEP 8: *Reassess to determine whether the amount to administer makes sense.*
If there are 40 mg/5 mL and the prescribed amount is 80 mg, it makes sense to administer 10 mL. The nurse should administer furosemide oral solution 10 mL PO daily.

Using Desired Over Have

STEP 1: *What is the unit of measurement to calculate?*
mL

STEP 2: *What is the dose needed? Dose needed = Desired.*
80 mg

STEP 3: *What is the dose available? Dose available = Have.*
40 mg

STEP 4: *Should the nurse convert the units of measurement?*
No

STEP 5: *What is the quantity of the dose available?*
5 mL

STEP 6: *Set up an equation and solve for X.*

$$\frac{\text{Desired} \times \text{Quantity}}{\text{Have}} = X$$

$$\frac{80 \text{ mg} \times 5 \text{ mL}}{40 \text{ mg}} = X \text{ mL}$$

$$10 = X$$

STEP 7: *Round if necessary.*

STEP 8: *Reassess to determine whether the amount to administer makes sense.*
If there are 40 mg/5 mL and the prescribed amount is 80 mg, it makes sense to administer 10 mL. The nurse should administer furosemide oral solution 10 mL PO daily.

Using Dimensional Analysis

STEP 1: *What is the unit of measurement to calculate?*
mL

STEP 2: *What quantity of the dose is available?*
5 mL

STEP 3: *What is the dose available? Dose available = Have.*
40 mg

STEP 4: *What is the dose needed? Dose needed = Desired.*
80 mg

STEP 5: *Should the nurse convert the units of measurement?*
No

STEP 6: *Set up an equation of factors and solve for X.*

$$X = \frac{\text{Quantity}}{\text{Have}} \times \frac{\text{Conversion (Have)}}{\text{Conversion (Desired)}} \times \frac{\text{Desired}}{}$$

$$X \text{ mL} = \frac{5 \text{ mL}}{40 \text{ mg}} \times \frac{80 \text{ mg}}{}$$

$$X = 10$$

STEP 7: *Round if necessary.*

STEP 8: *Reassess to determine whether the amount to administer makes sense.*
If there are 40 mg/5 mL and the prescribed amount is 80 mg, it makes sense to administer 10 mL. The nurse should administer furosemide oral solution 10 mL PO daily.

 NCLEX® Connection: Pharmacological Therapies, Dosage Calculation

4. **125** mL/hr

Using Ratio and Proportion, Desired Over Have, and Dimensional Analysis

STEP 1: *What is the unit of measurement to calculate?*
mL/hr

STEP 2: *What is the volume needed? Volume needed = Volume.*
750 mL

STEP 3: *What is the total infusion time? Time available = Time.*
6 hr

STEP 4: *Should the nurse convert the units of measurement?*
No

STEP 5: *Set up an equation and solve for X.*

$$\frac{\text{Volume (mL)}}{\text{Time (hr)}} = X$$

$$\frac{750 \text{ mL}}{6 \text{ hr}} = X \text{ mL/hr}$$

$$125 = X$$

STEP 6: *Round if necessary.*

STEP 7: *Reassess to determine whether the IV flow rate makes sense.*
If the amount prescribed is D_5W 750 mL IV to infuse over 6 hr, it makes sense to administer 125 mL/hr. The nurse should set the IV pump to deliver D_5W 750 mL at 125 mL/hr.

 NCLEX® Connection: Pharmacological Therapies, Dosage Calculation

5. **2 tablets**

Using Ratio and Proportion

STEP 1: *What is the unit of measurement to calculate?*
tablet

STEP 2: *What is the dose needed? Dose needed = Desired.*
2 mg

STEP 3: *What is the dose available? Dose available = Have.*
1 mg

STEP 4: *Should the nurse convert the units of measurement?*
No

STEP 5: *What is the quantity of the dose available?*
1 tablet

STEP 6: *Set up an equation and solve for X.*

$$\frac{Have}{Quantity} = \frac{Desired}{X}$$

$$\frac{1\,mg}{1\,tablet} = \frac{2\,mg}{X\,tablet(s)}$$

$$X = 2$$

STEP 7: *Round if necessary.*

STEP 8: *Reassess to determine whether the amount to give makes sense.*
If there is 1 mg/tablet and the prescribed amount is 2 mg, it makes sense to give 2 tablets. The nurse should administer haloperidol 2 tablets PO every 12 hr.

Using Desired Over Have

STEP 1: *What is the unit of measurement to calculate?*
tablet

STEP 2: *What is the dose needed? Dose needed = Desired.*
2 mg

STEP 3: *What is the dose available? Dose available = Have.*
1 mg

STEP 4: *Should the nurse convert the units of measurement?*
No

STEP 5: *What is the quantity of the dose available?*
1 tablet

STEP 6: *Set up an equation and solve for X.*

$$\frac{Desired \times Quantity}{Have} = X$$

$$\frac{2\,mg \times 1\,tablet}{1\,mg} = X\,tablet(s)$$

$$2 = X$$

STEP 7: *Round if necessary.*

STEP 8: *Reassess to determine whether the amount to give makes sense.*
If there is 1 mg/tablet and the prescribed amount is 2 mg, it makes sense to give 2 tablets. The nurse should administer haloperidol 2 tablets PO every 12 hr.

Using Dimensional Analysis

STEP 1: *What is the unit of measurement to calculate?*
tablet

STEP 2: *What quantity of the dose is available?*
1 tablet

STEP 3: *What is the dose available? Dose available = Have.*
1 mg

STEP 4: *What is the dose needed? Dose needed = Desired.*
2 mg

STEP 5: *Should the nurse convert the units of measurement?*
No

STEP 6: *Set up an equation of factors and solve for X.*

$$X = \frac{Quantity}{Have} \times \frac{Conversion\,(Have)}{Conversion\,(Desired)} \times Desired$$

$$X\,tablet(s) = \frac{1\,tablet}{1\,mg} \times \frac{2\,mg}{}$$

$$X = 2$$

STEP 7: *Round if necessary.*

STEP 8: *Reassess to determine whether the amount to give makes sense.*
If there is 1 mg/tablet and the prescribed amount is 2 mg, it makes sense to give 2 tablets. The nurse should administer haloperidol 2 tablets PO every 12 hr.

 NCLEX® Connection: Pharmacological Therapies, Dosage Calculation

6. **4** mL

Using Ratio and Proportion

STEP 1: *What is the unit of measurement to calculate?*
kg

STEP 2: *Set up an equation and solve for X.*

$$\frac{2.2 \text{ lb}}{1 \text{ kg}} = \frac{\text{Client weight in lb}}{X \text{ kg}}$$

$$\frac{2.2 \text{ lb}}{1 \text{ kg}} = \frac{44 \text{ lb}}{X \text{ kg}}$$

X = 20

STEP 3: *Round if necessary.*

STEP 4: *Reassess to determine whether the equivalent makes sense.*
If 1 kg = 2.2 lb, it makes sense that 44 lb = 20 kg.

STEP 5: *What is the unit of measurement to calculate?*
mg

STEP 6: *Set up an equation and solve for X.*
mg x kg/day = X
20 mg x 20 kg = 400 mg

STEP 7: *Round if necessary.*

STEP 8: *Reassess to determine whether the amount makes sense.*
If the prescribed amount is 20 mg/kg/day divided in equal doses every 12 hr and the preschool child weighs 20 kg, it makes sense to give 400 mg/day, or 200 mg every 12 hr.

STEP 9: *What is the unit of measurement to calculate?*
mL

STEP 10: *What is the dose needed? Dose needed = Desired.*
200 mg

STEP 11: *What is the dose available? Dose available = Have.*
250 mg

STEP 12: *Should the nurse convert the units of measurement?*
No

STEP 13: *What is the quantity of the dose available?*
5 mL

STEP 14: *Set up an equation and solve for X.*

$$\frac{\text{Have}}{\text{Quantity}} = \frac{\text{Desired}}{X}$$

$$\frac{250 \text{ mg}}{5 \text{ mL}} = \frac{200 \text{ mg}}{X \text{ mL}}$$

X = 4

STEP 15: *Round if necessary.*

STEP 16: *Reassess to determine whether the amount to give makes sense.*
If there are 250 mg/5 mL and the prescribed amount is 200 mg, it makes sense to give 4 mL. The nurse should administer amoxicillin suspension 4 mL PO every 12 hr.

Using Desired Over Have

STEP 1: *What is the unit of measurement to calculate?*
kg

STEP 2: *Set up an equation and solve for X.*

$$\frac{2.2 \text{ lb}}{1 \text{ kg}} = \frac{\text{Client weight in lb}}{X \text{ kg}}$$

$$\frac{2.2 \text{ lb}}{1 \text{ kg}} = \frac{44 \text{ lb}}{X \text{ kg}}$$

X = 20

STEP 3: *Round if necessary.*

STEP 4: *Reassess to determine whether the equivalent makes sense.*
If 1 kg = 2.2 lb, it makes sense that 44 lb = 20 kg.

STEP 5: *What is the unit of measurement to calculate?*
mg

STEP 6: *Set up an equation and solve for X.*
mg x kg/day = X
20 mg x 20 kg = 400 mg

STEP 7: *Round if necessary.*

STEP 8: *Reassess to determine whether the amount makes sense.*
If the prescribed amount is 20 mg/kg/day divided in equal doses every 12 hr and the preschool child weighs 20 kg, it makes sense to give 400 mg/day, or 200 mg every 12 hr.

STEP 9: *What is the unit of measurement to calculate?*
mL

STEP 10: *What is the dose needed? Dose needed = Desired.*
200 mg

STEP 11: *What is the dose available? Dose available = Have.*
250 mg

STEP 12: *Should the nurse convert the units of measurement?*
No

STEP 13: *What is the quantity of the dose available?*
5 mL

STEP 14: *Set up an equation and solve for X.*

$$\frac{\text{Desired x Quantity}}{\text{Have}} = X$$

$$\frac{200 \text{ mg x 5 mL}}{250 \text{ mg}} = X \text{ mL}$$

4 = X

STEP 15: *Round if necessary.*

STEP 16: *Reassess to determine whether the amount to give makes sense.*
If there are 250 mg/5 mL and the prescribed amount is 200 mg, it makes sense to give 4 mL. The nurse should administer amoxicillin suspension 4 mL PO every 12 hr.

Using Dimensional Analysis

STEP 1: *What is the unit of measurement to calculate?*
kg

STEP 2: *Set up an equation and solve for X.*

$$\frac{2.2\ lb}{1\ kg} = \frac{Client\ weight\ in\ lb}{X\ kg}$$

$$\frac{2.2\ lb}{1\ kg} = \frac{44\ lb}{X\ kg}$$

X = 20

STEP 3: *Round if necessary.*

STEP 4: *Reassess to determine whether the equivalent makes sense.*
If 1 kg = 2.2 lb, it makes sense that 44 lb = 20 kg.

STEP 5: *What is the unit of measurement to calculate?*
mg

STEP 6: *Set up an equation and solve for X.*
mg x kg/day = X
20 mg x 20 kg = 400

STEP 7: *Round if necessary.*

STEP 8: *Reassess to determine whether the amount makes sense.*
If the prescribed amount is 20 mg/kg/day divided in equal doses every 12 hr and the preschool child weighs 20 kg, it makes sense to give 400 mg/day, or 200 mg every 12 hr.

STEP 9: *What is the unit of measurement to calculate?*
mL

STEP 10: *What quantity of the dose is available?*
5 mL

STEP 11: *What is the dose available?*
Dose available = Have.
250 mg

STEP 12: *What is the dose needed?*
Dose needed = Desired.
200 mg

STEP 13: *Should the nurse convert the units of measurement?*
No

STEP 14: *Set up an equation of factors and solve for X.*

$$X = \frac{Quantity}{Have} \times \frac{Conversion\ (Have)}{Conversion\ (Desired)} \times \frac{Desired}{}$$

$$X\ mL = \frac{5\ mL}{250\ mg} \times \frac{200\ mg}{}$$

X = 4

STEP 15: *Round if necessary.*

STEP 16: *Reassess to determine whether the amount to give makes sense.*
If there are 250 mg/5 mL and the prescribed amount is 200 mg, it makes sense to give 4 mL. The nurse should administer amoxicillin suspension 4 mL PO every 12 hr.

 NCLEX® Connection: Pharmacological Therapies, Dosage Calculation

7. **0.8** mL

Using Ratio and Proportion

STEP 1: *What is the unit of measurement to calculate?*
mL

STEP 2: *What is the dose needed? Dose needed = Desired.*
15,000 units

STEP 3: *What is the dose available? Dose available = Have.*
20,000 units

STEP 4: *Should the nurse convert the units of measurement?*
No

STEP 5: *What is the quantity of the dose available?*
1 mL

STEP 6: *Set up an equation and solve for X.*

$$\frac{\text{Have}}{\text{Quantity}} = \frac{\text{Desired}}{X}$$

$$\frac{20{,}000 \text{ units}}{1 \text{ mL}} = \frac{15{,}000 \text{ units}}{X \text{ mL}}$$

$$X = 0.75$$

STEP 7: *Round if necessary.*
0.75 = 0.8

STEP 8: *Reassess to determine whether the amount to administer makes sense.*
If there are 20,000 units/mL and the prescribed amount is 15,000 units, it makes sense to administer 0.8 mL. The nurse should administer heparin injection 0.8 mL subcutaneously every 12 hr.

Using Desired Over Have

STEP 1: *What is the unit of measurement to calculate?*
mL

STEP 2: *What is the dose needed? Dose needed = Desired.*
15,000 units

STEP 3: *What is the dose available? Dose available = Have.*
20,000 units

STEP 4: *Should the nurse convert the units of measurement?*
No

STEP 5: *What is the quantity of the dose available?*
1 mL

STEP 6: *Set up an equation and solve for X.*

$$\frac{\text{Desired} \times \text{Quantity}}{\text{Have}} = X$$

$$\frac{15{,}000 \text{ units} \times 1 \text{ mL}}{20{,}000 \text{ units}} = X \text{ mL}$$

$$0.75 = X$$

STEP 7: *Round if necessary.*
0.75 = 0.8

STEP 8: *Reassess to determine whether the amount to administer makes sense.*
If there are 20,000 units/mL and the prescribed amount is 15,000 units, it makes sense to administer 0.8 mL. The nurse should administer heparin injection 0.8 mL subcutaneously every 12 hr.

Using Dimensional Analysis

STEP 1: *What is the unit of measurement to calculate?*
mL

STEP 2: *What quantity of the dose is available?*
1 mL

STEP 3: *What is the dose available? Dose available = Have.*
20,000 units

STEP 4: *What is the dose needed? Dose needed = Desired.*
15,000 units

STEP 5: *Should the nurse convert the units of measurement?*
No

STEP 6: *Set up an equation of factors and solve for X.*

$$X = \frac{\text{Quantity}}{\text{Have}} \times \frac{\text{Conversion (Have)}}{\text{Conversion (Desired)}} \times \frac{\text{Desired}}{}$$

$$X \text{ mL} = \frac{1 \text{ mL}}{20{,}000 \text{ units}} \times \frac{15{,}000 \text{ units}}{}$$

$$X = 0.75$$

STEP 7: *Round if necessary.*
0.75 = 0.8

STEP 8: *Reassess to determine whether the amount to administer makes sense.*
If there are 20,000 units/mL and the prescribed amount is 15,000 units, it makes sense to administer 0.8 mL. The nurse should administer heparin injection 0.8 mL subcutaneously every 12 hr.

 NCLEX® Connection: Pharmacological Therapies, Dosage Calculation

8. **6.5** mL

Using Ratio and Proportion

STEP 1: *What is the unit of measurement to calculate?*
mL

STEP 2: *What is the dose needed? Dose needed = Desired.*
650 mg

STEP 3: *What is the dose available? Dose available = Have.*
500 mg

STEP 4: *Should the nurse convert the units of measurement?*
No

STEP 5: *What is the quantity of the dose available?*
5 mL

STEP 6: *Set up an equation and solve for X.*

$$\frac{Have}{Quantity} = \frac{Desired}{X}$$

$$\frac{500 \text{ mg}}{5 \text{ mL}} = \frac{650 \text{ mg}}{X \text{ mL}}$$

X = 6.5

STEP 7: *Round if necessary.*

STEP 8: *Reassess to determine whether the amount to administer makes sense.*
If there are 500 mg/5 mL and the prescribed amount is 650 mg, it makes sense to administer 6.5 mL. The nurse should administer acetaminophen liquid 6.5 mL PO every 6 hr PRN for pain.

Using Desired Over Have

STEP 1: *What is the unit of measurement to calculate?*
mL

STEP 2: *What is the dose needed? Dose needed = Desired.*
650 mg

STEP 3: *What is the dose available? Dose available = Have.*
500 mg

STEP 4: *Should the nurse convert the units of measurement?*
No

STEP 5: *What is the quantity of the dose available?*
5 mL

STEP 6: *Set up an equation and solve for X.*

$$\frac{Desired \times Quantity}{Have} = X$$

$$\frac{650 \text{ mg} \times 5 \text{ mL}}{500 \text{ mg}} = X \text{ mL}$$

6.5 = X

STEP 7: *Round if necessary.*

STEP 8: *Reassess to determine whether the amount to administer makes sense.*
If there are 500 mg/5 mL and the prescribed amount is 650 mg, it makes sense to administer 6.5 mL. The nurse should administer acetaminophen liquid 6.5 mL PO every 6 hr PRN for pain.

Using Dimensional Analysis

STEP 1: *What is the unit of measurement to calculate?*
mL

STEP 2: *What quantity of the dose is available?*
5 mL

STEP 3: *What is the dose available? Dose available = Have.*
500 mg

STEP 4: *What is the dose needed? Dose needed = Desired.*
650 mg

STEP 5: *Should the nurse convert the units of measurement?*
No

STEP 6: *Set up an equation of factors and solve for X.*

$$X = \frac{Quantity}{Have} \times \frac{Conversion \text{ (Have)}}{Conversion \text{ (Desired)}} \times \frac{Desired}{}$$

$$X \text{ mL} = \frac{5 \text{ mL}}{500 \text{ mg}} \times \frac{650 \text{ mg}}{}$$

X = 6.5

STEP 7: *Round if necessary.*

STEP 8: *Reassess to determine whether the amount to administer makes sense.*
If there are 500 mg/5 mL and the prescribed amount is 650 mg, it makes sense to administer 6.5 mL. The nurse should administer acetaminophen liquid 6.5 mL PO every 6 hr PRN for pain.

 NCLEX® Connection: Pharmacological Therapies, Dosage Calculation

chapter 4

Overview

- IV therapy involves administering fluids via an IV catheter for the purpose of providing medications; supplementing fluid intake; or giving fluid replacement, electrolytes, or nutrients.
- Large-volume IV infusions are administered on a continuous basis.
- An IV medication may be mixed in a large volume of fluid and given as a continuous IV infusion; mixed in a small amount of solution and given intermittently (intermittent IV bolus); or given in a small amount of solution, concentrated or diluted, and injected over a short time (IV bolus dose).
- Be aware of the scope of practice for PNs. Generally, with special training or certification, PNs may perform venipuncture and insert IV catheters, but they may not administer IV medications. Nevertheless, they need to be aware of all the principles and techniques outlined in this chapter.

Indications and Risk Factors

- Advantages and Disadvantages of IV Therapy

ADVANTAGES	DISADVANTAGES
› Rapid effects	› Circulatory fluid overload is possible if the infusion is large and/or too rapid.
› Precise amounts	
› Less discomfort after initial insertion	› Immediate absorption leaves no time to correct errors.
› Control over therapeutic blood levels	› IV administration can cause irritation to the lining of the vein.
› Less irritation to subcutaneous and muscle tissue	› Failure to maintain surgical asepsis can lead to local infection and septicemia.

Description of Procedure

- The provider prescribes the type of IV fluid, volume to be infused, and either the rate at which the IV fluid should be infused or the total amount of time it should take for the fluid to be infused. The nurse regulates the IV infusion to ensure the appropriate amount is administered. This can be done with an IV pump or manually.
- Large-volume IV infusions are administered on a continuous basis, such as 0.9% sodium chloride IV to infuse at 100 mL/hr or 0.9% sodium chloride 1,000 mL to be given IV over 3 hr.
- A fluid bolus is a large amount of IV fluid given in a short period of time, usually less than 1 hr. It is given to rapidly replace fluid loss that could be caused by dehydration, shock, hemorrhage, burns, or trauma.
  - A large-gauge IV catheter (18-gauge or larger) is essential for maintaining the rapid rate necessary to give a fluid bolus to an adult.

- Methods to administer IV medication infusions:
  - Mix medication in a large volume of fluid (500 to 1,000 mL) and administer as continuous IV infusion.
  - Use premixed solution bags or solutions that have been prepared by the pharmacist.
  - Intermittent IV bolus administration
    - Some medications, such as antibiotics, are given intermittently in a small amount of solution (25 to 250 mL) through a continuous IV system, or with saline or heparin lock systems.
    - The medications infuse for short periods of time and are given on a scheduled basis.
    - These infusions can be administered by a secondary IV bag or bottle or tandem setup, volume-control administration set, or mini-infusion pump.
  - IV bolus dose administration
    - The medications are typically in small amounts of solution, concentrated or diluted, that can be injected over a short time in emergent and nonemergent situations.

    - Some medications, such as pain medications, are given directly into the peripheral IV or access port to achieve an immediate medication level in the bloodstream.

    - When caring for a client who has received IV bolus medications, observe for complications (localized redness, burning, or increasing pain).
    - Monitor for adverse effects of the medication, such as hypotension or respiratory depression. Observe for therapeutic effects, such as pain relief.
- Types of IV Access
  - IV access can be via a peripheral or central vein (central venous access device).
  - Central venous access devices can be peripherally inserted or directly inserted into the jugular or subclavian vein through venipuncture, or by surgical intervention with implantation of access ports for long-term use.

Guidelines for Safe IV Medication Administration

- When caring for clients who are receiving IV medications, be aware of the following safety guidelines.
  - Some medications, such as potassium chloride, can cause serious adverse reactions and should be infused with an electronic IV pump for accurate dosage control and never given by IV bolus.
  - IV medication should be in a new IV fluid container, not in an IV container that was already hanging.
  - IV medication must not infuse through tubing that is infusing blood, blood products, or parenteral nutritional solutions.
  - Multiple medications infusing through the same tubing must be compatible.
- Needlestick Prevention
  - Be familiar with IV insertion equipment.
  - Avoid using needles when needleless systems are available.
  - Use protective safety devices when available.
  - Dispose of needles immediately in designated puncture-resistant receptacles.
  - Do not break, bend, or recap needles.

- Special Considerations

- ○ Older adult clients, clients taking anticoagulants, or clients who have fragile veins
    - ▪ Avoid tourniquets. Use a blood pressure cuff instead.
    - ▪ Do not slap the extremity to visualize veins.
    - ▪ Apply traction to the skin below the vein to stabilize the vein.
    - ▪ Use a small gauge catheter when possible.
    - ▪ Instruct the client to hold his hand below the level of his heart.
    - ▪ Avoid using the back of the client's hand.
  - ○ Edema in extremities
    - ▪ Apply digital pressure over the selected vein to displace edema.
    - ▪ Apply pressure with an alcohol pad.
    - ▪ Perform cannulation quickly.
  - ○ Clients who are obese may require the use of anatomical landmarks to find veins.

- Preventing IV Infections
  - ○ Use standard precautions.
  - ○ Have IV sites changed when indicated or according to the facility's policy.
  - ○ Remove catheters as soon as they are no longer clinically indicated.
    - ▪ Ensure replacement of the catheter if any break in surgical aseptic technique is suspected, such as with emergency insertions.
  - ○ Use a sterile needle/catheter for each insertion attempt.
  - ○ Avoid writing on IV bags with pens or markers, because ink could contaminate the solution.
  - ○ Replace tubing immediately if contamination is known or suspected.
  - ○ Fluids should not hang longer than 24 hr unless it is a closed system.
  - ○ Wipe all ports with alcohol or an antiseptic swab before connecting IV lines or inserting a syringe to prevent the introduction of micro-organisms into the system.
  - ○ Never disconnect tubing for convenience or to position the client.
  - ○ Do not allow ports to remain exposed to air.
  - ○ Perform hand hygiene before and after handling the IV system.

Preprocedure

- Equipment
  - ○ Correct size catheter
    - ▪ 16-gauge for trauma clients, rapid fluid volume
    - ▪ 18-gauge for surgical clients, rapid blood administration
    - ▪ 20-gauge for adults
    - ▪ 22- to 24-gauge for older adults and children

- Correct tubing, including short extension tubing with a saline-filled syringe
- Infusion pump, if indicated
- Clean gloves
- Scissors or electric shaver for hair removal
- Tourniquet or blood pressure cuff
- IV dressing supplies

- Nursing Actions
  - Check the provider's prescription (solution, rate).
  - Check clients for allergies to products used in initiating and maintaining IV therapy (latex, tape, iodine).
  - Follow the rights of medication administration (including compatibilities of all IV solutions).
  - Perform hand hygiene.
  - Examine the solution to be infused for clarity, leaks, and expiration date.
  - Prime tubing as indicated.
  - Don clean gloves before insertion.
  - Observe extremities and veins. If hair removal is needed, clip it with scissors or shave it with an electric shaver.

- Client Education
  - Identify clients and explain the procedure.
  - Place clients in a comfortable position.

Intraprocedure

- Nursing Actions
  - Select vein by choosing:
    - Distal veins first on the nondominant hand.
    - A site that is not painful or bruised and will not interfere with activity.
    - A vein that is resilient with a soft, bouncy feeling.
  - Document in medical record
    - Date and time of insertion
    - Insertion site and appearance
    - Catheter size
    - Type of dressing
    - IV fluid and rate (if applicable)
    - Number, locations, and conditions of site-attempted cannulations
    - Client's response

Postprocedure

- Nursing Actions
  - Maintaining patency of IV access
    - Do not stop a continuous infusion or allow blood to back up into the catheter for any length of time. Clots can form at the tip of the needle or catheter and can become lodged against the vein wall, blocking the flow of fluid.
    - Instruct clients not to manipulate flow rate device, change settings on IV pump, or lie on the tubing.
    - Make sure the IV insertion site dressing is not too tight.
    - Flush intermittent IV catheters with appropriate solution after every medication administration or every 8 to 12 hr when not in use.
    - Monitor site and infusion rate at least every hour.

Complications

- Complications require notification of the provider and complete documentation. Remove the IV catheter and restart with new tubing and catheter.

INFILTRATION '	
Findings	› Pallor, local swelling at the site, decreased skin temperature around the site, damp dressing, slowed infusion
Treatment	› Stop the infusion and remove the catheter. › Elevate the extremity. › Encourage active range of motion. › Apply warm or cold compresses based on the type of solution that infiltrated the tissue. › Check with the provider to determine whether the client still needs IV therapy. If so, restart the infusion proximal to the site or in another extremity.
Prevention	› Carefully select site and catheter. › Secure the catheter.
EXTRAVASATION (INFILTRATION OF A VESICANT OR TISSUE-DAMAGING MEDICATION)	
Findings	› Pain, burning, redness, swelling
Treatment	› Stop the infusion and notify the provider. › Follow facility protocol, which may include infusing an antidote through the catheter before removal.
Prevention	› Closely monitor the IV site and dressing. › Always use an infusion pump.

PHLEBITIS/THROMBOPHLEBITIS

Findings	› Edema; throbbing, burning, or pain at the site; increased skin temperature; erythema; a red line up the arm with a palpable band at the vein site, slowed infusion
Treatment	› Promptly discontinue the infusion and remove the catheter. › Elevate the extremity. › Apply a cold compress to minimize the flow of blood, then apply a warm compress to increase circulation. › Check with the provider to determine whether the client still needs IV therapy. If so, restart the infusion in the opposite extremity. › If drainage is present, obtain a specimen from the site and send it and the catheter for culture.
Prevention	› Rotate IV sites when indicated or per policy. › Avoid the lower extremities. › Use hand hygiene. › Use surgical aseptic technique.

HEMATOMA

Findings	› Ecchymosis at site
Treatment	› Do not apply alcohol. › Apply pressure after IV catheter removal. › Use warm compress and elevation after bleeding stops.
Prevention	› Minimize tourniquet time. › Remove the tourniquet before starting IV infusion. › Maintain pressure after IV catheter removal.

CELLULITIS

Findings	› Pain; warmth; edema; induration; red streaking; fever, chills, and malaise
Treatment	› Promptly discontinue the infusion and remove catheter. › Elevate the extremity. › Apply warm compresses three to four times/day. › If drainage is present, obtain a specimen from the site and send it and the catheter for culture. › Administer: » Antibiotics. » Analgesics. » Antipyretics.
Prevention	› Rotate IV sites when indicated or per policy. › Avoid the lower extremities. › Use hand hygiene. › Use surgical aseptic technique.

FLUID OVERLOAD	
Findings	› Distended neck veins, increased blood pressure, tachycardia, shortness of breath, crackles in the lungs, edema
Treatment	› Slow the IV rate to keep the vein open in accordance with facility policy. › Raise the head of the bed. › Check vital signs. › Anticipate administration of diuretics.
Prevention	› Use an infusion pump. › Monitor I&O.
CATHETER EMBOLUS	
Findings	› Missing catheter tip when discontinued; severe pain at the site with migration, or no symptoms if no migration
Treatment	› Place the tourniquet high on the extremity to limit venous flow. › Prepare for removal under x-ray or via surgery. › Save the catheter after removal to determine the cause.
Prevention	› Do not reinsert the stylet into the catheter.

APPLICATION EXERCISES

1. A nurse is observing a client's IV site. Which of the following findings indicate phlebitis? (Select all that apply.)

_____ A. Tingling sensation below insertion site

_____ B. Tachycardia

_____ C. Palpable, hard mass above insertion site

_____ D. Cool, pale skin

_____ E. Pain at site

2. A nurse manager is reviewing facility policies for IV therapy management with the members of his team. The nurse manager should inform the team members that which of the following techniques will minimize the risk of catheter embolism?

A. Perform hand hygiene before and after IV insertion.

B. Rotate the IV sites at least every 72 hr.

C. Minimize tourniquet time.

D. Avoid reinserting the needle into an IV catheter.

3. A nurse is preparing to initiate IV therapy for an older adult client. Which of the following actions should the nurse plan to take?

A. Use a disposable razor to remove excess hair on the extremity.

B. Select the back of the client's hand to insert the IV catheter.

C. Distend the veins by using a blood pressure cuff.

D. Direct the client to raise his arm above his heart.

4. A nurse is caring for a client receiving dextrose 5% in water IV at 250 mL/hr. Which of the following findings indicate fluid overload? (Select all that apply.)

_____ A. Hypotension

_____ B. Bradycardia

_____ C. Shortness of breath

_____ D. Crackles heard in lungs

_____ E. Distended neck veins

5. A nurse is preparing to administer dextrose 5% in water 200 mL IV to infuse over 5 hr. The nurse should set the IV pump to deliver how many mL/hr? (Round the answer to the nearest whole number.)

6. A nurse on a medical-surgical unit is providing care for a group of clients who are receiving IV therapy. The nurse is monitoring the clients for related complications. Use ATI Active Learning Template: Nursing Skill to complete this item to include the following:

  A. Indications: Identify three indications for IV therapy.

  B. Complications: Identify four potential complications of IV therapy.

APPLICATION EXERCISES KEY

1. A. INCORRECT: A tingling sensation below the insertion site is a clinical manifestation of nerve damage.

   B. INCORRECT: Tachycardia is a clinical manifestation of fluid volume overload.

   C. **CORRECT:** A palpable, hard mass above the insertion site is a clinical manifestation of thrombophlebitis.

   D. INCORRECT: Cool, pale skin is a clinical manifestation of infiltration.

   E. **CORRECT:** Pain at the IV site is a clinical manifestation of thrombophlebitis.

   Ⓝ NCLEX® Connection: Physiological Adaptations, Unexpected Response to Therapies

2. A. INCORRECT: The nurse manager should remind the members of the team to perform hand hygiene to prevent infection, but this technique does not reduce the risk of catheter embolism.

   B. INCORRECT: The nurse manager should remind the members of the team to rotate IV sites at least every 72 hr to prevent phlebitis, but this technique does not minimize the risk of catheter embolism.

   C. INCORRECT: The nurse manager should remind the members of the team to minimize tourniquet time, but this technique does not minimize the risk of catheter embolism.

   D. **CORRECT:** The nurse manager should remind the members of the team to avoid reinserting a needle into an IV catheter. This action can result in severing the end of the catheter and consequently cause a catheter embolism.

   Ⓝ NCLEX® Connection: Pharmacological Therapies, Medication Administration

3. A. INCORRECT: The nurse should remove excess hair by clipping it with scissors. Shaving with a disposable razor can cause skin damage that can lead to infection.

   B. INCORRECT: In most instances, the nurse inserts the IV catheter into a distal site, such as the back of the client's hand. However, when inserting an IV catheter for an older adult, the nurse should select a site on the arm because older adults typically have fragile veins in the backs of their hands.

   C. **CORRECT:** The nurse should distend the veins using a blood pressure cuff to reduce overfilling of the vein, which can result in a hematoma.

   D. INCORRECT: The nurse should direct the client to hold his arm below the level of his heart to distend the vein.

   Ⓝ NCLEX® Connection: Pharmacological Therapies, Medication Administration

4. A. INCORRECT: Due to an excess of fluid in the cardiovascular system, hypertension is a clinical manifestation of fluid volume overload.

    B. INCORRECT: Due to an increase in fluid in the cardiovascular system, tachycardia is a clinical manifestation of fluid volume overload.

    C. **CORRECT:** Due to an excess of fluid in the cardiovascular system, shortness of breath is a manifestation of fluid volume overload.

    D. **CORRECT:** Due to an excess of fluid in the cardiovascular system, crackles in the lungs is a manifestation of fluid volume overload.

    E. **CORRECT:** Due to an excess of fluid in the cardiovascular system, distended neck veins is a manifestation of fluid volume overload.

    Ⓝ NCLEX® Connection: Physiological Adaptations, Unexpected Response to Therapies

5. **40** mL/hr

Using Ratio and Proportion, Desired Over Have, and Dimensional Analysis

    STEP 1: *What is the unit of measurement to calculate?*
    mL/hr

    STEP 2: *What is the volume needed? Volume needed = Volume.*
    200 mL

    STEP 3: *What is the total infusion time? Time available = Time.*
    5 hr

    STEP 4: *Should the nurse convert the units of measurement?*
    No (mL = mL)
    No (hr = hr)

    STEP 5: *Set up an equation and solve for X.*

    $$\frac{Volume\ (mL)}{Time\ (hr)} = X$$

    $$\frac{200\ mL}{5\ hr} = X\ mL/hr$$

    $$40 = X$$

    STEP 6: *Round if necessary.*

    STEP 7: *Reassess to determine whether the IV flow rate makes sense.*
    If the amount prescribed is 200 mL to infuse over 5 hr, it makes sense to administer 40 mL/hr. The nurse should set the IV pump to deliver dextrose 5% in water 200 mL at 40 mL/hr.

    Ⓝ NCLEX® Connection: Pharmacological Therapies, Dosage Calculation

6. *Using the ATI Active Learning Template: Nursing Skill*

    A. Indications for IV therapy
    - To administer medications
    - To supplement fluid intake
    - To replace electrolytes and nutrients

    B. Complications of IV therapy
    - Infiltration
    - Extravasation
    - Cellulitis
    - Fluid overload
    - Catheter embolus
    - Hematoma
    - Phlebitis/thrombophlebitis

    Ⓝ NCLEX® Connection: Pharmacological Therapies, Medication Administration

chapter 5

Overview

- To ensure safe medication administration and prevent errors, the nurse must know why a medication is prescribed and the intended therapeutic effect. In addition, the nurse must be aware of potential side and adverse effects, interactions, contraindications, and precautions.

- Every medication has the potential to cause side effects and adverse effects. Side effects are expected, and they occur when the medication is given at a therapeutic dose. Discontinuation of the medication is usually not warranted. Adverse effects are undesired, inadvertent, and unexpected dangerous effects of the medication. Adverse effects can occur at both therapeutic and higher-than-therapeutic doses.

- Medications are chemicals that affect the body. When more than one medication is given, there is a potential for an interaction. In addition, medications can interact with foods.

- Contraindications and precautions of specific medications refer to client conditions that make it unsafe or potentially harmful to administer these medications.

- Response to medications differs for individuals based on multiple factors, such as age, gender, disease process, and ethnic and genetic variations. These factors can cause many expected and unexpected adverse effects.

Adverse Medication Effects

- These effects can be classified according to body systems.

ADVERSE MEDICATION EFFECTS	NURSING INTERVENTIONS/CLIENT EDUCATION
› Central nervous system (CNS) effects can result from either CNS stimulation (excitement) or CNS depression.	› If CNS stimulation is expected, clients can be at risk for seizures, and precautions should be taken. › If CNS depression is likely, advise clients not to drive or participate in other activities that can be dangerous.
› Extrapyramidal symptoms (EPS) (abnormal body movements) include involuntary fine-motor tremors, rigidity, uncontrollable restlessness, and acute dystonias (spastic movements and/or muscle rigidity affecting the head, neck, eyes, facial area, and limbs). These can occur within a few hours or take months to develop.	› EPS are more often associated with medications affecting the CNS, such as those that treat mental health disorders.
› Anticholinergic effects are a result of muscarinic receptor blockade. Most effects are in the eyes, smooth muscle, exocrine glands, and heart.	› Advise clients to relieve dry mouth by sipping on liquids, wear sunglasses to manage photophobia, and reduce urinary retention by urinating before taking the medication.

ADVERSE MEDICATION EFFECTS	NURSING INTERVENTIONS/CLIENT EDUCATION
› Cardiovascular effects involve blood vessels and the heart.	› Antihypertensives can cause orthostatic hypotension. › Instruct clients about signs of orthostatic hypotension (lightheadedness, dizziness). If these occur, advise clients to sit or lie down and to minimize orthostatic hypotension by getting up and changing position slowly.
› Gastrointestinal (GI) effects can result from local irritation of the GI tract. Stimulation of the vomiting center also results in adverse effects.	› NSAIDs can cause GI upset. Advise clients to take these medications with food.
› Hematologic effects are relatively common and potentially life-threatening with some groups of medications.	› Bone marrow depression/suppression generally is associated with anticancer medications and hemorrhagic disorders with anticoagulants and thrombolytics. Inform clients taking anticoagulants about bleeding (bruising, discolored urine/stool, petechiae, bleeding gums). Tell clients to notify the provider if these effects occur.
› Hepatotoxicity can occur with many medications. Because most medications are metabolized in the liver, the liver is particularly vulnerable to drug-induced injury. Damage to liver cells can impair metabolism of many medications, causing medication accumulation in the body and producing adverse effects. Many medications can alter normal values of liver function tests with no obvious clinical signs of liver dysfunction.	› When two or more medications that are hepatotoxic are combined, the risk for liver damage is increased. › Liver function tests are indicated when clients start a medication known to be hepatotoxic and periodically thereafter. › Monitor clients for manifestations of hepatotoxicity, such as nausea, vomiting, jaundice, and anorexia.
› Nephrotoxicity can occur with some of medications, but it is primarily the result of certain antimicrobial agents and NSAIDs. Damage to the kidneys can interfere with medication excretion, leading to medication accumulation and adverse effects.	› Aminoglycosides injure cells in the renal tubules of the kidney. Monitor serum creatinine and BUN, as well as peak and trough medication levels for clients taking medication that is nephrotoxic.
› Toxicity is an adverse medication effect that is severe and potentially life-threatening. It can be caused by an excessive dose, but it also can occur at therapeutic dose levels.	› Liver damage will occur with an acetaminophen (Tylenol) overdose. There is a greater risk of liver damage with chronic alcohol use. Acetylcysteine can help minimize liver damage.
› Allergic reaction occurs when an individual develops an immune response to a medication. The individual has been previously exposed to the medication and has developed antibodies.	› Allergic reactions range from minor to serious. Withhold the medication and notify the provider of the client's previous reaction to penicillin. › Treat mild rashes and hives with diphenhydramine. › Before administering any medications, obtain a complete medication history.

ADVERSE MEDICATION EFFECTS	NURSING INTERVENTIONS/CLIENT EDUCATION
› Anaphylactic reaction is a life-threatening, immediate allergic reaction that causes respiratory distress, severe bronchospasm, and cardiovascular collapse.	› Treat with epinephrine, bronchodilators, and antihistamines. Provide respiratory support, and inform the provider.
› Immunosuppression is a decreased or absent immune response.	› Immunosuppressant medications, such as glucocorticoids, can mask the usual manifestations of infection, such as fever. › Monitor clients taking an immunosuppressant, such as a glucocorticoid, for delayed wound healing and subtle manifestations of infection, such as sore throat. › Advise clients who take an immunosuppressant to avoid contact with a person who has a communicable disease.

Drug-Drug Interactions

- Consequences of Drug-Drug Interactions

TYPE OF INTERACTION	NURSING IMPLICATIONS/INTERVENTIONS
Increase therapeutic effects	› Some medications are given together to increase therapeutic effects. Opioid analgesics are often prescribed with nonopioids, such as NSAIDs, to manage cancer pain. Clients who have asthma are instructed to use albuterol (Proventil-HFA), a beta$_2$-adrenergic agonist inhaler, 5 min prior to using beclomethasone (QVAR), a glucocorticoid inhaler, to increase the absorption of beclomethasone.
Increase adverse effects	› When clients take two medications that have the same adverse effect, the risk of these effects increases. Diazepam (Valium) and hydrocodone bitartrate 5 mg/acetaminophen 500 mg (Co-Gesic) both have CNS depressant effects. Clients who take both have an increased risk for CNS depression.
Decrease therapeutic effects	› One medication can increase the metabolism of a second medication and therefore decrease the serum level and effectiveness of the second medication. For example, phenytoin (Dilantin) increases hepatic medication-metabolizing enzymes that affect warfarin (Coumadin) and thereby decreases the serum level and the effect of warfarin.
Decrease adverse effects	› One medication can be given to counteract the adverse effects of another medication. Ondansetron hydrochloride (Zofran), an antiemetic, can be administered to counteract the effects of nausea and vomiting for clients receiving chemotherapy.
Increase serum levels, leading to toxicity	› One medication can decrease the metabolism of a second medication and therefore increase the serum level of the second medication. This can lead to toxicity. Fluconazole (Diflucan) inhibits hepatic medication-metabolizing enzymes that affect aripiprazole (Abilify) and thereby increases serum levels of this medication.

- Over-The-Counter (OTC) Medications

INTERACTIONS	NURSING IMPLICATIONS/INTERVENTIONS
› Ingredients in OTC medications can interact with other OTC or prescription medications.	› Obtain a complete medication history. › Instruct clients to follow the manufacturer's recommendation for dosage.
› Inactive ingredients, such as dyes, alcohol, or preservatives, can cause adverse reactions.	
› Potential for overdose exists because of the use of several preparations (including prescription medications) with similar ingredients.	
› Interactions of certain prescription and OTC medications can interfere with therapeutic effects.	› Advise clients to use caution and to check with the provider before using any OTC preparations such as antacids, laxatives, decongestants, or cough syrups. For example, antacids can interfere with the absorption of ranitidine (Zantac) and other medications. Advise clients to take antacids 1 hr apart from other medications.

Medication-Food Interactions

- Food can alter medication absorption and/or contain substances that react with some medications.

- Examples

  - Consuming foods that contain tyramine while taking monoamine oxidase inhibitors (MAOIs) can lead to hypertensive crisis. Clients taking MAOIs should be aware of foods containing tyramine, such as cheese and processed meats, and avoid them.

  - Vitamin K can decrease the therapeutic effects of warfarin (Coumadin) and place clients at risk for developing blood clots. Clients taking warfarin should include a consistent amount of vitamin K in their diet.

  - Tetracycline can interact with a chelating agent, such as milk, and form an insoluble, unabsorbable compound. Instruct clients not to take tetracycline within 2 hr of consuming dairy products.

  - Grapefruit juice seems to act by inhibiting medication metabolism in the small bowel, thus increasing the amount of medication available for absorption of some oral medications. This increases either the therapeutic effects or the adverse reactions. Clients should be instructed not to drink grapefruit juice if they are taking such a medication.

Contraindications and Precautions

- A specific medication can be contraindicated based on the client's condition. For example, penicillins are contraindicated for a client who has an allergy to this medication.

- Precautions should be taken for a client who is more likely to have an adverse reaction than another client. Morphine (Duramorph) depresses respiratory function, so it should be used with caution for clients who have asthma or impaired respiratory function.

- The U.S. Food and Drug Administration places medications in categories based on risk to a fetus.

  - Category A: There is no evidence of risk to the fetus during pregnancy based on adequate and well-controlled studies.

  - Category B: There is no evidence of risk to animal fetuses based on studies, but there are no adequate and well-controlled studies in pregnant women.

  - Category C: Adverse effects have been demonstrated on animal fetuses. There are no adequate and well-controlled studies in pregnant women, but use of the medication during pregnancy can be warranted based on the potential benefits.

  - Category D: Adverse effects have been demonstrated on human fetuses based on data from investigational or marketing experience, but use of the medication during pregnancy can be warranted based on the potential benefits.

  - Category X: Adverse effects have been demonstrated on animal and human fetuses based on studies and data from investigational or marketing experience. The use of the medication is contraindicated during pregnancy because the risks outweigh the potential benefits.

APPLICATION EXERCISES

1. A nurse is reinforcing teaching for a client who has a new prescription for a tetracycline antibiotic to treat Lyme disease. The nurse should remind the client to eliminate which of the following from her diet for the duration of treatment?

    A. Milk products

    B. Green, leafy vegetables

    C. Grapefruit juice

    D. Processed meats

2. A nurse is preparing to administer an IM dose of penicillin to a client who has a new prescription. The client states she took penicillin 3 years ago and developed a rash. Which of the following is an appropriate nursing action?

    A. Administer the prescribed dose.

    B. Withhold the medication.

    C. Ask the provider to change the prescription to an oral form.

    D. Administer an oral antihistamine at the same time.

3. A nurse is reinforcing discharge instructions for a client who has a new prescription for an antihypertensive medication. Which of the following is an appropriate statement by the nurse?

    A. "Be sure to limit your potassium intake while taking the medication."

    B. "You should check your blood pressure every 8 hr while taking this medication."

    C. "Your medication dosage will be increased if you develop tachycardia."

    D. "Change positions slowly when you move from sitting to standing."

4. A nurse is reviewing a client's health record and notes that a previous medication caused permanent extrapyramidal effects. The nurse recognizes that the medication affected the client's

    A. cardiovascular system.

    B. immune system.

    C. central nervous system.

    D. gastrointestinal system.

5. A nurse is caring for a client who is taking oral oxycodone (Percolone), an opioid analgesic. The client states he is also taking ibuprofen (Advil), an NSAID, in three recommended doses daily. The interaction between these two medications will cause which of the following?

    A. A decrease in serum levels of ibuprofen, possibly leading to a need for increased doses of this medication

    B. A decrease in serum levels of oxycodone, possibly leading to a need for increased doses of this medication

    C. An increase in the expected therapeutic effect of both medications

    D. An increase in expected adverse effects for both medications

6. A nurse in a family practice clinic is reviewing with a newly licensed nurse the risks involved in taking medications during pregnancy. Use the ATI Active Learning Template: Basic Concept to describe the U.S. Food and Drug Administration's fetal risk categories for classifying medications.

APPLICATION EXERCISES KEY

1. A. **CORRECT:** Tetracycline can interact with a chelating agent, such as milk, and form an insoluble, unabsorbable compound. Clients should not take tetracycline within 2 hr of consuming dairy products.

    B. INCORRECT: Green, leafy vegetables are a good source of vitamin K, which can decrease the therapeutic effects of anticoagulants but does not affect tetracycline use.

    C. INCORRECT: Grapefruit juice seems to act by inhibiting medication metabolism and raising blood levels of some drugs, but it does not affect tetracycline use.

    D. INCORRECT: Consuming foods that contain tyramine, such as processed meats, can cause a hypertensive crisis in clients who take monoamine oxidase inhibitors. Tyramine does not affect tetracycline use.

    Ⓝ NCLEX® Connection: Pharmacological Therapies, Adverse Effects/Contraindications/ Side Effects/Interactions

2. A. INCORRECT: Administering the IM penicillin in the prescribed dosage could cause a severe reaction and is not the appropriate action.

    B. **CORRECT:** The nurse should withhold the medication and notify the provider of the client's previous reaction to penicillin so that an alternative antibiotic can be prescribed. Allergic reactions to penicillin can range from mild to severe anaphylaxis, and prior sensitization should be reported to the provider.

    C. INCORRECT: Administering the penicillin orally rather than intramuscularly would not prevent a reaction and is not the appropriate nursing action.

    D. INCORRECT: Giving the penicillin along with an oral antihistamine would not prevent a reaction from occurring and is not the appropriate nursing action.

    Ⓝ NCLEX® Connection: Safety and Infection Control, Accident/Error/Injury Prevention

3. A. INCORRECT: Potassium can actually lower blood pressure, so clients who have hypertension should eat plenty of fresh fruits and vegetables.

    B. INCORRECT: Clients should check their blood pressure daily on a regular basis when taking an antihypertensive medication, but every 8 hr is unnecessary.

    C. INCORRECT: Tachycardia is an adverse effect that would not warrant an increase in a dose of medication.

    D. **CORRECT:** Orthostatic hypotension is a common adverse effect of antihypertensive medications. The client should move slowly to a sitting or standing position and should sit or lie down if lightheadedness or dizziness occurs.

    Ⓝ NCLEX® Connection: Pharmacological Therapies, Medication Administration

4. A. INCORRECT: Medications affecting the cardiovascular system generally do not cause extrapyramidal effects.

    B. INCORRECT: Medications affecting the immune system generally do not cause extrapyramidal effects.

    C. **CORRECT:** The nurse should realize that extrapyramidal effects are movement disorders that can be caused by some of central nervous system medications, such as typical antipsychotic medications.

    D. INCORRECT: Medications affecting the gastrointestinal system generally do not cause extrapyramidal effects.

    ⓝ NCLEX® Connection: Pharmacological Therapies, Adverse Effects/Contraindications/ Side Effects/Interactions

5. A. INCORRECT: Taking these medications together does not cause a decrease in serum levels of ibuprofen.

    B. INCORRECT: Taking these medications together does not cause a decrease in serum levels of oxycodone.

    C. **CORRECT:** These medications work together to increase the pain-relieving effects of both medications. Oxycodone is an opioid analgesic, and ibuprofen is an NSAID. They work by different mechanisms, but relieve pain better when taken together.

    D. INCORRECT: Adverse effects of oxycodone and ibuprofen are not increased when the medications are taken together.

    ⓝ NCLEX® Connection: Pharmacological Therapies, Adverse Effects/Contraindications/ Side Effects/Interactions

6. *Using the ATI Active Learning Template: Basic Concept*
    - Fetal Risk Categories for Classifying Medications
      ○ Category A: There is no evidence of risk to the fetus during pregnancy based on adequate and well-controlled studies.
      ○ Category B: There is no evidence of risk to animal fetuses based on studies, but there are no adequate and well-controlled studies in pregnant women.
      ○ Category C: Adverse effects have been demonstrated on animal fetuses. There are no adequate and well-controlled studies in pregnant women, but use of the medication during pregnancy can be warranted based on the potential benefits.
      ○ Category D: Adverse effects have been demonstrated on human fetuses based on data from investigational or marketing experience, but use of the medication during pregnancy can be warranted based on the potential benefits.
      ○ Category X: Adverse effects have been demonstrated on animal and human fetuses based on studies and data from investigational or marketing experience. The use of the medication is contraindicated during pregnancy because the risks outweigh the potential benefits.

    ⓝ NCLEX® Connection: Pharmacological Therapies, Adverse Effects/Contraindications/ Side Effects/Interactions

UNIT 2   Medications Affecting the Nervous System

CHAPTERS

› Anxiety Disorders
› Depressive Disorders
› Bipolar Disorders
› Psychotic Disorders
› Medications for Children and Adolescents with Mental Health Issues
› Substance Use Disorders
› Chronic Neurologic Disorders
› Eye and Ear Disorders
› Miscellaneous Central Nervous System Medications
› Sedative-Hypnotics

NCLEX® CONNECTIONS

When reviewing the chapters in this unit, keep in mind the relevant sections of the NCLEX® outline, in particular:

Client Needs: Pharmacological Therapies

› Relevant topics/tasks include:
  » Adverse Effects/Contraindications/Side Effects/Interactions
    › Monitor the client for actual and potential adverse effects of medications.
  » Expected Actions/Outcomes
    › Evaluate the client's response to medications (adverse reactions, interactions, therapeutic effects).
  » Medication Administration
    › Administer medication by the oral route.
    › Administer a subcutaneous, intradermal, or intramuscular medication.

chapter 6

Overview

- The major medications used to treat anxiety disorders
  - Benzodiazepine sedative hypnotic anxiolytics, such as alprazolam (Xanax)
  - Atypical anxiolytic/nonbarbiturate anxiolytics, such as buspirone
  - Selected antidepressants
    - Paroxetine (Paxil), a selective serotonin reuptake inhibitor (SSRI)
    - Sertraline (Zoloft), an SSRI
- Other classifications (in detail in other chapters of this review module)
  - Other antidepressants
    - Venlafaxine, a serotonin-norepinephrine reuptake inhibitor (SNRI)
    - Amitriptyline, a tricyclic antidepressant (TCA)
    - Clomipramine (Anafranil), a TCA
  - Antihistamines, such as hydroxyzine (Vistaril)
  - Beta-blockers, such as propranolol (Inderal)
  - Anticonvulsants, such as gabapentin (Neurontin)
- In addition to anxiety disorders, these medications are used to treat trauma- and stressor-related disorders, as well as obsessive-compulsive and related disorders.

MEDICATION CLASSIFICATION: SEDATIVE HYPNOTIC ANXIOLYTIC – BENZODIAZEPINE

- Select Prototype Medication: alprazolam (Xanax)
- Other Medications
  - Diazepam (Valium)
  - Lorazepam (Ativan)
  - Chlordiazepoxide (Librium)
  - Clorazepate (Tranxene)
  - Oxazepam
  - Clonazepam (Klonopin)

Purpose

- Expected Pharmacological Action
    - Benzodiazepines enhance the inhibitory effects of gamma-aminobutyric acid in the CNS. Relief from anxiety occurs rapidly following administration.
- Therapeutic Uses
    - Generalized anxiety disorder (GAD) and panic disorder
    - Other uses for benzodiazepines
        - Seizure disorders
        - Insomnia
        - Muscle spasm
        - Alcohol withdrawal (for prevention and treatment of acute manifestations)
        - Induction of anesthesia
        - Amnesic prior to surgery or procedures

Complications

ADVERSE EFFECTS	NURSING INTERVENTIONS/CLIENT EDUCATION
› CNS depression (sedation, lightheadedness, ataxia, decreased cognitive function)	› Advise clients to observe for CNS depression and to notify the provider if effects occur. › Advise clients to avoid hazardous activities (driving, operating heavy equipment/machinery).
› Anterograde amnesia (difficulty recalling events that occur after dosing)	› Advise clients to observe for manifestations and to notify the provider if effects occur.
› Acute toxicity › Oral toxicity (drowsiness, lethargy, confusion) › IV toxicity (can lead to respiratory depression, severe hypotension, or cardiorespiratory arrest)	› For oral toxicity, use gastric lavage, followed by activated charcoal or saline cathartics. › For IV toxicity, clients will require IV flumazenil to counteract sedation and reverse adverse effects. › Monitor vital signs, maintain a patent airway, and provide fluids to maintain blood pressure. › Have resuscitation equipment available.
› Paradoxical response (insomnia, excitation, euphoria, anxiety, rage)	› Advise clients to watch for manifestations and to notify the provider if these occur.
› Manifestations of withdrawal include anxiety, insomnia, diaphoresis, tremors, lightheadedness.	› Advise clients that withdrawal effects are not common with short-term use. › Advise clients who have been taking diazepam regularly and in high doses to taper the dose over several weeks.

Contraindications/Precautions

- Most benzodiazepines are Pregnancy Risk Category D medications.
- Benzodiazepines are Schedule IV medications according to the Controlled Substances Act.
- Sleep apnea, respiratory depression, and glaucoma are contraindications for benzodiazepines.
- Use benzodiazepines cautiously with clients who have liver disease or a history of mental illness or a substance use disorder.

- Benzodiazepines are generally for short-term use due to the risk for dependence.

Interactions

MEDICATION/FOOD INTERACTIONS	NURSING INTERVENTIONS/CLIENT EDUCATION
› CNS depressants (alcohol, barbiturates, opioids) can result in respiratory depression.	› Advise clients to avoid alcohol and other substances that cause CNS depression. › Advise clients to avoid hazardous activities (driving, operating heavy equipment/machinery).

Nursing Administration

- Advise clients to take the medication as prescribed and to avoid abrupt discontinuation of treatment to prevent withdrawal manifestations.
- Clients who have taken benzodiazepines regularly for long periods and in higher doses should taper the dose over several weeks.
- Administer the medication with meals or snacks if gastrointestinal (GI) upset occurs.
- Advise clients to swallow sustained-release tablets and to avoid chewing or crushing the tablets.
- Inform clients about the possible development of dependence during and after treatment and to notify the provider if indications of withdrawal occur.

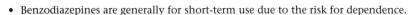

MEDICATION CLASSIFICATION: ATYPICAL ANXIOLYTIC/NONBARBITURATE ANXIOLYTIC

- Select Prototype Medication: buspirone

Purpose

- Expected Pharmacological Action
  - The exact antianxiety mechanism of this medication is unknown. This medication binds to serotonin and dopamine receptors. Dependence is much less likely than with other anxiolytics, and buspirone does not result in sedation or potentiate the effects of other CNS depressants.
- Therapeutic Uses
  - Panic disorder
  - Social anxiety disorder
  - Obsessive-compulsive and related disorders
  - Trauma- and stressor-related disorders, such as posttraumatic stress disorder (PTSD)

Complications

ADVERSE EFFECTS	NURSING INTERVENTIONS/CLIENT EDUCATION
› Dizziness, nausea, headache, lightheadedness, agitation	› Advise the client to take with food to decrease nausea. › Inform the client that most adverse effects are self-limiting.

Contraindications/Precautions

- Buspirone is a Pregnancy Risk Category B medication.
- Breastfeeding is a contraindication for buspirone.
- Use buspirone cautiously with older adult clients and clients who have liver or kidney dysfunction.
- Clients may not take buspirone concurrently with monoamine oxidase inhibitor (MAOI) antidepressants or for 14 days after stopping use. Hypertensive crisis can result.

Interactions

MEDICATION/FOOD INTERACTIONS	NURSING INTERVENTIONS/CLIENT EDUCATION
› Erythromycin, ketoconazole, St. John's wort, and grapefruit juice can increase the effects of buspirone.	› Advise clients to avoid the use of these antimicrobial agents. › Advise clients to avoid herbal preparations containing St. John's wort. › Advise clients to avoid drinking grapefruit juice.

Nursing Administration

- Advise clients to take the medication with meals to prevent gastric irritation.
- Inform clients that effects do not occur immediately. It can take 1 week to notice the first therapeutic effects and 3 to 6 weeks for the full benefit. Clients should take the medication on a regular basis, not PRN.
- Instruct clients that tolerance, dependence, and withdrawal effects are not an issue with this medication.

MEDICATION CLASSIFICATION: SELECTIVE SEROTONIN REUPTAKE INHIBITORS (SSRI ANTIDEPRESSANTS)

- Select Prototype Medication: paroxetine (Paxil)
- Other Medications
  - Sertraline (Zoloft)
  - Escitalopram (Lexapro)
  - Fluoxetine (Prozac)
  - Fluvoxamine (Luvox)

Purpose

- Expected Pharmacological Action
  - Paroxetine selectively inhibits serotonin reuptake, allowing more serotonin to stay at the junction of the neurons.
  - Paroxetine does not block uptake of dopamine or norepinephrine.
  - Paroxetine produces CNS stimulation, which can cause insomnia.
  - Paroxetine has a long effective half-life. Up to 4 weeks are necessary to produce therapeutic medication levels.
- Therapeutic Uses
  - Paroxetine
    - GAD
    - Panic disorder
      - □ Decreases both the frequency and intensity of panic attacks, and also prevents anticipatory anxiety about attacks
    - Obsessive-compulsive disorder (OCD)
      - □ Reduces manifestations by increasing serotonin
    - Social anxiety disorder
    - Trauma- and stressor-related disorders
    - Depressive disorders
  - Sertraline treats panic disorder, OCD, social anxiety disorder, and PTSD.
  - Escitalopram treats GAD and OCD.
  - Fluoxetine treats panic disorder and OCD.
  - Fluvoxamine treats OCD and social anxiety disorder.

Complications

ADVERSE EFFECTS	NURSING INTERVENTIONS/CLIENT EDUCATION
› Early adverse effects (first few days/weeks): nausea, diaphoresis, tremor, fatigue, drowsiness	› Instruct clients to report adverse effects to the provider. › Instruct clients to take the medication as prescribed. › Inform clients that these effects should soon subside.
› Later adverse effects (after 5 to 6 weeks of therapy): sexual dysfunction (impotence, delayed or absent orgasm, delayed or absent ejaculation, decreased sexual interest)	› Instruct clients to report problems with sexual function (managed with dose reduction, medication holiday, changing medications).
› Weight gain	› Advise clients to follow a well-balanced diet and exercise regularly.
› GI bleeding	› Use caution with clients who have a history of GI bleeding or ulcers and with clients taking other medications that affect blood coagulation. › Advise clients to report indications of bleeding such as dark stool or coffee-ground emesis.
› Hyponatremia (more likely in older adult clients taking diuretics)	› Obtain baseline serum sodium, and monitor level periodically throughout treatment.
› Serotonin syndrome » Agitation, confusion, disorientation, difficulty concentrating, anxiety, hallucinations, hyperreflexia, incoordination, tremors, fever, diaphoresis » Usually begins 2 to 72 hr after initiation of treatment » Resolves with stopping the medication	› Watch for and advise clients to report any of these manifestations, which could indicate a life-threatening problem.
› Bruxism: grinding and clenching of teeth, usually during sleep	› Report bruxism to the provider, who may » Switch the client to another class of medication. » Treat bruxism with low-dose buspirone. » Advise the client to use a mouth guard during sleep.
› Withdrawal syndrome » Nausea, sensory disturbances, anxiety, tremor, malaise, unease » Minimal with tapering the medication slowly	› Advise clients that, after a long period of use, tapering it slowly avoids withdrawal syndrome. › Advise clients not to discontinue use abruptly.

Contraindications/Precautions

- Paroxetine is a Pregnancy Risk Category D medication.

- Concurrent use of MAOIs or TCAs is a contraindication for paroxetine.

- Clients taking paroxetine should avoid alcohol.

- Use paroxetine cautiously with clients who have liver or kidney dysfunction, seizure disorders, or a history of GI bleeding.

Interactions

MEDICATION/FOOD INTERACTIONS	NURSING INTERVENTIONS/CLIENT EDUCATION
› Use of MAOIs or TCAs can cause serotonin syndrome.	› Educate the client about this combination.

Nursing Administration

- Advise clients to take medications with food. Taking them in the morning minimizes sleep disturbances.

- Instruct clients to take the medication on a daily basis to establish therapeutic plasma levels.

- Assist with medication regimen adherence by informing clients that it can take up to 4 weeks to achieve therapeutic effects from an SSRI.

Nursing Evaluation of Medication Effectiveness

- Depending on the therapeutic intent, clients demonstrate effectiveness by

  - Maintaining an expected sleep pattern

  - Verbalizing feeling less anxious and more relaxed

  - Being better able to participate in social and occupational interactions

APPLICATION EXERCISES

1. A provider prescribes sertraline (Zoloft) for a client who has social anxiety disorder. The nurse reinforcing teaching with the client knows she understands how to take this medication when the client makes which of the following statements?

    A. "I'll be sure to take this medication on an empty stomach."

    B. "I might feel a little drowsy at first, but it should go away."

    C. "If I get headaches, I'll take aspirin."

    D. "I should start feeling less anxious in a week or two."

2. A nurse is caring for a client who is to begin taking escitalopram (Lexapro) for treatment of generalized anxiety disorder. Which of the following statements by the client indicates understanding of the use of this medication?

    A. "I will take the medication at bedtime."

    B. "I will need follow a low-sodium diet while taking this medication."

    C. "I need to discontinue this medication slowly."

    D. "I probably won't desire intimacy during the first days of treatment."

3. A nurse is reinforcing teaching with a client who has a new prescription to start buspirone in place of diazepam (Valium). The client has a history of panic disorder and cirrhosis of the liver. The client asks why his provider is making the medication change. Which of the following statements is an appropriate response by the nurse?

    A. "Diazepam can cause seizures as an adverse effect."

    B. "Diazepam does not treat panic disorder."

    C. "Buspirone is a safe medication for clients who have liver dysfunction."

    D. "Buspirone has less risk for dependence than other treatment options."

4. A nurse working in a mental health clinic is caring for a client who has obsessive-compulsive disorder and recently started a new prescription for buspirone. The client tells the nurse that the medication has not helped him sleep and that he is still having obsessive compulsions. Which of the following statements is an appropriate response by the nurse?

    A. "It may take several weeks before you feel like the medication is helping."

    B. "Take the medication just before bedtime to promote sleep."

    C. "You should take the medication on an as-needed basis when you have obsessive urges."

    D. "Your provider may need to increase your dose if you develop tolerance."

5. A nurse is caring for a client who takes paroxetine (Paxil) to treat posttraumatic stress disorder. The client states that he grinds his teeth during the night, which causes jaw pain. The nurse should identify which of the following as possible measures to manage the client's bruxism? (Select all that apply.)

_____ A. Concurrent administration of buspirone

_____ B. Administration of a different SSRI

_____ C. Use of a mouth guard

_____ D. Changing to a different class of antianxiety medication

_____ E. Increasing the dose of paroxetine

6. A nurse is monitoring a client 4 hr after receiving an initial dose of fluoxetine (Prozac). The nurse is concerned that the client is developing serotonin syndrome. Use the ATI Active Learning Template: Systems Disorder and the Mental Health Nursing Review Module to complete this item to include the following sections:

A. Description of Disorder/Disease Process

B. Assessment: Objective and Subjective – Identify at least six expected findings.

C. Assessment: Risk Factors – Describe at least one risk factor.

APPLICATION EXERCISES KEY

1.   A. INCORRECT: Clients may take sertraline with food.

     B. **CORRECT:** Nausea, diaphoresis, tremor, fatigue, and drowsiness are common when clients first start taking sertraline, but these effects should soon subside.

     C. INCORRECT: Sertraline can cause gastrointestinal bleeding. Clients taking it should avoid medications that affect blood coagulation, such as aspirin.

     D. INCORRECT: It can take about 4 weeks for the client to reach therapeutic serum levels of sertraline.

     Ⓝ NCLEX® Connection: Pharmacological Therapies, Medication Administration

2.   A. INCORRECT: The client should take escitalopram in the morning to minimize sleep disturbances.

     B. INCORRECT: The client is at risk for hyponatremia while taking escitalopram.

     C. **CORRECT:** When discontinuing escitalopram, the client should taper the medication slowly according to a prescribed tapered dosing schedule to reduce the risk of withdrawal syndrome.

     D. INCORRECT: Sexual dysfunction, including decreased libido, is a late adverse effect that is possible after 5 to 6 weeks of treatment with escitalopram.

     Ⓝ NCLEX® Connection: Pharmacological Therapies, Medication Administration

3.   A. INCORRECT: Diazepam treats seizure activity and does not cause seizures as an adverse effect.

     B. INCORRECT: Both buspirone and diazepam treat panic disorder.

     C. INCORRECT: Buspirone requires caution with clients who have liver dysfunction.

     D. **CORRECT:** Buspirone is preferable to diazepam for long-term use due to the decreased risk for dependence.

     Ⓝ NCLEX® Connection: Pharmacological Therapies, Expected Actions/Outcomes

4. A. **CORRECT:** It can take 3 to 6 weeks for the client to feel the full therapeutic benefit of buspirone.

    B. INCORRECT: Buspirone does not have any sedative effects and therefore will not promote sleep.

    C. INCORRECT: The client should take buspirone on a regular basis rather than an as-needed basis.

    D. INCORRECT: Buspirone does not cause tolerance.

    (N) NCLEX® Connection: Pharmacological Therapies, Expected Actions/Outcomes

5. A. **CORRECT:** Concurrent administration of a low dose of buspirone is an effective measure to manage the adverse effects of paroxetine.

    B. INCORRECT: Other SSRIs also have bruxism as an adverse effect. Therefore, this is not an effective measure.

    C. **CORRECT:** Using a mouth guard during sleep can decrease the risk for oral damage resulting from bruxism.

    D. **CORRECT:** Changing to different class of antianxiety medication that does not have the adverse effect of bruxism is an effective measure.

    E. INCORRECT: Increasing the dose of paroxetine can worsen the adverse effect of bruxism. Therefore, this is not an effective measure.

    (N) NCLEX® Connection: Pharmacological Therapies, Adverse Effects/Contraindications/ Side Effects/Interactions

6. *Using the ATI Active Learning Template: Systems Disorder*

    A. Description of Disorder/Disease Process
    • Serotonin syndrome is a potentially life-threatening complication that usually begins 2 to 72 hr after initiation of treatment with an SSRI. The syndrome resolves when the medication is discontinued.

    B. Assessment: Objective and Subjective

• Agitation	• Anxiety	• Tremors
• Confusion	• Hallucinations	• Fever
• Disorientation	• Hyperreflexia	• Diaphoresis
• Difficulty concentrating	• Incoordination	

    C. Assessment: Risk Factors
    • Onset of treatment with an SSRI within the last 2 to 72 hr
    • Concurrent use of an SSRI with an MAOI
    • Concurrent use of an SSRI with a TCA

    (N) NCLEX® Connection: Pharmacological Therapies, Adverse Effects/Contraindications/ Side Effects/Interactions

chapter 7

Overview

- Depressive disorders are a widespread problem, ranking high among causes of disability.
- Clients who have major depression can require hospitalization with close observation and suicide precautions until the antidepressant medications reach their peak effect.
- Antidepressant mediations include the following.
  - Selective serotonin inhibitors (SSRIs)
  - Atypical antidepressants
  - Tricyclic antidepressants (TCAs)
  - Monoamine oxidase inhibitors (MAOIs)

MEDICATION CLASSIFICATION:
SELECTIVE SEROTONIN REUPTAKE INHIBITORS (SSRIs)

- Select Prototype Medication: fluoxetine (Prozac)
- Other Medications
  - Citalopram (Celexa)
  - Escitalopram (Lexapro)
  - Paroxetine (Paxil)
  - Sertraline (Zoloft)
  - Vilazodone (Viibryd)

Purpose

- Expected pharmacological action
  - SSRIs selectively block reuptake of the monoamine neurotransmitter serotonin in the synaptic space, thereby intensifying the effects of serotonin.
- Therapeutic Uses
  - Major depression
  - Obsessive-compulsive disorders
  - Bulimia nervosa
  - Premenstrual dysphoric disorders
  - Panic disorders
  - Posttraumatic stress disorder

Complications

ADVERSE EFFECTS	NURSING INTERVENTIONS/CLIENT EDUCATION
› Sexual dysfunction (no orgasm, impotence, decreased libido)	› Warn clients of possible adverse effects and to notify the provider if intolerable. › Instruct client about ways to manage sexual dysfunction, such as lowering the dosage, discontinuing medication temporarily (medication holiday), and using adjunct medications to improve sexual function (sildenafil [Viagra] and buspirone). › Inform clients that an atypical antidepressant such as bupropion (Wellbutrin) has fewer sexual dysfunction adverse effects.
› CNS stimulation (inability to sleep, agitation, anxiety)	› Advise clients to notify the provider for dosage adjustment. › Advise clients to take the medication in the morning. › Advise clients to avoid caffeinated beverages. › Teach relaxation techniques to promote sleep.
› Weight loss early in therapy; weight gain with long-term treatment	› Monitor weight. › Encourage clients to participate in regular exercise and to follow a healthy, well-balanced diet.

› Serotonin syndrome can begin 2 to 72 hr after starting treatment and can be life-threatening.
› Manifestations include the following.
  » Mental confusion, difficulty concentrating
  » Fever
  » Agitation
  » Anxiety
  » Hallucinations
  » Incoordination, hyperreflexia
  » Diaphoresis
  » Tremors
	› Advise clients to observe for manifestations, and, if any occur, to notify the provider and withhold the medication.

› Withdrawal syndrome resulting in headache, nausea, visual disturbances, anxiety, dizziness, and tremors	› Instruct clients to taper the dose gradually.
› Hyponatremia (more likely in older adult clients taking diuretics)	› Obtain baseline serum sodium, and monitor level periodically throughout treatment.
› Rash	› Advise clients that a rash is treatable with an antihistamine or withdrawal of medication.

ADVERSE EFFECTS	NURSING INTERVENTIONS/CLIENT EDUCATION
› Drowsiness, faintness, lightheadedness	› Advise clients that these adverse effects are not common, but can occur. › Advise clients to avoid driving if these effects occur.
› Gastrointestinal (GI) bleeding	› Use caution with clients who have a history of GI bleeding and ulcers and with those taking other medications that affect blood coagulation.
› Bruxism	› Advise clients to report to the provider. › Advise clients to use a mouth guard. › Changing to a different classification of antidepressants or adding a low dose of buspirone can decrease this adverse effect.

Contraindications/Precautions

- Most of these medications are Pregnancy Risk Category C.
  - Fluoxetine (Category C) and paroxetine (Category D) increase the risk of birth defects. Late in pregnancy, use of SSRIs increases the risk of withdrawal symptoms or pulmonary hypertension in the newborn.
- Concurrent use of MAOIs or tricyclic antidepressants (TCAs) is a contraindication for SSRIs.
- Use cautiously with clients who have liver and renal dysfunction, cardiac disease, seizure disorders, diabetes, ulcers, or a history of GI bleeding.

Interactions

MEDICATION/FOOD INTERACTIONS	NURSING INTERVENTIONS/CLIENT EDUCATION
› MAOIs, TCAs, and St. John's wort increase the risk of serotonin syndrome.	› Clients should stop taking MAOIs for 14 days prior to starting an SSRI. If already taking fluoxetine, the client should wait 5 weeks before starting an MAOI. › Avoid concurrent use of TCAs and St. John's wort.
› Fluoxetine can displace warfarin (Coumadin) from bound protein and result in increased warfarin levels.	› Monitor PT and INR. › Check for indications of bleeding and the need for dosage adjustment.
› Fluoxetine can increase the levels of TCAs and lithium.	› Avoid concurrent use.
› Fluoxetine suppresses platelet aggregation and thus taking NSAIDs or anticoagulants with fluoxetine increases the risk of bleeding.	› Advise clients to monitor for indications of bleeding (bruising, hematuria) and to notify the provider if they occur.

MEDICATION CLASSIFICATION: ATYPICAL ANTIDEPRESSANTS

- Select Prototype Medication: bupropion HCl (Wellbutrin)

Purpose

- Expected Pharmacological Action
    - Action is not fully understood. However, it likely acts by inhibiting dopamine uptake.
- Therapeutic Uses
    - Treatment of depression
    - Alternative to SSRIs for clients unable to tolerate sexual dysfunction effects of SSRIs
    - Aid to quit smoking
    - Prevention of seasonal pattern depression

Complications

ADVERSE EFFECTS	NURSING INTERVENTIONS/CLIENT EDUCATION
› Headache, dry mouth, GI distress, constipation, increased heart rate, nausea, restlessness, and insomnia	› Advise clients to observe for effects and to notify the provider if intolerable. › Treat headache with mild analgesic. › Advise clients to sip fluids to treat dry mouth and to increase dietary fiber to prevent constipation.
› Suppresses appetite and often causes weight loss	› Monitor weight and food intake.
› Seizures	› Avoid administering to clients at risk for seizures, such as a client who has a head injury. › Monitor for seizures, and treat accordingly.

Contraindications/Precautions

- Bupropion is a Pregnancy Risk Category B medication.
- MAOI use is a contraindication for bupropion.
- Seizure disorders are a contraindication for bupropion.

Interactions

MEDICATION/FOOD INTERACTIONS	NURSING INTERVENTIONS/CLIENT EDUCATION
› MAOIs such as phenelzine increase the risk of toxicity.	› Clients should stop taking MAOIs 2 weeks prior to beginning treatment with bupropion.

OTHER ATYPICAL ANTIDEPRESSANTS

PHARMACOLOGICAL ACTION	NURSING IMPLICATIONS
Venlafaxine, duloxetine (Cymbalta)	
› These medications inhibit serotonin and norepinephrine reuptake, thereby increasing the amount of these neurotransmitters available in the brain for impulse transmission. There is also a minimal amount of dopamine blockade.	› Adverse effects include headache, nausea, agitation, anxiety, and sleep disturbances. › Monitor for hyponatremia, especially in older adult clients. › Monitor for weight loss. › Monitor for increases in diastolic pressure. › Discuss ways to manage interference with sexual functioning. › Advise clients not to stop taking the medication abruptly.
Mirtazapine (Remeron)	
› This medication increases the release of serotonin and norepinephrine, thereby increasing the amount of neurotransmitters available for impulse transmission.	› Therapeutic effects can occur sooner with less sexual dysfunction than with SSRIs. › Clients generally tolerate mirtazapine well, but some develop sleepiness that can be exacerbated by other CNS depressants (alcohol, benzodiazepines), weight gain, and elevated cholesterol.
Reboxetine (Edronax)	
› This medication selectively inhibits the reuptake of norepinephrine, thereby increasing the amount of neurotransmitters available for impulse transmission.	› This medication has results similar to SSRIs. › Clients generally tolerate reboxetine well, but some develop dry mouth, decreased blood pressure, constipation, sexual dysfunction, and urinary hesitancy or retention. › Weight gain and sleepiness do not occur. › Clients should not combine this medication with an MAOI.
Trazodone (Desyrel)	
› This medication has moderate selective blockade of serotonin receptors, which allows more serotonin to be available for impulse transmission.	› This medication is usually used with another antidepressant agent. Sedation is a potential problem; this medication can help clients who have insomnia caused by an SSRI. › Priapism is a potential adverse effect. Instruct clients to seek medical attention immediately if this occurs.

MEDICATION CLASSIFICATION: TRICYCLIC ANTIDEPRESSANTS (TCAs)

- Select Prototype Medication: amitriptyline
- Other Medications
  - Imipramine (Tofranil)
  - Doxepin (Silenor)
  - Nortriptyline (Aventyl)
  - Amoxapine
  - Trimipramine (Surmontil)

Purpose

- Expected Pharmacological Action
  - These medications block reuptake of norepinephrine and serotonin in the synaptic space, thereby intensifying the effects of these neurotransmitters.
- Therapeutic Uses
  - Depression
  - Depressive episodes of bipolar disorders
  - Other Uses
    - Neuropathic pain
    - Fibromyalgia
    - Anxiety disorders
    - Insomnia

Complications

ADVERSE EFFECTS	NURSING INTERVENTIONS/CLIENT EDUCATION
› Orthostatic hypotension	› Instruct clients about the effects of postural hypotension (lightheadedness, dizziness). If these occur, advise the client to sit or lie and to change positions slowly.
	› Monitor blood pressure and heart rate for clients in the hospital for orthostatic changes before administration and 1 hr after. For a significant decrease in blood pressure and/or increase in heart rate, do not administer the medication, and notify the provider.
› Anticholinergic effects » Dry mouth » Blurred vision » Photophobia » Urinary hesitancy or retention » Constipation » Tachycardia	› Instruct clients about ways to minimize anticholinergic effects. » Chewing gum » Sipping water » Wearing sunglasses when outdoors » Eating foods high in fiber » Participating in regular exercise » Increasing fluid intake to at least 2 to 3 L a day from beverages and food sources » Urinating just before taking medication › Advise the client to notify the provider if effects persist.
› Sedation	› This effect usually diminishes over time. › Advise clients to avoid hazardous activities such as driving if sedation is excessive. › Advise clients to take medication at bedtime to minimize daytime sleepiness and to promote sleep.

ADVERSE EFFECTS	NURSING INTERVENTIONS/CLIENT EDUCATION
› Toxicity resulting in cholinergic blockade and cardiac toxicity, causing dysrhythmias, mental confusion, and agitation, followed by seizures, coma, and possible death	› Obtain baseline ECG. › Monitor vital signs. › Monitor for signs of toxicity. › Notify the provider if signs of toxicity occur.
› Decreased seizure threshold	› Monitor clients who have seizure disorders.
› Excessive sweating	› Inform clients of this effect. Assist clients with frequent linen changes.

Contraindications/Precautions

- TCAs are Pregnancy Risk Category C medications.

- Seizure disorders are a contraindication for TCAs.

- Use cautiously with clients who have coronary artery disease; diabetes mellitus; liver, kidney, and respiratory disorders; urinary retention and obstruction; angle-closure glaucoma; benign prostatic hyperplasia; and hyperthyroidism.

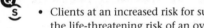

- Clients at an increased risk for suicide should receive a 1-week supply of medication at a time due to the life-threatening risk of an overdose.

Interactions

MEDICATION/FOOD INTERACTIONS	NURSING INTERVENTIONS/ CLIENT EDUCATION
› Concurrent use with MAOIs or St. John's wort can lead to serotonin syndrome. › Antihistamines and other anticholinergic agents have additive anticholinergic effects. › Increased effects of epinephrine, dopamine (direct-acting sympathomimetics) occur because TCAs block uptake into the nerve terminals, and they remain for a longer amount of time in the synaptic space. › TCAs decrease the effects of ephedrine and amphetamine (indirect-acting sympathomimetics) because they block uptake into the nerve terminals, and they are unable to reach their site of action.	› Avoid concurrent use.
› Alcohol, benzodiazepines, opioids, and antihistamines cause additive CNS depression.	› Advise clients to avoid other CNS depressants.

MEDICATION CLASSIFICATION: MONOAMINE OXIDASE INHIBITORS (MAOIs)

- Select Prototype Medication: phenelzine (Nardil)
- Other Medications
  - Isocarboxazid (Marplan)
  - Tranylcypromine (Parnate)
  - Selegiline (Emsam) – transdermal MAOI

Purpose

- Expected Pharmacological Action
  - These medications block MAO in the brain, thereby increasing the amount of norepinephrine, dopamine, and serotonin available for transmission of impulses. An increased amount of these neurotransmitters at nerve endings intensifies responses and relieves depression.
- Therapeutic Uses
  - Depression
  - Bulimia nervosa

Complications

ADVERSE EFFECTS	NURSING INTERVENTIONS/CLIENT EDUCATION
› CNS stimulation (anxiety, agitation, mania, or hypomania)	› Advise clients to observe for effects and notify the provider if they occur.
› Orthostatic hypotension	› Monitor BP and heart rate for orthostatic changes. Withhold the medication and notify the provider of significant changes. Instruct the client to change positions slowly.
› Hypertensive crisis resulting from intake of dietary tyramine › Severe hypertension occurs as a result of intensive vasoconstriction and stimulation of the heart. › Clients will most likely develop headache, nausea, and increased heart rate and blood pressure.	› Monitor clients who receive phentolamine (Regitine) IV, a rapid-acting alpha-adrenergic blocker or nifedipine (Procardia) SL. › Provide continuous cardiac monitoring and respiratory support.
› Local rash with transdermal preparation	› Choose a clean, dry area for each application. › Apply a topical glucocorticoid on the affected area.

Contraindications/Precautions

- MAOIs are Pregnancy Risk Category C medications.
- SSRI therapy, pheochromocytoma, heart failure, cardiovascular and cerebral vascular disease, and severe renal insufficiency are contraindications for MAOIs.
- Use cautiously with clients who have diabetes mellitus, seizure disorders, and those taking TCAs.
- Use of carbamazepine (Tegretol) or oxcarbazepine (Trileptal) is a contraindication for transdermal selegiline because those medications can increase blood levels of the MAOI.

Interactions

MEDICATION/FOOD INTERACTIONS	NURSING INTERVENTIONS/CLIENT EDUCATION
› Indirect-acting sympathomimetic medications (ephedrine, amphetamine) promote the release of norepinephrine and can lead to hypertensive crisis.	› Instruct clients to avoid over-the-counter decongestants and cold remedies, which frequently contain medications with sympathomimetic action.
› Use of tricyclic antidepressants can lead to hypertensive crisis.	› Use MAOIs and TCAs cautiously.
› Use of SSRIs can lead to serotonin syndrome.	› Avoid concurrent use.
› Antihypertensives have an additive hypotensive effect.	› Monitor BP. › Notify the provider about dosage reduction for a significant drop in BP.
› Use of meperidine (Demerol) can lead to hyperpyrexia.	› Use an alternative analgesic.
› Tyramine-rich foods can lead to hypertensive crisis. Clients will most likely develop headache, nausea, increased heart rate, and increased BP.	› Determine clients' ability to adhere strictly to dietary restrictions. › Instruct clients to notify the provider if manifestations occur. › Provide clients with written instructions regarding foods and beverages to avoid. › Tyramine-rich foods include aged cheese, pepperoni, salami, avocados, figs, bananas, smoked fish, protein dietary supplements, soups, soy sauce, some beers, and red wine. › Advise clients to avoid taking any medications without approval of the provider.
› Concurrent use of vasopressors (phenylethylamine, caffeine) can result in hypertension.	› Advise clients to avoid foods that contain these agents (caffeinated beverages, chocolate, fava beans, ginseng).

Nursing Administration

- Instruct clients to take these medications as prescribed on a daily basis to establish therapeutic plasma levels.

- Assist with medication regimen adherence by informing clients that it can take 1 to 3 weeks to begin to feel therapeutic effects. Full therapeutic effects can take 2 to 3 months.

- Instruct clients to continue therapy after achieving therapeutic effects. Sudden discontinuation of medication can result in relapse.

- Advise clients that therapy usually continues for 6 months after resolution of symptoms and can continue for a year or longer.

- Evaluate clients for suicide risk. Antidepressant medications can increase the risk for suicide particularly during initial treatment. Antidepressant-induced suicide typically affects clients younger than age 25.

- For SSRIs
    - Advise clients to take medication in the morning to minimize sleep disturbances.
    - Advise clients to take medication with food to minimize GI disturbances.
    - Obtain baseline sodium levels for older adult clients taking diuretics, and monitor periodically.

- For atypical antidepressants
    - For all atypical antidepressant medications, avoid use with MAOIs.
    - Advise clients taking bupropion for prevention of seasonal pattern depression to take medication beginning in the autumn each year and gradually taper the dose and discontinue it by spring.

- For TCAs
    - Monitor for toxicity (cardiac dysrhythmias).
    - Administer at bedtime due to sedation and risk for orthostatic hypotension.

- For MAOIs
    - Give clients a list of tyramine-rich food so they can avoid hypertensive crises.
    - Advise clients to avoid taking any other prescription or nonprescription medications unless the provider approves.

Nursing Evaluation of Medication Effectiveness

- Depending on therapeutic intent, clients demonstrate effectiveness by:
    - Verbalization of improvement in mood.
    - Ability to perform ADLs.
    - Improved sleeping and eating habits.
    - Increased interaction with peers.

APPLICATION EXERCISES

1. A nurse is caring for a client who has a new prescription for phenelzine (Nardil) for the treatment of depression. Which of the following indicates that the client has developed an adverse effect of this medication?

    A. Orthostatic hypotension

    B. Hearing loss

    C. Gastrointestinal bleeding

    D. Weight loss

2. A nurse is reinforcing teaching with a client who has a new prescription for amitriptyline for treatment of depression. Which of the following instructions should the nurse include? (Select all that apply.)

_____ A. Expect therapeutic effects in 24 to 48 hr.

_____ B. Stop taking the medication after a week of improved mood.

_____ C. Change positions slowly to minimize dizziness.

_____ D. Decrease dietary fiber intake to control diarrhea.

_____ E. Chew gum to prevent dry mouth.

3. A nurse is providing follow-up dietary teaching for a client who has a new prescription for phenelzine (Nardil). When reviewing the client's dietary log, which of the following foods on the log suggests a need for further reinforcement of teaching?

    A. Cottage cheese

    B. Banana bread

    C. Apple pie

    D. Grilled steak

4. A nurse is reinforcing discharge teaching with a client who is to begin taking fluoxetine (Prozac) for posttraumatic stress disorder. Which of the following statements is appropriate for the nurse to include?

    A. "You may have a decreased desire for intimacy while taking this medication."

    B. "You should take this medication at bedtime to help promote sleep."

    C. "You will have fewer urinary adverse effects if you urinate just before taking this medication."

    D. "You'll need to wear sunglasses when outdoors due to the light sensitivity this medication causes."

5. A nurse is caring for a client who has been taking sertraline (Zoloft) for the past 2 days. Which of the following findings should alert the nurse to the possibility that the client is developing serotonin syndrome?

    A. Bruising

    B. Fever

    C. Abdominal pain

    D. Rash

6. A nurse working in an urgent care center is caring for a client who reports headaches, nausea, and a "fast heartbeat." The client reports taking tranylcypromine (Parnate) for the treatment of depression and that he ate pepperoni pizza shortly before the manifestations began. Use the ATI Active Learning Template: Systems Disorder and the ATI Mental Health Review Module to complete this item to include the following sections:

    A. Description of Disorder/Disease Process

    B. Assessment: Objective and Subjective – Identify at least three expected findings.

    C. Patient-Centered Care: Medications – Identify at least one medication appropriate for treatment.

    D. Management of Client Care: Client Education – Identify four dietary sources of tyramine the client should avoid.

APPLICATION EXERCISES KEY

1. A. **CORRECT:** Orthostatic hypotension is an adverse of effect of MAOIs, including phenelzine.

    B. INCORRECT: Phenelzine is more likely to cause blurred vision than hearing loss.

    C. INCORRECT: Clients taking phenelzine are at risk for multiple adverse effects. However, these do not include GI bleeding.

    D. INCORRECT: Clients taking phenelzine are at risk for weight gain rather than weight loss.

    Ⓝ NCLEX® Connection: Pharmacological Therapies, Adverse Effects/Contraindications/ Side Effects/Interactions

2. A. INCORRECT: Therapeutic effects take several weeks of amitriptyline therapy to develop.

    B. INCORRECT: Stopping amitriptyline abruptly can result in relapse.

    C. **CORRECT:** Changing positions slowly helps prevent orthostatic hypotension, which is an adverse effect of amitriptyline.

    D. INCORRECT: Clients should increase dietary fiber to prevent constipation, which is an adverse effect of amitriptyline.

    E. **CORRECT:** Chewing gum can minimize dry mouth, which is an adverse effect of amitriptyline.

    Ⓝ NCLEX® Connection: Pharmacological Therapies, Medication Administration

3. A. INCORRECT: The client should avoid aged rather than cottage cheese, which contains little or no tyramine.

    B. **CORRECT:** Clients taking phenelzine, an MAOI, should avoid foods containing tyramine. Bananas and yeast products contain tyramine.

    C. INCORRECT: Apple pie contains little or no tyramine.

    D. INCORRECT: The client should avoid aged meats rather than grilled steak, which contains little or no tyramine.

    Ⓝ NCLEX® Connection: Pharmacological Therapies, Medication Administration

4. A. **CORRECT:** Decreased libido is a potential adverse effect of fluoxetine and other SSRIs.

    B. INCORRECT: Clients should take fluoxetine in the morning due to CNS stimulation.

    C. INCORRECT: Clients taking a TCA, rather than fluoxetine, should void prior to taking the medication due to the potential for urinary hesitancy or retention.

    D. INCORRECT: Clients taking a TCA, rather than fluoxetine, should wear sunglasses when outdoors due to the potential for photophobia.

    (N) NCLEX® Connection: Pharmacological Therapies, Adverse Effects/Contraindications/ Side Effects/Interactions

5. A. INCORRECT: Bleeding can result if an SSRI is administered with warfarin (Coumadin). However, this is not an indication of serotonin syndrome.

    B. **CORRECT:** Fever is a manifestation of serotonin syndrome, which can result from taking an SSRI such as sertraline.

    C. INCORRECT: Abdominal pain is not an indication of serotonin syndrome. Common manifestations include confusion, disorientation, hallucinations, and incoordination.

    D. INCORRECT: A localized rash is associated with transdermal preparation. However, it is not an indication of serotonin syndrome.

    (N) NCLEX® Connection: Pharmacological Therapies, Adverse Effects/Contraindications/ Side Effects/Interactions

6. *Using the ATI Active Learning Template: Systems Disorder*

    A. Description of Disorder/Disease Process
    - Hypertensive crisis results from intensive vasoconstriction due to the intake of dietary tyramine while taking an MAOI.

    B. Assessment: Objective and Subjective
    - Severe hypertension
    - Headache
    - Nausea
    - Increased heart rate

    C. Patient-Centered Care: Medications
    - Phentolamine (Regitine) IV, a rapid-acting alpha-adrenergic blocker
    - Nifedipine (Procardia SL), a calcium channel blocker

    D. Management of Client Care: Client Education
    - Aged cheeses
    - Smoked or preserved fish or meats, such as pepperoni and salami
    - Avocados
    - Figs
    - Bananas
    - Protein dietary supplements
    - Soups containing meat extracts
    - Soy sauce
    - Some beers
    - Red wine

    (N) NCLEX® Connection: Pharmacological Therapies, Adverse Effects/Contraindications/ Side Effects/Interactions

chapter 8

Overview

- Bipolar disorders are managed primarily with mood-stabilizing medications such as lithium carbonate (Lithobid).
- Other medications used to treat bipolar disorders include the following.
  - Antiepileptic medications
    - Valproic acid (Depakote)
    - Carbamazepine (Tegretol, Equetro)
    - Lamotrigine (Lamictal)
  - Atypical antipsychotics – These can be useful in early treatment to promote sleep and to decrease anxiety and agitation. These medications also demonstrate mood-stabilizing properties.
  - Anxiolytics – Clonazepam (Klonopin) and lorazepam (Ativan) can be useful in treating acute mania and managing the psychomotor agitation of mania.
  - Antidepressants – Medications such as bupropion (Wellbutrin) and sertraline (Zoloft) can be useful during the depressive phase, typically in combination with a mood stabilizer to prevent rebound mania.

MEDICATION CLASSIFICATION: MOOD STABILIZER

- Select Prototype Medication: lithium carbonate

Purpose

- Expected Pharmacological Action
  - Lithium produces neurochemical changes in the brain, including serotonin receptor blockade.
  - There is evidence that lithium can decrease neuronal atrophy and increase neuronal growth.
- Therapeutic Uses
  - Lithium treats bipolar disorders. It controls episodes of acute mania, helps prevent the return of mania or depression, and decreases the incidence of suicide.
  - Other uses
    - Alcohol use disorder
    - Bulimia nervosa
    - Psychotic disorders

Complications

- Effects with therapeutic lithium levels (some effects will resolve within a few weeks)

ADVERSE EFFECTS	NURSING INTERVENTIONS/CLIENT EDUCATION
› Gastrointestinal (GI) distress (nausea, diarrhea, abdominal pain)	› Inform clients that effects are usually transient. › Administer medication with meals or milk.
› Fine hand tremors that can interfere with purposeful motor skills and can be exacerbated by factors such as stress and caffeine	› Administer beta-adrenergic blocking agents such as propranolol (Inderal). › Adjust to the lowest possible dosage, give in divided doses, or use long-acting formulations. › Advise clients to report an increase in tremors.
› Polyuria, mild thirst	› Use a potassium-sparing diuretic, such as spironolactone (Aldactone). › Instruct clients to consume 2,000 to 3,000 mL of fluid from beverages and food sources.
› Weight gain	› Assist clients to follow a healthy diet and regular exercise regimen.
› Renal toxicity	› Monitor I&O. › Request a prescription for a lower dose. › Check baseline kidney function, and monitor kidney function.
› Goiter and hypothyroidism with long-term treatment	› Obtain baseline T_3, T_4, and TSH levels prior to starting treatment, and then annually. › Advise clients to monitor for manifestations of hypothyroidism (cold, dry skin; decreased heart rate; weight gain). › Administer levothyroxine (Synthroid) to manage hypothyroid effects.
› Bradydysrhythmia, hypotension, and electrolyte imbalances	› Encourage clients to consume adequate fluids.

- Lithium toxicity

LITHIUM LEVEL	CLINICAL MANIFESTATIONS	NURSING INTERVENTIONS/CLIENT EDUCATION
Early indications		
Less than 1.5 mEq/L	› Diarrhea, nausea, vomiting, thirst, polyuria, muscle weakness, fine hand tremor, slurred speech	› Advise clients to withhold medication and notify the provider. › Administer the new dosage based on serum lithium levels.
Advanced indications		
1.5 to 2.0 mEq/L	› Ongoing gastrointestinal distress, including nausea, vomiting, and diarrhea; mental confusion; poor coordination; coarse tremors	› Advise clients to withhold medication and notify the provider. › Administer the new dosage based on serum lithium levels. › If manifestations are severe, it can be necessary to promote excretion.

LITHIUM LEVEL	CLINICAL MANIFESTATIONS	NURSING INTERVENTIONS/CLIENT EDUCATION
Severe toxicity		
2.0 to 2.5 mEq/L	› Extreme polyuria with dilute urine, tinnitus, blurred vision, ataxia, seizures, severe hypotension leading to coma and possibly death from respiratory complications	› Give alert clients an emetic. › Perform gastric lavage; monitor clients receiving urea, mannitol, or aminophylline to increase the rate of excretion.
Greater than 2.5 mEq/L	› Rapid progression of symptoms leading to coma and death	› Hemodialysis

Contraindications/Precautions

- Lithium is a Pregnancy Risk Category D medication. It is teratogenic, especially during the first trimester.
- Discourage clients from breastfeeding if lithium therapy is necessary.
- Use cautiously with clients who have renal dysfunction, heart disease, sodium depletion, or dehydration.

Interactions

MEDICATION/FOOD INTERACTIONS	NURSING INTERVENTIONS/CLIENT EDUCATION
› Sodium is excreted with the use of diuretics. Reduced serum sodium decreases lithium excretion, which can lead to toxicity.	› Monitor clients for indications of toxicity. › Advise clients to observe for indications of toxicity and to notify the provider. › Encourage clients to consume a diet adequate in sodium, and to drink 2,000 mL to 3,000 mL of water each day from food and beverage sources.
› Concurrent use of NSAIDs (ibuprofen [Motrin] and celecoxib [Celebrex]) will increase renal reabsorption of lithium, leading to toxicity.	› Avoid the use of some NSAIDs. › Use aspirin as a mild analgesic.
› Anticholinergics (antihistamines, tricyclic antidepressants) can induce urinary retention and polyuria, leading to abdominal discomfort.	› Advise clients to avoid medications with anticholinergic effects.

Nursing Administration

- Monitor plasma lithium levels. At initiation of treatment, check levels every 2 to 3 days and then every 1 to 3 months. Older adult clients often require more frequent monitoring. Obtain blood for lithium levels in the morning, usually 12 hr after the last dose.

  - During initial treatment of a manic episode, levels should be between 0.8 and 1.4 mEq/L.

  - Maintenance level range is between 0.4 and 1.0 mEq/L.

  - Plasma levels above 1.5 mEq/L can result in toxicity.

- Care for clients who have a toxic plasma lithium level in an acute care setting, and provide supportive measures. Hemodialysis can be indicated.

- Advise clients that effects begin within 7 to 14 days.

- Advise clients to take lithium as prescribed, in two to three doses daily due to its short half-life. Taking lithium with food will help decrease GI distress.

- Encourage clients to adhere to laboratory appointments to monitor lithium effectiveness and adverse effects. Emphasize the high risk of toxicity due to the narrow therapeutic range.

- Reinforce nutritional counseling. Stress the importance of adequate fluid and sodium intake.

- Instruct clients to monitor for clinical manifestations of toxicity and when to contact the provider. Clients should withhold medication and seek medical attention for diarrhea, vomiting, or excessive sweating.

MEDICATION CLASSIFICATION: MOOD-STABILIZING ANTIEPILEPTIC DRUGS (AEDs)

- Select Prototype Medications

  - Carbamazepine (Tegretol, Equetro)

    - Tegretol and Equetro are the same formulation of carbamazepine, and both are effective for bipolar disorder. However, only Equetro is approved for this use.

  - Valproic acid (Depakote)

  - Lamotrigine (Lamictal)

Purpose

- Expected Pharmacological Action

  - AEDs help treat and manage bipolar disorders by various mechanisms.

    - Slowing the entrance of sodium and calcium back into the neuron, thus extending the time it takes for the nerve to return to its active state

    - Potentiating the inhibitory effects of gamma-aminobutyric acid (GABA)

    - Inhibiting glutamic acid (glutamate), which in turn suppresses CNS excitation

- Therapeutic Uses

  - Treatment of manic and depressive episodes, and prevention of relapse of mania and depressive episodes. Especially useful for clients who have mixed mania and rapid cycling bipolar disorders.

Complications

CARBAMAZEPINE	
Adverse Effects	**Nursing Interventions/Client Education**
› Minimal effect on cognitive function › Nystagmus, double vision, vertigo, staggering gait, headache	› Administer low doses initially, with gradual increases in dosage. › Inform clients that CNS effects should subside within a few weeks. › Administer the medication at bedtime.
› Blood dyscrasias (leukopenia, anemia, thrombocytopenia)	› Obtain a baseline CBC and platelets, and perform ongoing monitoring. › Observe for indications of bruising and bleeding of gums. › Monitor for sore throat, fatigue, and other indications of infection.
› Teratogenesis	› Advise clients to avoid use in pregnancy.
› Hypo-osmolarity (promotes secretion of ADH, which inhibits water excretion by the kidneys and places clients with heart failure at risk for fluid overload)	› Monitor serum sodium. › Monitor for edema, decrease in urine output, and hypertension.
› Skin disorders (dermatitis, rash, Stevens-Johnson syndrome)	› Treat mild reactions with anti-inflammatory or antihistamine medications. › Advise clients to wear sunscreen. › Instruct clients to notify the provider if they develop a Stevens-Johnson syndrome rash and to withhold the medication.

LAMOTRIGINE	
Adverse Effects	**Nursing Interventions/Client Education**
› Common effects include double or blurred vision, dizziness, headache, nausea, and vomiting.	› Caution clients about performing activities requiring concentration.
› Serious skin rashes including Stevens-Johnson syndrome	› Instruct clients to withhold medication and notify the provider if they develop a rash.

VALPROIC ACID

Adverse Effects	Nursing Interventions/Client Education
› GI effects (nausea, vomiting, indigestion)	› Inform clients that manifestations are usually self-limiting. › Advise clients to take the medication with food or switch to enteric-coated pills.
› Hepatotoxicity as evidenced by anorexia, nausea, vomiting, fatigue abdominal pain, jaundice	› Obtain baseline liver function, and monitor liver function regularly. › Advise clients to observe for manifestations and to notify the provider if they occur. › Be aware that this medication is inappropriate for children younger than 2 years old. › Be aware that clients should take the lowest effective dose.
› Pancreatitis (nausea, vomiting, and abdominal pain)	› Advise clients to observe for manifestations and to withhold the medication and notify the provider immediately if they occur. › Monitor amylase levels.
› Thrombocytopenia	› Advise clients to observe for manifestations such as bruising, and to notify the provider if these occur. › Monitor platelet counts.
› Teratogenesis	› Advise the client to avoid use in pregnancy.

Contraindications/Precautions

- These are Pregnancy Risk Category D medications and can result in birth defects.
- Bone marrow suppression and bleeding disorders are contraindications for carbamazepine.
- Liver disorders are contraindications for valproic acid.

Interactions

CARBAMAZEPINE

Medication/Food Interactions	Nursing Interventions/Client Education
› Concurrent use of carbamazepine causes a decrease in the effects of oral contraceptives and warfarin (Coumadin) because of stimulation of hepatic drug-metabolizing enzymes.	› Advise clients to use an alternate form of birth control. › Monitor for therapeutic effects of warfarin. › Request dosage adjustments.
› Grapefruit juice inhibits metabolism, thus increasing carbamazepine levels.	› Advise clients to avoid grapefruit juice.
› Phenytoin and phenobarbital decrease the effects of carbamazepine by stimulating metabolism.	› Monitor phenytoin and phenobarbital levels. › Request dosage adjustments.

LAMOTRIGINE	
Medication/Food Interactions	Nursing Interventions/Client Education
› Carbamazepine, phenytoin, and phenobarbital promote liver drug-metabolizing enzymes, thereby decreasing the effect of lamotrigine.	› Monitor for therapeutic effects. › Request dosage adjustments.
› Valproic acid inhibits medication-metabolizing enzymes and thus increases the half-life of lamotrigine.	› Monitor for adverse effects. › Request dosage adjustments.

VALPROIC ACID	
Medication/Food Interactions	Nursing Interventions/Client Education
› Concurrent use of valproic acid increases the levels of phenytoin and phenobarbital.	› Monitor phenytoin and phenobarbital levels. › Request dosage adjustments.

Nursing Evaluation of Medication Effectiveness

- Depending on therapeutic intent, clients demonstrate effectiveness by:
  - ○ Relief from acute mania (flight of ideas, obsessive talking, agitation) and depression (fatigue, poor appetite, psychomotor retardation).
  - ○ Verbalization of improvement in mood.
  - ○ Ability to perform ADLs.
  - ○ Improved sleeping and eating habits.
  - ○ More interaction with peers.

APPLICATION EXERCISES

1. A nurse is reviewing laboratory findings and notes that a client's plasma lithium level is 2.1 mEq/L. Which of the following is an appropriate action by the nurse?

    A. Perform immediate gastric lavage.

    B. Prepare the client for hemodialysis.

    C. Administer an additional oral dose of lithium.

    D. Request a stat repeat of the laboratory test.

2. A nurse is caring for a client who has a new prescription for lithium carbonate (Lithobid). When reinforcing teaching about ways to prevent lithium toxicity, the nurse should advise the client to do which of the following?

    A. Avoid the use of acetaminophen for headaches.

    B. Restrict intake of foods rich in sodium.

    C. Decrease fluid intake to less than 1,500 mL daily

    D. Limit aerobic activity in hot weather.

3. A nurse in a primary care clinic is collecting data from a client who takes lithium carbonate (Lithobid) for the treatment of bipolar disorder. The nurse should recognize which of the following findings as a possible indication of toxicity from this medication?

    A. Severe hypertension

    B. Coarse tremors

    C. Constipation

    D. Urinary retention

4. A nurse is caring for a client who has a new prescription for valproic acid (Depakote). The nurse should instruct the client that while taking this medication he will need which of the following laboratory tests periodically? (Select all that apply.)

    _____ A. Thrombocyte count

    _____ B. Hematocrit

    _____ C. Amylase

    _____ D. Liver function tests

    _____ E. Potassium

5. A nurse is reinforcing teaching with a female client who has bipolar disorder about her new prescription for lithium carbonate (Lithobid). Which of the following is appropriate for the nurse to include? (Select all that apply.)

_____ A. Expect amenorrhea as an adverse effect of this medication.

_____ B. Take an antidepressant with lithium during phases of mania.

_____ C. Take this medication with food or a glass of milk.

_____ D. Avoid pregnancy while taking this medication.

_____ E. Have thyroid function tests prior to lithium therapy.

6. A nurse is reinforcing discharge instructions with a client who has a new diagnosis of bipolar disorder. The client has a new prescription for lithium carbonate (Lithobid) 600 mg PO three times a day. Use the ATI Active Learning Template: Medication to complete this item to include three side or adverse effects the nurse should include in the information.

APPLICATION EXERCISES KEY

1. A. **CORRECT:** Gastric lavage is appropriate for a client who has severe toxicity, with a plasma lithium level of 2.1 mEq/L. This action will lower the client's lithium level.

    B. INCORRECT: Hemodialysis is appropriate for a client who has a plasma lithium level above 2.5 mEq/L.

    C. INCORRECT: Administering an additional dose of lithium will worsen the level of toxicity.

    D. INCORRECT: There is no indication that the client needs another laboratory test, and this action can delay treatment.

    N NCLEX® Connection: Pharmacological Therapies, Adverse Effects/Contraindications/ Side Effects/Interactions

2. A. INCORRECT: The client should use acetaminophen, rather than NSAIDs, such as ibuprofen, for headaches because NSAIDs interact with lithium and can cause increased blood levels of lithium.

    B. INCORRECT: The client should increase, rather than decrease, sodium intake to reduce the risk for toxicity.

    C. INCORRECT: The client should increase, rather than decrease, fluid intake to reduce the risk for toxicity.

    D. **CORRECT:** The client should avoid activities that have the potential to cause sodium/water depletion, which can increase the risk for toxicity.

    N NCLEX® Connection: Pharmacological Therapies, Medication Administration

3. A. INCORRECT: Severe hypotension, rather than hypertension, is an indication of toxicity.

    B. **CORRECT:** Coarse tremors are an indication of toxicity.

    C. INCORRECT: Diarrhea, rather than constipation, is a sign of toxicity.

    D. INCORRECT: Polyuria, rather than retention, is a sign of toxicity.

    N NCLEX® Connection: Pharmacological Therapies, Adverse Effects/Contraindications/ Side Effects/Interactions

4. A. **CORRECT:** Treatment with valproic acid can result in thrombocytopenia. The nurse should monitor the client's thrombocyte count.

B. INCORRECT: Treatment with valproic acid does not affect hematocrit.

C. **CORRECT:** Treatment with valproic acid can result in pancreatitis. The nurse should monitor the client's amylase.

D. **CORRECT:** Treatment with valproic acid can result in hepatotoxicity. The nurse should monitor the client's liver function.

E. INCORRECT: Treatment with valproic acid does not affect potassium.

Ⓝ NCLEX® Connection: Pharmacological Therapies, Medication Administration

5. A. INCORRECT: Lithium carbonate does not cause amenorrhea, although it can cause oliguria.

B. INCORRECT: An antidepressant, combined with lithium, is effective during phases of depression rather than mania.

C. **CORRECT:** Taking lithium with food or a glass of milk can help reduce gastrointestinal distress.

D. **CORRECT:** Lithium is a Pregnancy Risk Category D medication that is teratogenic, especially during the first trimester. The client should avoid pregnancy while taking this medication.

E. **CORRECT:** Because lithium can cause goiter and hypothyroidism, the nurse should check the client's thyroid function prior to lithium therapy.

Ⓝ NCLEX® Connection: Pharmacological Therapies, Medication Administration

6. *Using the ATI Active Learning Template: Medication*
   - Side/Adverse Effects
     - Gastrointestinal distress – nausea, diarrhea, abdominal pain
     - Fine hand tremors
     - Polyuria
     - Mild thirst
     - Weight gain
     - Renal toxicity
     - Goiter and hypothyroidism
     - Bradydysrhythmias
     - Hypotension
     - Electrolyte imbalances

   Ⓝ NCLEX® Connection: Pharmacological Therapies, Adverse Effects/Contraindications/ Side Effects/Interactions

chapter 9

Overview

- Schizophrenia spectrum disorders are the primary reason for the administration of antipsychotic medications.
  - The clinical course of schizophrenia usually involves acute exacerbations with intervals of semiremission.
  - Medications treat:
    - Positive symptoms related to behavior, thought, and speech (agitation, delusions, hallucinations, tangential speech patterns).
    - Negative symptoms (social withdrawal, lack of emotion, lack of energy [anergia], flattened affect, decreased motivation, decreased pleasure in activities).
  - Goals of psychopharmacological treatment for schizophrenia spectrum and other psychotic disorders
    - Suppressing acute episodes.
    - Preventing acute recurrence.
    - Maintaining the highest possible level of functioning.
- First-generation (conventional) antipsychotic medications control mainly the positive symptoms, such as hallucinations, delusions, and bizarre behavior of psychotic disorders. These medications are for clients who are:
  - Using them successfully and can tolerate the adverse effects.
  - Violent or particularly aggressive.
- Second-generation (atypical) antipsychotic agents are medications of choice for clients receiving initial treatment and for treating breakthrough episodes of clients receiving conventional medication therapy, because they are more effective with fewer adverse effects.
  - Advantages of atypical antipsychotic agents
    - Relief of both the positive and negative symptoms of schizophrenia
    - Decrease in affective manifestations (depression, anxiety) and suicidal behavior
    - Improvement of neurocognitive deficits, such as poor memory
    - Fewer or no extrapyramidal side effects (EPSs), including tardive dyskinesia (TD), because of less dopamine blockade
    - Fewer anticholinergic adverse effects because most atypical antipsychotics, with the exception of clozapine (Clozaril), cause little or no blockade of cholinergic receptors
    - Less relapse

MEDICATION CLASSIFICATION:
ANTIPSYCHOTICS – FIRST-GENERATION (CONVENTIONAL)

- Select Prototype Medication: chlorpromazine – low potency
- Other Medications
  - Haloperidol (Haldol) – high potency
  - Fluphenazine – high potency
  - Thiothixene (Navane) – high potency
  - Perphenazine – medium potency

Purpose

- Expected Pharmacological Action
  - Block dopamine (D_2), acetylcholine, histamine, and norepinephrine (NE) receptors in the brain and periphery.
  - Inhibit psychotic manifestations, believed to be a result of D_2 blockade in the brain.
- Therapeutic Uses
  - Acute and chronic psychotic disorders
  - Schizophrenia spectrum disorders
  - Bipolar disorders (primarily the manic phase)
  - Tourette's disorder
  - Prevention of nausea/vomiting through blocking dopamine in the chemoreceptor trigger zone of the medulla

Complications

ADVERSE EFFECTS	NURSING INTERVENTIONS/CLIENT EDUCATION
Extrapyramidal side effects (EPSs)	
› Acute dystonia	
› Clinical findings include severe spasms of tongue, neck, face, or back. This is a crisis situation that requires rapid treatment.	› Monitor for acute dystonia between 5 hr to 5 days after administration of the first dose. › Treat with anticholinergic agents, such as benztropine (Cogentin) or diphenhydramine. Use oral doses for less acute effects. The client will need IM or IV doses for serious effects.
› Parkinsonism	
› Clinical findings include bradykinesia, rigidity, shuffling gait, drooling, and tremors.	› Observe for parkinsonism within 1 month of initiation of therapy. › Treat with benztropine, diphenhydramine, or amantadine (Symmetrel). If manifestations return after stopping the medications, the provider can prescribe an atypical antipsychotic.

ADVERSE EFFECTS	NURSING INTERVENTIONS/CLIENT EDUCATION
Extrapyramidal side effects (EPSs)	
› Akathisia	
› The client is unable to stand still or sit, and is continually pacing and agitated.	› Observe for akathisia within 2 months of the initiation of treatment. › Manage effects with a beta-blocker, benzodiazepine, or anticholinergic medication.
› Tardive dyskinesia (TD)	
› Manifestations include involuntary movements of the tongue and face, such as lip-smacking, which cause speech and eating disturbances. › TD can also include involuntary movements of arms, legs, or trunk.	› TD is a late EPS that can develop months to years after the start of therapy, and can improve following medication change or be permanent. › Clients should take the lowest dosage possible to control manifestations. › Evaluate after 12 months of therapy and then every 3 months. If indications of TD appear, the provider should lower the dosage or switch to an atypical agent.
Other adverse effects	
› Neuroleptic malignant syndrome	
› Manifestations include sudden high-grade fever, blood pressure fluctuations, dysrhythmias, muscle rigidity, and changes in level of consciousness developing into coma.	› Stop antipsychotic medication. › Monitor vital signs. › Apply cooling blankets. › Administer antipyretics (aspirin, acetaminophen). › Increase fluid intake. › Administer diazepam (Valium) to control anxiety. › Administer dantrolene (Dantrium) to induce muscle relaxation. › Wait 2 weeks before resuming therapy. Consider requesting an atypical agent.
› Anticholinergic effects	
› Dry mouth › Blurred vision › Photophobia › Urinary hesitancy/retention › Constipation › Tachycardia	› Suggest strategies to decrease anticholinergic effects. » Chewing gum » Sipping water » Avoiding hazardous activities » Wearing sunglasses when outdoors » Eating foods high in fiber » Participating in regular exercise » Consuming 2 to 3 L of water daily from food and beverage sources » Urinating just before taking the medication
› Neuroendocrine effects	
› Effects include gynecomastia (breast enlargement), galactorrhea, and menstrual irregularities.	› Advise clients to observe for manifestations and to notify the provider if these occur.

ADVERSE EFFECTS	NURSING INTERVENTIONS/CLIENT EDUCATION
Other adverse effects	
› Seizures	
› The greatest risk for developing seizures is existing seizure disorders.	› Advise clients to report seizure activity to the provider. › An increase in antiseizure medication can be necessary.
› Skin effects	
› Effects include photosensitivity resulting in severe sunburn, and contact dermatitis from handling medications.	› Advise clients to avoid excessive exposure to sunlight, to use sunscreen, and to wear protective clothing. › Advise clients to avoid direct contact with the medication.
Additional effects	
› Orthostatic hypotension	› Clients should develop tolerance in 2 to 3 months. › In the hospital setting, monitor blood pressure and heart rate for orthostatic changes. For a significant decrease in blood pressure or increase in heart rate, do not administer the medication, and notify the provider. › Instruct clients about the signs of orthostatic hypotension (lightheadedness, dizziness). If these occur, advise the client to sit or lie and to get up and change positions slowly.
› Sedation	› Inform clients that effects should diminish within a few weeks. › Clients can take this medication at bedtime to avoid daytime sleepiness. › Advise clients not to drive until sedation has subsided.
› Sexual dysfunction (common in both males and females)	› Inform clients of possible adverse effects. › Encourage clients to report adverse effects to the provider. › The client can need a lower dosage or a high-potency agent.
› Agranulocytosis	› Advise clients to observe for indications of infection (fever, sore throat), and to notify the provider if these occur. › If indications of infection appear, obtain a baseline WBC. If the results indicate infection, withhold the medication and inform the provider.
› Severe dysrhythmias	› Obtain a baseline ECG and potassium level prior to treatment and periodically throughout the treatment period. › Avoid concurrent use with other medications that prolong the QT interval.

Contraindications/Precautions

- Coma, severe depression, Parkinson's disease, prolactin-dependent cancer of the breast, and severe hypotension are contraindications for conventional antipsychotics.
- Dementia in older clients is a contraindication for conventional antipsychotics.
- Use cautiously with clients who have glaucoma, paralytic ileus, prostate enlargement, heart disorders, liver or kidney disease, and seizure disorders.

Interactions

MEDICATION/FOOD INTERACTIONS	NURSING INTERVENTIONS/CLIENT EDUCATION
› Concurrent use of anticholinergic agents with other anticholinergic medications will increase anticholinergic effects.	› Advise clients to avoid over-the-counter medications that contain anticholinergic agents, such as sleep aids.
› Alcohol, opioids, and antihistamines have additive CNS depressant effects.	› Advise clients to avoid alcohol and other medications that cause CNS depression. › Advise clients to avoid hazardous activities, such as driving.
› By activating dopamine receptors, levodopa counteracts the effects of antipsychotic agents.	› Avoid concurrent use of levodopa and other direct dopamine receptor agonists.

Nursing Administration

- Use the Abnormal Involuntary Movement Scale (AIMS) to screen for the presence of EPS.
- Observe clients to differentiate between EPS and worsening of the psychotic disorder.
- Administer anticholinergics, beta-blockers, and benzodiazepines to control early EPS. If adverse effects are intolerable, the provider can switch the client to a low-potency or an atypical antipsychotic agent.
- Inform clients that antipsychotic medications do not cause addiction.
- Advise clients to take the medication as prescribed and to take it on a regular schedule.
- Inform clients that they might notice some therapeutic effects within a few days, but significant improvement can take 2 to 4 weeks, and possibly several months for full effects.
- Consider depot preparations administered IM once every 2 to 4 weeks for clients who have difficulty with adherence. Explain that depot preparations are lower dosages, which will decrease the risk of adverse effects and the development of tardive dyskinesia.
- Start administration with twice-a-day dosing, then switch to daily dosing at bedtime to decrease daytime drowsiness and promote sleep.

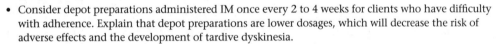

MEDICATION CLASSIFICATION: ANTIPSYCHOTICS – SECOND-GENERATION (ATYPICAL)

- Select Prototype Medication: risperidone (Risperdal)
- Other Medications
  - Olanzapine (Zyprexa)
  - Quetiapine (Seroquel)
  - Aripiprazole (Abilify)
  - Ziprasidone (Geodon)
  - Clozapine (Clozaril)
  - Asenapine (Saphris)
  - Lurasidone (Latuda)
  - Paliperidone (Invega)
  - Iloperidone (Fanapt)

Purpose

- Expected Pharmacological Action – These antipsychotic agents work mainly by blocking serotonin, and to a lesser degree, dopamine receptors. These medications also block receptors for norepinephrine, histamine, and acetylcholine.

- Therapeutic Uses

    ○ Schizophrenia spectrum disorders (negative and positive symptoms)

    ○ Psychotic episodes induced by levodopa therapy

    ○ Relief of psychotic manifestations in other disorders such as bipolar disorders

- Formulations

    ○ Tablets

    ○ Quick-dissolving tablets

    ○ Oral solution

    ○ IM depot preparation (Risperdal Consta)

Complications

ADVERSE EFFECTS	NURSING INTERVENTIONS/CLIENT EDUCATION
› New onset of diabetes mellitus or loss of glucose control in clients who have diabetes	› Obtain baseline fasting blood glucose and monitor throughout treatment. › Instruct clients to report indications (increased thirst, urination, and appetite).
› Weight gain	› Advise clients to follow a healthy low-calorie diet, engage in regular exercise, and monitor weight gain.
› Hypercholesterolemia with increased risk for hypertension and other cardiovascular disease	› Monitor cholesterol, triglycerides, and blood glucose for any significant weight gain.
› Orthostatic hypotension	› Monitor blood pressure and heart rate for orthostatic changes. Instruct clients to change positions slowly.
› Anticholinergic effects such as urinary hesitancy or retention, dry mouth	› Monitor for effects and report occurrence to the provider. › Inform clients about measures to relieve dry mouth, such as sipping fluids.
› Agitation, dizziness, sedation, and sleep disruption	› Monitor for effects and report to the provider if they occur. › Administer alternative medication if prescribed.
› Mild EPS, such as tremor	› Monitor for and instruct clients to recognize EPS. › Use AIMS assessment to screen for EPS.

Contraindications/Precautions

- Risperidone is a Pregnancy Risk Category C medication.
- Dementia is a contraindication for risperidone.
- All atypical antipsychotic medications can cause death related to cerebrovascular accident or infection.
- Clients should avoid drinking alcohol.
- Use cautiously with clients who have cardiovascular or cerebrovascular disease, seizures, or diabetes mellitus. Obtain a fasting blood glucose for clients who have diabetes, and monitor blood glucose carefully.
- Other atypical antipsychotic agents

OLANZAPINE	
Formulations	› Tablets
	› Short-acting injectable
	› Extended-release injection
Complications	› Olanzapine has a low risk of EPS.
	› Olanzapine has a high risk for diabetes mellitus, weight gain, and dyslipidemia.
	› Other adverse effects include sedation, orthostatic hypotension, and anticholinergic effects.

QUETIAPINE	
Formulations	› Tablets
	› Extended-release tablets
Complications	› Quetiapine has a low risk of EPS.
	› Quetiapine has a moderate risk for diabetes mellitus, weight gain, and dyslipidemia.
	› Other effects include cataracts, sedation, orthostatic hypotension, and anticholinergic effects.
	› Clients should have a screening eye examination and then every 6 months.

ARIPIPRAZOLE	
Formulations	› Tablets
	› Orally disintegrating tablets
	› Oral solution
	› Short-acting injectable
Complications	› Aripiprazole has low or no risk of EPS, diabetes mellitus, weight gain, dyslipidemia, hypotension, and anticholinergic effects.
	› Other adverse effects include headache, anxiety, insomnia, sedation, and gastrointestinal upset.

ZIPRASIDONE	
Comments	› Affects both dopamine and serotonin; useful for clients who have concurrent depression
Formulations	› Capsules › Short-acting injectable
Complications	› Ziprasidone has a low risk of EPS, diabetes mellitus, weight gain, and dyslipidemia. › Other effects include sedation, orthostatic hypotension, anticholinergic effects, and rash. › ECG changes and QT prolongation can lead to torsades de pointes.
CLOZAPINE	
Comments	› The first atypical antipsychotic developed › Despite its effectiveness for schizophrenia spectrum disorders, it is no longer considered a first-line medication because of its adverse effects.
Formulations	› Tablets › Orally disintegrating tablets
Complications	› Clozapine has a low risk of EPS, but a high risk of weight gain, diabetes mellitus, and dyslipidemia. › Agranulocytosis can occur. Obtain a baseline WBC and monitor weekly. › Monitor for infection (fever, sore throat, mouth lesions), and notify the provider if manifestations occur. › Other adverse effects include sedation, orthostatic hypotension, and anticholinergic effects.
PALIPERIDONE	
Formulations	› Extended-release tablets › Extended-release injection
Complications	› Paliperidone has a high risk for diabetes mellitus, weight gain, and dyslipidemia. › Other adverse effects include sedation, prolonged QT interval, orthostatic hypotension, anticholinergic effects, and mild EPS.
ASENAPINE	
Formulations	› Sublingual tablets
Complications	› Adverse effects include drowsiness, prolonged QT interval, and EPS (higher doses). › Causes temporary numbing of the mouth. › Asenapine has a low risk of diabetes mellitus, weight gain, dyslipidemia, and anticholinergic effects.

ILOPERIDONE	
Formulations	› Tablets
Complications	› Common adverse effects include dry mouth, sedation, fatigue, and nasal congestion.
	› Iloperidone has a significant risk for weight gain, prolonged QT interval, and orthostatic hypotension.
	» Advise following the titration schedule during initial therapy to minimize hypotension.
	› Iloperidone has a low risk for diabetes mellitus, dyslipidemia, and EPS.

LURASIDONE	
Formulations	› Tablets
Complications	› Common adverse effects include sedation, akathisia, parkinsonism, agitation, and anxiety.
	› Lurasidone has a low risk for diabetes mellitus, weight gain, and dyslipidemia.
	› Lurasidone does not cause anticholinergic effects.

Interactions

MEDICATION/FOOD INTERACTIONS	NURSING INTERVENTIONS/CLIENT EDUCATION
› Immunosuppressive medications, such as anticancer medications, can further suppress immune function in clients taking clozapine.	› Avoid use in clients taking clozapine.
› Alcohol, opioids, and antihistamines have additive CNS depressant effects.	› Advise clients to avoid alcohol and medications that cause CNS depression. › Advise clients to avoid hazardous activities, such as driving.
› By activating dopamine receptors, levodopa counteracts the effects of antipsychotic agents.	› Avoid concurrent use of levodopa and other direct dopamine receptor agonists.
› Tricyclic antidepressants, amiodarone (Cordarone), and clarithromycin (Biaxin) prolong the QT interval and thus increase the risk of cardiac dysrhythmias for clients taking ziprasidone.	› Atypical antipsychotics that prolong the QT interval should not be used concurrently with other medications that have the same effect.
› Barbiturates and phenytoin (Dilantin) stimulate hepatic medication-metabolizing enzymes and thereby decrease drug levels of aripiprazole, quetiapine, and ziprasidone.	› Monitor medication effectiveness.
› Fluconazole (Diflucan) inhibits hepatic medication-metabolizing enzymes and thereby increases levels of aripiprazole, quetiapine, and ziprasidone.	› Monitor for adverse effects or toxicity.

Nursing Administration

- Administer by oral or IM route. For clients who have difficulty with adherence to an oral regimen, risperidone is available as a depot injection (Risperdal Consta) administered IM once every 2 weeks. Therapeutic effect occurs 4 to 6 weeks after the first depot injection. Clients often require oral preparations until depot injections are effective.

- Explain to clients that they will receive low doses initially, with gradual increases.

- Use oral disintegrating tablets for clients who might attempt to "cheek" (or pocket) tablets or have difficulty swallowing them.

- Advise clients taking asenapine to avoid eating or drinking for 10 min after each dose.

- Administer lurasidone with food to increase absorption.

- The cost of antipsychotic medications can be a factor for some clients. Evaluate the need for case management intervention.

Nursing Evaluation of Medication Effectiveness

- Depending on therapeutic intent, clients demonstrate effectiveness by:
  - Improvement of manifestations (hallucinations, delusions, anxiety, hostility).
  - Improvement in the ability to perform ADLs.
  - Improvement in the ability to interact socially with peers.
  - Improvement in sleeping and eating habits.

APPLICATION EXERCISES

1. A nurse is reinforcing teaching with a client who has schizophrenia about strategies for coping with the anticholinergic effects of fluphenazine. Which of the following should the nurse suggest to the client to minimize anticholinergic effects?

    A. Take the medication in the morning to prevent insomnia.

    B. Chew gum to moisten the mouth.

    C. Use cooling measures to decrease fever.

    D. Take an antacid to relieve nausea.

2. A nurse is collecting data from a male client who recently began taking haloperidol (Haldol). Which of the following findings is the highest priority to report to the provider?

    A. Shuffling gait

    B. Neck spasms

    C. Drowsiness

    D. Impotence

3. A nurse is reinforcing discharge teaching for a client who has a new prescription for clozapine (Clozaril). Which of the following statements is appropriate for the nurse to include?

    A. "You should have a high-carbohydrate snack between meals and at bedtime."

    B. "You are likely to develop hand tremors if you take this medication for a long period of time."

    C. "You may feel temporary numbness of your mouth after each dose."

    D. "You should have your white blood cell count monitored every week."

4. A nurse performs an Abnormal Involuntary Movement Scale (AIMS) screening for a client who began taking loxapine 2 years ago for the treatment of schizophrenia. Findings include lip smacking, tongue protrusion, and facial grimacing. The nurse should suspect which of the following?

    A. Parkinsonism

    B. Tardive dyskinesia

    C. Anticholinergic effects

    D. Akathisia

5. A nurse is preparing to collect data at a follow-up visit of a client who takes chlorpromazine (Thorazine) for the treatment of schizophrenia. The nurse should expect to find the greatest improvement in which of the following manifestations? (Select all that apply.)

_____ A. Disorganized speech

_____ B. Bizarre behavior

_____ C. Impaired social interactions

_____ D. Hallucinations

_____ E. Decreased motivation

6. A nurse is caring for a client who has neuroleptic malignant syndrome. Use the ATI Active Learning Template: Systems Disorder to complete this item to include the following sections:

A. Description of Disorder/Disease Process

B. Data Collection: Identify at least four expected objective findings.

C. Medications: Identify two medications appropriate for treatment and their purpose.

D. Nursing Care: Identify at least three appropriate interventions.

APPLICATION EXERCISES KEY

1. A. INCORRECT: Insomnia is not an anticholinergic effect. Blurred vision, photophobia, urinary hesitancy and retention, constipation, and tachycardia are common anticholinergic effects.

    B. **CORRECT:** Chewing gum can help the client cope with dry mouth, a potential anticholinergic effect of fluphenazine.

    C. INCORRECT: Fever is not an anticholinergic effect. Blurred vision, photophobia, urinary hesitancy and retention, constipation, and tachycardia are common anticholinergic effects.

    D. INCORRECT: Nausea is not an anticholinergic effect. Blurred vision, photophobia, urinary hesitancy and retention, constipation, and tachycardia are common anticholinergic effects.

    N NCLEX® Connection: Pharmacological Therapies, Adverse Effects/Contraindications/ Side Effects/Interactions

2. A. INCORRECT: Shuffling gait is an indication of parkinsonism and requires reporting to the provider. However, this is not the greatest risk to the client and is therefore not the priority finding.

    B. **CORRECT:** Neck spasms are an indication of acute dystonia, which is a crisis situation requiring rapid treatment. This is the greatest risk to the client and is therefore the priority finding.

    C. INCORRECT: Drowsiness is an adverse effect of haloperidol and requires reporting to the provider. However, this is not the greatest risk to the client and is therefore not the priority finding.

    D. INCORRECT: Sexual dysfunction is an adverse effect of haloperidol and requires reporting to the provider. However, this is not the greatest risk to the client and is therefore not the priority finding.

    N NCLEX® Connection: Pharmacological Therapies, Adverse Effects/Contraindications/ Side Effects/Interactions

3. A. INCORRECT: Clozapine increases the client's risk of developing diabetes mellitus and weight gain. It is not appropriate to increase carbohydrate intake.

    B. INCORRECT: Clozapine has a low risk of EPS such as hand tremors.

    C. INCORRECT: Asenapine, rather than clozapine, causes temporary numbing of the mouth.

    D. **CORRECT:** Due to the risk for fatal agranulocytosis, weekly monitoring of the client's WBC count is essential during clozapine therapy.

    N NCLEX® Connection: Pharmacological Therapies, Medication Administration

4.   A. INCORRECT: These findings do not indicate parkinsonism, which is most common during the first month of therapy.

    B. **CORRECT:** These findings indicate tardive dyskinesia, which can occur months to years after the initiation of therapy.

    C. INCORRECT: These findings do not indicate an anticholinergic effect. Dry mouth, blurred vision, photophobia, urinary hesitancy and retention, constipation, and tachycardia are common anticholinergic effects.

    D. INCORRECT: These findings do not indicate akathisia, which is most common during the first 2 months of therapy.

    Ⓝ NCLEX® Connection: Pharmacological Therapies, Adverse Effects/Contraindications/ Side Effects/Interactions

5.   A. **CORRECT:** A client who takes a conventional antipsychotic medication, such as chlorpromazine, should have the greatest improvement in positive symptoms such as disorganized speech.

    B. **CORRECT:** A client who takes a conventional antipsychotic medication, such as chlorpromazine, should have the greatest improvement in positive symptoms such as bizarre behavior.

    C. INCORRECT: Conventional antipsychotic medications, such as chlorpromazine, have less effect on negative symptoms, such as impaired social interactions.

    D. **CORRECT:** A client who takes a conventional antipsychotic medication, such as chlorpromazine, should have the greatest improvement in positive symptoms such as hallucinations.

    E. INCORRECT: Conventional antipsychotic medications, such as chlorpromazine, have less effect on negative symptoms, such as decreased motivation.

    Ⓝ NCLEX® Connection: Pharmacological Therapies, Expected Actions/Outcomes

6. *Using the ATI Active Learning Template: Systems Disorders*

   A. Description of Disorder/Disease Process

   - Neuroleptic malignant syndrome is a potential adverse effect of first-generation (conventional) antipsychotic medications that most commonly occurs within the first 2 weeks of treatment.

   B. Data Collection

   - Sudden high fever
   - Blood pressure fluctuations
   - Dysrhythmias
   - Muscle rigidity
   - Changes in level of consciousness
   - Coma

   C. Medications

   - Aspirin – antipyretic
   - Acetaminophen (Tylenol) – antipyretic
   - Dantrolene (Dantrium) – induces muscle relaxation

   D. Nursing Care

   - Notify the provider immediately.
   - Withhold the conventional antipsychotic medication.
   - Monitor vital signs.
   - Apply cooling blankets.
   - Increase fluid intake.
   - Discuss with the provider the need to wait 2 weeks before resuming therapy.
   - Discuss with the provider the possible need to switch to an atypical agent.

   (N) NCLEX® Connection: Pharmacological Therapies, Adverse Effects/Contraindications/ Side Effects/Interactions

chapter 10

CHAPTER 10 **Medications for Children and Adolescents with Mental Health Issues**

Overview

- Various medications are used to manage behavioral disorders in children and adolescents. Parents should understand that pharmacological management is most effective when accompanied by techniques to modify behavior.

- Medications include tricyclic antidepressants, antipsychotics, nonbarbiturate anxiolytics, CNS stimulants, and norepinephrine selective reuptake inhibitors.

MEDICATION CLASSIFICATION: CNS STIMULANTS

- Select Prototypes and Other Medications

MEDICATION	SHORT-ACTING	INTERMEDIATE-ACTING	LONG-ACTING
Methylphenidate	› Ritalin, Methylin	› Ritalin SR, Methylin ER	› Ritalin LA, Concerta, Daytrana (transdermal)
Dexmethylphenidate	› Focalin		› Focalin XR
Dextroamphetamine	› Dexedrine		› Dexedrine spansule
Amphetamine mixture	› Adderall		› Adderall XR
Lisdexamfetamine dimesylate			› Vyvanse

Purpose

- Expected Pharmacological Action
  - These medications raise the levels of norepinephrine, serotonin, and dopamine into the CNS.
- Therapeutic Uses
  - ADHD
  - Conduct disorder

Complications

ADVERSE EFFECTS	NURSING INTERVENTIONS/CLIENT EDUCATION
› CNS stimulation (insomnia, restlessness)	› Advise clients to observe for effects and notify the provider if they occur. › Administer the last dose before 4 p.m.
› Weight loss	› Monitor the client's weight and compare to baseline weight. › Administer medication immediately before or after meals. › Promote good nutrition in children. › Encourage children to eat at regular meal times and avoid unhealthy foods for snacks.
› Cardiovascular effects (dysrhythmias, chest pain, high blood pressure) › Increased risk of sudden death in clients who have heart abnormalities	› Monitor vital signs and ECG. › Advise clients to observe for effects and to notify the provider if they occur.
› Development of psychotic manifestations such as hallucinations, paranoia	› Instruct clients to report manifestations immediately and to discontinue the medication if they occur.
› Withdrawal reaction	› Advise clients to not stop taking medication suddenly. Doing so can lead to depression and severe fatigue.
› Hypersensitivity skin reaction to transdermal methylphenidate (hives, papules)	› Remove the patch and notify the provider.

Contraindications/Precautions

- These medications are contraindicated in clients who have a history of substance use disorder, cardiovascular disorders, severe anxiety, and psychosis.

Interactions

MEDICATION/FOOD INTERACTIONS	NURSING INTERVENTIONS/ CLIENT EDUCATION
› Concurrent use of MAOIs can cause hypertensive crisis.	› Avoid concurrent use.
› Concurrent use of caffeine can increase CNS stimulant effects.	› Instruct clients to avoid foods and beverages that contain caffeine.
› Methylphenidate inhibits metabolism of phenytoin (Dilantin), warfarin (Coumadin), and phenobarbital, leading to increased serum levels.	› Monitor clients for adverse effects (CNS depression, indications of bleeding). › Concurrent use of these medications is done with caution.
› OTC cold and decongestant medications with sympathomimetic action can increase CNS stimulant effects.	› Instruct clients to avoid use of OTC medications.

Nursing Administration

- Advise clients to swallow sustained-release tablets whole and to not chew or crush the tablets.

- Instruct clients about the importance of administering the medication on a regular schedule.

- Instruct clients who use transdermal medication (Daytrana) to place the patch on one hip daily in the morning and leave it in place no longer than 9 hr. Alternate hips daily.

- Instruct parents and clients that ADHD is not cured by medication. Management with an overall treatment plan that includes family therapy and cognitive therapy will improve outcomes.

- Instruct parents that these medications have special handling procedures controlled by federal law. Handwritten prescriptions are required for medication refills.

- Instruct parents in safety and storage of medications.

- Advise parents that these medications have a high potential for development of a substance use disorder, especially in adolescents.

Nursing Evaluation of Medication Effectiveness

- Depending on therapeutic intent, effectiveness can be evidenced by:

  - Improvement of manifestations of ADHD, such as increased ability to focus and complete tasks, interact with peers, and manage impulsivity.

  - Improved ability to stay awake.

MEDICATION CLASSIFICATION: NOREPINEPHRINE SELECTIVE REUPTAKE INHIBITOR

- Select Prototype Medication: atomoxetine (Strattera)

Purpose

- Expected Pharmacological Action

  - Block reuptake of norepinephrine at synapses in the CNS. Atomoxetine is not a stimulant medication.

- Therapeutic Use

  - ADHD

Complications

- Atomoxetine is usually tolerated well with minimal adverse effects.

ADVERSE EFFECTS	NURSING INTERVENTIONS/CLIENT EDUCATION
› Appetite suppression, weight loss, growth suppression	› Monitor the client's weight and compare to baseline weight. › Administer medication right before meals. › Encourage children to eat at regular meal times and avoid unhealthy foods for snacks.
› GI effects (nausea and vomiting)	› Advise client to take medication with food if GI effects occur.
› Suicidal ideation (in children and adolescents)	› Monitor for indications of depression. › Advise clients to report change in mood, excessive sleeping, agitation, and irritability.
› Hepatotoxicity	› Advise client to report indications of liver damage (influenza-like manifestations, yellowing skin, abdominal pain).

Contraindications/Precautions

- Use cautiously in clients who have cardiovascular disorders.

Interactions

MEDICATION/FOOD INTERACTIONS	NURSING INTERVENTIONS
› Concurrent use of MAOIs an cause hypertensive crisis.	› Avoid concurrent use.
› Paroxetine (Paxil), fluoxetine (Prozac), or quinidine gluconate (Quinidine Dura-Tabs) inhibit hepatic metabolizing enzymes, thereby increasing levels of atomoxetine.	› Instruct clients to watch for and report increased adverse reactions of atomoxetine. › Dosage of atomoxetine may need to be reduced if used concurrently with these medications.

Nursing Administration

- Note any changes in the child's behavior related to dosing and timing of medications.
- Administer the medication in a daily dose in the morning, or in two divided doses (morning and afternoon), with or without food.
- Instruct clients that therapeutic effects can take at 1 to 3 weeks to fully develop.

Nursing Evaluation of Medication Effectiveness

- Depending on therapeutic intent, effectiveness can be evidenced by improvement of manifestations of ADHD, such as increase in ability to focus and complete tasks, interact with peers, and manage impulsivity.

MEDICATION CLASSIFICATION: TRICYCLIC ANTIDEPRESSANTS (TCAs)

- Select Prototype Medication: desipramine (Norpramin)
- Other Medications
  - Imipramine (Tofranil)
  - Clomipramine (Anafranil)

Purpose

- Expected Pharmacological Action
  - These medications block reuptake of the monoamine neurotransmitters norepinephrine and serotonin in the synaptic space, thereby intensifying the effects that these neurotransmitters produce.
- Therapeutic Uses in Children
  - Depression
  - Autism spectrum disorder
  - ADHD
  - Panic, school phobia, separation anxiety disorder
  - OCD

Complications

ADVERSE EFFECTS	NURSING INTERVENTIONS/CLIENT EDUCATION
› Orthostatic hypotension	› Monitor blood pressure with first dose. Instruct client to change positions slowly.
› Anticholinergic effects » Dry mouth » Blurred vision » Photophobia » Urinary hesitancy or retention » Constipation » Tachycardia	› Instruct clients about ways to minimize anticholinergic effects. » Chewing sugarless gum » Sipping on water » Avoiding hazardous activities » Wearing sunglasses when outdoors » Eating foods high in fiber » Participating in regular exercise » Increasing fluid intake to at least 2 to 3 L/day from beverages or food sources » Voiding just before taking medication › Advise clients to notify the provider if anticholinergic effects are intolerable.
› Weight gain	› Monitor the client's weight. › Encourage clients to participate in regular exercise and to follow a healthy, low-calorie diet.

ADVERSE EFFECTS	NURSING INTERVENTIONS/CLIENT EDUCATION
› Sedation	› Advise clients that this adverse effect usually diminishes over time. › Advise clients to avoid hazardous activities such as driving if sedation is excessive. › Advise clients to take medication at bedtime to minimize daytime sleepiness and to promote sleep.
› Toxicity resulting in cholinergic blockade and cardiac toxicity evidenced by dysrhythmias, mental confusion, and agitation, followed by seizures and coma	› Give clients who are acutely ill a 1-week supply of medication. › Obtain the client's baseline ECG. › Monitor vital signs frequently. › Monitor clients for toxicity and notify the provider if indications of toxicity occur.
› Decreased seizure threshold	› Monitor clients who have seizure disorders.
› Excessive sweating	› Inform clients of this adverse effect and assist with frequent linen changes.

Contraindications/Precautions

- Use cautiously in clients who have seizure disorders; diabetes; liver, kidney and respiratory disorders; and hyperthyroidism.

Interactions

MEDICATION/FOOD INTERACTIONS	NURSING INTERVENTIONS/ CLIENT EDUCATION
› Concurrent use of monoamine oxidase inhibitors (MAOIs) causes hypertension.	› Avoid concurrent use with TCAs.
› Antihistamines and other anticholinergic agents have additive anticholinergic effects.	
› TCAs block uptake of epinephrine and NE (direct-acting sympathomimetics) in the synaptic space, leading to decreased intensity of their effects.	
› TCAs inhibit uptake of ephedrine and amphetamine (indirect-acting sympathomimetics), and reduce their ability to get to the site of action in the nerve terminal, leading to decreased responses to these medications.	
› Alcohol, benzodiazepines, opioids, and antihistamines cause additive CNS depression when used concurrently.	› Advise clients to avoid other CNS depressants.

Nursing Administration

- Instruct the client's parents to administer this medication as prescribed on a daily basis to establish therapeutic plasma levels.

- Assist with medication regimen compliance by informing clients and parents that it can take 1 to 3 weeks to experience therapeutic effects. Full therapeutic effects can take 2 to 3 months.

- Instruct clients and parents about the importance of continuing therapy after improvement in manifestations. Sudden discontinuation of the medication can result in relapse.

- Give only a week's worth of medication at a time for an acutely ill client.

Nursing Evaluation of Medication Effectiveness

- Depending on therapeutic intent, effectiveness can be evidenced by the following:
  - For depression
    - Verbalizing improvement in mood
    - Improved sleeping and eating habits
    - Increased interaction with peers
  - For autism spectrum disorder: Decreased anger and compulsive behavior
  - For ADHD: Less hyperactivity, greater ability to pay attention

---

MEDICATION CLASSIFICATION: ALPHA$_2$-ADRENERGIC AGONISTS

- Select Prototype Medication: guanfacine (Intuniv)
- Other Medication: clonidine (Kapvay)

Purpose

- Expected Pharmacological Action
  - The action of alpha$_2$-adrenergic agonists is not completely understood. However, they are known to activate presynaptic alpha$_2$-adrenergic receptors within the brain.
- Therapeutic Use
  - ADHD

ADVERSE EFFECTS	NURSING INTERVENTIONS/CLIENT EDUCATION
› CNS effects (sedation, drowsiness, fatigue)	› Monitor for these adverse effects and report their occurrence to the provider. › Advise the client to avoid hazardous activities.
› Cardiovascular effects (hypotension, bradycardia)	› Monitor blood pressure and pulse especially during initial treatment. › Advise the client not to abruptly discontinue medication which can cause rebound hypertension.
› Weight gain	› Monitor the client's weight. › Encourage the client to participate in regular exercise and to follow a healthy, well-balanced diet.

Contraindications/Precautions

- Extended-release clonidine is contraindicated for children less than 6 years old.
- Use cautiously in clients who have cardiac disease.

Interactions

MEDICATION/FOOD INTERACTIONS	NURSING INTERVENTIONS/CLIENT EDUCATION
› CNS depressants, including alcohol, can increase CNS effects.	› Avoid concurrent use.
› Antihypertensives can worsen hypotension.	› Avoid concurrent use.
› Foods with high fat content will increase guanfacine absorption.	› Advise clients to avoid taking medication with a high-fat meal.

Nursing Administration

- Determine any use of alcohol and CNS depressants, especially with adolescent clients.
- Instruct clients to not chew, crush, or split extended-release preparations.
- Monitor blood pressure and pulse at baseline, with initial treatment, and with each dosage change.
- Advise clients to avoid abrupt discontinuation of medication which can result in rebound hypertension. Medication should be tapered according to a prescribed dosage schedule when discontinuing treatment.

Nursing Evaluation of Medication Effectiveness

- Depending on therapeutic intent, effectiveness can be evidenced by improvement of manifestations of ADHD, such as increase in ability to focus and complete tasks, interact with peers, and manage impulsivity.

MEDICATION CLASSIFICATION: ANTIPSYCHOTICS – ATYPICAL

- Select Prototype Medication: risperidone (Risperdal)
- Other Medication: olanzapine (Zyprexa)

Purpose

- Expected Pharmacological Action
    - These antipsychotic agents work mainly by blocking serotonin, and to a lesser degree, dopamine receptors. These medications also block receptors for norepinephrine, histamine, and acetylcholine.
- Therapeutic Uses
    - Autism spectrum disorder
    - Conduct disorder
    - Posttraumatic stress disorder (PTSD)
    - Relief of psychotic manifestations

Complications

ADVERSE EFFECTS	NURSING INTERVENTIONS/CLIENT EDUCATION
› New onset of diabetes mellitus or loss of glucose control in clients who have diabetes	› Obtain the client's baseline fasting blood glucose and monitor periodically throughout treatment. › Instruct clients to report indications such as increased thirst, urination, and appetite.
› Weight gain	› Advise clients to follow a healthy, low-calorie diet, engage in regular exercise, and monitor weight gain.
› Hypercholesterolemia with increased risk for hypertension and other cardiovascular disease	› Monitor cholesterol, triglycerides, and blood glucose if weight gain is more than 14 kg (30 lb).
› Orthostatic hypotension	› Monitor blood pressure with first dose. Instruct clients to change positions slowly.
› Anticholinergic effects (urinary hesitancy or retention, dry mouth)	› Monitor for these adverse effects and report their occurrence to the provider. › Encourage clients to use measures to relieve dry mouth, such as sipping fluids throughout the day.
› Agitation, dizziness, sedation, and sleep disruption	› Monitor for these adverse effects and report their occurrence to the provider. › Administer an alternative medication if prescribed.
› Mild extrapyramidal adverse effects, such as tremor	› Monitor for and reinforce teaching to clients to recognize extrapyramidal adverse effects. These are usually dose-related.

Contraindications/Precautions

- Be aware of possible alcohol use in the adolescent client. Instruct clients to avoid the use of alcohol.
- Use cautiously in clients who have cardiovascular disease, seizures, or diabetes mellitus. Obtain a baseline fasting glucose for clients who have diabetes mellitus, and monitor carefully.

Interactions

MEDICATION/FOOD INTERACTIONS	NURSING INTERVENTIONS/CLIENT EDUCATION
› Alcohol, opioids, and antihistamines cause additive CNS depressant effects.	› Advise clients to avoid alcohol and other medications that cause CNS depression. › Advise clients to avoid hazardous activities, such as driving.
› By activating dopamine receptors, levodopa counteracts effects of antipsychotic agents.	› Avoid concurrent use of levodopa and other direct dopamine receptor agonists.
› Tricyclic antidepressants, amiodarone (Cordarone), and clarithromycin (Biaxin) prolong QT interval and thus increase the risk of cardiac dysrhythmias.	› Avoid concurrent use.
› Barbiturates and phenytoin (Dilantin) promote hepatic drug-metabolizing enzymes, thereby decreasing drug levels of quetiapine.	› Monitor medication effectiveness.
› Medications that inhibit CYP3A4, such as fluconazole (Diflucan), inhibit hepatic drug-metabolizing enzymes, thereby increasing drug levels of aripiprazole, quetiapine, and ziprasidone.	› Monitor for adverse effects.

Nursing Administration

- Administer by oral or IM route.
  - Risperidone is available in an oral solution and quick-dissolving tablets for ease in administration.
  - Olanzapine is available in an orally disintegrating tablet for ease in administration.
- Advise clients that low doses of medication are given initially and are then gradually increased.

Nursing Evaluation of Medication Effectiveness

- Depending on therapeutic intent, effectiveness is evidenced by the following.
  - For autism spectrum disorder: reduction of hyperactivity and improvement in mood
  - For conduct disorder: decrease in aggressiveness
  - For PTSD
    - Decrease in aggressiveness and reduction of flashbacks
    - Improvement of psychosis (prevention of acute psychotic manifestations and absence of hallucinations, delusions, anxiety, and hostility)
    - Improvement in ability to perform ADLs
    - Improvement in ability to interact socially with peers
    - Improvement of sleeping and eating habits

APPLICATION EXERCISES

1. A nurse is reinforcing teaching to the parents of a child who has a new prescription for desipramine (Norpramin) about possible adverse effects. The nurse should instruct the parents that which of the following adverse effects is the highest priority to report to the provider?

   A. Diaphoresis

   B. Confusion

   C. Blurred vision

   D. Dizziness

2. A nurse is reinforcing teaching to an adolescent client who has a new prescription for clomipramine (Anafranil) for OCD. Which of the following should the nurse teach the client in order to minimize an adverse effect of his medication?

   A. Wear sunglasses when outdoors.

   B. Check temperature daily while taking this medication.

   C. Take medication first thing in the morning before eating.

   D. Add extra calories to the diet as between-meal snacks.

3. A nurse is caring for a school-age child who recently began a prescription for atomoxetine (Strattera). For which of the following possible complications should the nurse monitor the child?

   A. Renal toxicity

   B. Liver damage

   C. Seizure activity

   D. Adrenal insufficiency

4. A nurse is caring for a school-age child who has a new prescription for methylphenidate (Concerta) to treat ADHD. Which of the following should the nurse instruct the client and family about this medication?

   A. Apply the patch once daily at bedtime.

   B. Take the medication orally once daily in the morning.

   C. Take a second dose of the medication orally at bedtime.

   D. Apply the patch on awakening and remove at bedtime.

5. A nurse is reinforcing teaching to a school-age child and his parents about a new prescription for lisdexamfetamine dimesylate (Vyvanse). Which of the following is appropriate for the nurse to include in the teaching? (Select all that apply.)

_____ A. An adverse effect of this medication is CNS stimulation.

_____ B. Administer the medication 1 hr before breakfast.

_____ C. Monitor blood pressure while taking this medication.

_____ D. Therapeutic effects of this medication will take 1 to 3 weeks to fully develop.

_____ E. This medication raises the levels of dopamine into the brain.

6. A nurse working in a pediatric mental health clinic is caring for a client who has a new prescription for risperidone (Risperdal) for the treatment of conduct disorder. Use the Medication ATI Active Learning Template to complete this item to include the following sections:

A. Side/Adverse Effects: Identify at least four adverse effects of this medication.

B. Nursing Interventions/Client Education: Identify at least four nursing interventions to prevent or minimize the adverse effects of this medication.

APPLICATION EXERCISES KEY

1. A. INCORRECT: Diaphoresis is an adverse effect and should be reported. However, it does not pose the greatest risk to the client and is therefore not the highest priority to report to the provider.

   B. **CORRECT:** Confusion is an indication of toxicity, which is the greatest risk to the client and is therefore the highest priority to report to the provider.

   C. INCORRECT: Blurred vision is an adverse effect and should be reported. However, it does not pose the greatest risk to the client and is therefore not the highest priority to report to the provider.

   D. INCORRECT: Dizziness is an adverse effect and should be reported. However, it does not pose the greatest risk to the client and is therefore not the highest priority to report to the provider.

   Ⓝ NCLEX® Connection: Pharmacological Therapies, Adverse Effects/Contraindications/ Side Effects/Interactions

2. A. **CORRECT:** Wearing sunglasses when outdoors will decrease photophobia, an anticholinergic effect associated with TCA use.

   B. INCORRECT: Checking the client's temperature daily is not necessary while taking a TCA.

   C. INCORRECT: Taking the medication at bedtime rather than in the morning is appropriate to prevent daytime sleepiness.

   D. INCORRECT: Following a low-calorie diet plan rather than adding extra calories as snacks will help prevent weight gain, a common adverse effect of TCAs.

   Ⓝ NCLEX® Connection: Pharmacological Therapies, Adverse Effects/Contraindications/ Side Effects/Interactions

3. A. INCORRECT: Renal toxicity is not a complication expected when taking atomoxetine.

   B. **CORRECT:** Liver damage is a potential complication of atomoxetine. The nurse should monitor for manifestations such as jaundice, upper abdominal tenderness, darkening of urine, and elevated liver enzymes.

   C. INCORRECT: Seizure activity is not a complication expected when taking atomoxetine.

   D. INCORRECT: Adrenal insufficiency is not a complication expected when taking atomoxetine.

   Ⓝ NCLEX® Connection: Pharmacological Therapies, Adverse Effects/Contraindications/ Side Effects/Interactions

4. A. INCORRECT: A transdermal patch of methylphenidate is available. However, Concerta is an oral formulation.

    B. **CORRECT:** Concerta is a long-acting formulation of methylphenidate that is taken orally once daily in the morning.

    C. INCORRECT: Concerta is a once-daily medication that should be taken in the morning to decrease CNS stimulation at bedtime.

    D. INCORRECT: A transdermal patch of methylphenidate is available. However, Concerta is an oral formulation.

    Ⓝ NCLEX® Connection: Pharmacological Therapies, Medication Administration

5. A. **CORRECT:** An adverse effect of Vyvanse is CNS stimulation such as insomnia and restlessness.

    B. INCORRECT: Administer Vyvanse immediately before or after a meal due to appetite suppression.

    C. **CORRECT:** Monitoring the client's blood pressure is appropriate due to potential cardiovascular effects of Vyvanse.

    D. INCORRECT: Atomoxetine (Strattera), rather than Vyvanse, takes 1 to 3 weeks to fully develop therapeutic effects.

    E. **CORRECT:** Vyvanse, a CNS stimulant, works by raising the levels of norepinephrine, serotonin, and dopamine into the CNS.

    Ⓝ NCLEX® Connection: Pharmacological Therapies, Adverse Effects/Contraindications/ Side Effects/Interactions

6. *Using the ATI Active Learning Template: Medication*

    A. Side/Adverse Effects
    - New onset of diabetes mellitus or loss of glucose control in clients who have diabetes.
    - Weight gain
    - Hypercholesterolemia
    - Orthostatic hypotension
    - Anticholinergic effects (urinary hesitancy or retention, dry mouth)
    - Agitation
    - Dizziness
    - Sedation
    - Sleep disruption
    - Tremors

    B. Nursing Interventions/Client Education
    - Obtain the client's fasting blood glucose prior to and periodically throughout treatment.
    - Instruct the client to report indications of diabetes mellitus, including increased thirst, urination, and appetite.
    - Advise clients to follow a healthy, low-calorie diet.
    - Recommend regular exercise.
    - Monitor weight throughout treatment.
    - Monitor cholesterol and triglycerides especially if weight gain is more than 30 lb.
    - Monitor blood pressure with first dose and instruct client to change positions slowly.
    - Encourage the client to sip fluids throughout the day.

    Ⓝ NCLEX® Connection: Pharmacological Therapies, Adverse Effects/Contraindications/ Side Effects/Interactions

chapter 11

Overview

- Abstinence syndrome occurs when clients abruptly withdraw from a substance on which they are physically dependent.

- Withdrawing from a substance that has the potential to cause addiction can cause abstinence syndrome. Manifestations of abstinence syndrome can be distressing and can lead to coma and death.

- Major substances associated with substance use disorder include alcohol, cannabis, hallucinogens, inhalants, opioids, sedatives/hypnotics, stimulants, and tobacco.

- Substance withdrawal varies with the substance and can produce a variety of manifestations, including gastrointestinal distress, neurological and behavioral changes, cardiovascular changes, and seizures.

MEDICATIONS TO SUPPORT WITHDRAWAL/ABSTINENCE FROM ALCOHOL

- Effects of withdrawal usually start within 4 to 12 hr of the last intake of alcohol, peak after 24 to 48 hr, and subside within 5 to 7 days, unless alcohol withdrawal delirium occurs.

- Manifestations include nausea; vomiting; tremors; restlessness and inability to sleep; depressed mood or irritability; increased heart rate, blood pressure, respiratory rate, and temperature; and tonic-clonic seizures. Illusions also are common.

- Alcohol withdrawal delirium can occur 2 to 3 days after cessation of alcohol intake, can last 2 to 3 days, and is a medical emergency. Findings include severe disorientation, psychotic manifestations (hallucinations), severe hypertension, and cardiac dysrhythmias that can progress to death.

Detoxification

BENZODIAZEPINES	
Examples	› Chlordiazepoxide (Librium), diazepam (Valium), lorazepam (Ativan)
Intended Effects	› Maintenance of vital signs within expected ranges › Decrease in the risk of seizures › Decrease in the intensity of withdrawal manifestations
Nursing Interventions/ Client Education	› Administer around the clock or PRN. › Use chlordiazepoxide only if the client is able to tolerate oral intake. Otherwise, the client will need IV diazepam and lorazepam. The client later may take diazepam and lorazepam orally. › Measure baseline vital signs. › Monitor vital signs and neurological status. › Provide seizure precautions (padded side rails and suction equipment at the bedside).

ADJUNCT MEDICATIONS	
Examples	› Carbamazepine (Tegretol), clonidine (Catapres), propranolol (Inderal)
Intended Effects	› Decrease in seizures – carbamazepine › Depression of autonomic response (decrease in blood pressure, heart rate) – clonidine and propranolol › Decrease in craving – propranolol
Nursing Interventions/ Client Education	› Provide seizure precautions (padded side rails, suction equipment at the bedside). › Measure baseline vital signs, and continue to monitor them.

Abstinence Maintenance (Following Detoxification)

DISULFIRAM (ANTABUSE)	
Intended Effects	› Disulfiram is a daily oral medication that is a type of aversion (behavioral) therapy. › Concurrent use of disulfiram and alcohol will cause acetaldehyde syndrome. › Effects include nausea, vomiting, weakness, sweating, palpitations, and hypotension. › Acetaldehyde syndrome can progress to respiratory depression, cardiovascular suppression, seizures, and death.
Nursing Interventions/ Client Education	› Inform clients of the potential dangers of drinking any alcohol. › Advise clients to avoid any products that contain alcohol (cough syrups, mouthwash, aftershave lotion). › Monitor frequent liver function tests to detect hepatotoxicity. › Encourage clients to wear a medical alert bracelet. › Encourage clients to participate in a 12-step self-help program. › Advise clients that medication effects (potential for acetaldehyde syndrome with alcohol ingestion) persist for 2 weeks following discontinuation of disulfiram.

NALTREXONE (VIVITROL)	
Intended Effects	› Naltrexone is a pure opioid antagonist that suppresses the craving and pleasurable effects of alcohol (also used for opioid withdrawal).
Nursing Interventions/ Client Education	› Take an accurate history to determine whether clients are also dependent on opioids. Concurrent use of naltrexone and opiates increases the risk for an opiate overdose. › Advise clients to take the medication with meals to decrease gastrointestinal distress. › Suggest monthly IM injections for clients who have difficulty adhering to the regimen.

ACAMPROSATE (CAMPRAL)	
Intended Effects	› Acamprosate decreases unpleasant effects resulting from abstinence (anxiety, restlessness).
Nursing Interventions/ Client Education	› Inform clients that diarrhea can result. › Advise clients to maintain adequate fluid intake and to receive adequate rest. › Advise clients to avoid use in pregnancy.

MEDICATIONS TO SUPPORT WITHDRAWAL/ABSTINENCE FROM OPIOIDS

- Characteristic withdrawal syndrome occurs within 1 hr to several days after cessation of substance use.
- Clinical findings include agitation, insomnia, influenza-like manifestations, rhinorrhea, yawning, sweating, and diarrhea.
- Manifestations are not life-threatening, although suicidal ideation can occur.

METHADONE (DOLOPHINE) SUBSTITUTION	
Intended Effects	› Methadone is an oral opioid agonist that replaces the opioid to which the client is addicted. › This will prevent abstinence syndrome and eliminate the client's need to obtain illegal substances. › It is used for withdrawal and long-term maintenance. › Dependence transfers from the illegal opioid to methadone.
Nursing Interventions/ Client Education	› Inform clients that slow tapering of the methadone dose is essential for detoxification. › Encourage clients to participate in a 12-step self-help program. › Inform clients that they must obtain the medication from an approved treatment center.

CLONIDINE (CATAPRES)	
Intended Effects	› Clonidine assists with withdrawal effects related to autonomic hyperactivity (diarrhea, nausea, vomiting). › Clonidine therapy does not reduce the craving for opioids.
Nursing Interventions/ Client Education	› Measure baseline vital signs. › Advise clients to avoid activities that require mental alertness until drowsiness subsides. › Encourage clients to chew gum or suck on hard candy and to sip small amounts of water or suck on ice chips to treat dry mouth.

BUPRENORPHINE (BUPRENEX)	
Intended Effects	› Buprenorphine is an agonist-antagonist opioid that promotes detoxification and maintenance. › It decreases feelings of craving and can help with maintaining adherence.
Nursing Interventions/ Client Education	› Inform clients that they must obtain the medication from an approved treatment center. › Buprenorphine is available in sublingual, IM, or IV formulations.

MEDICATIONS TO SUPPORT WITHDRAWAL/ABSTINENCE FROM NICOTINE

- Abstinence syndrome causes irritability, nervousness, restlessness, insomnia, and difficulty concentrating.

BUPROPION (ZYBAN)	
Intended Effects	› Bupropion decreases nicotine craving and manifestations of withdrawal.
Nursing Interventions/ Client Education	› To treat dry mouth, encourage clients to chew gum or suck on hard candy and to sip small amounts of water or suck on ice chips. › Advise clients to avoid caffeine and other CNS stimulants to control insomnia.

NICOTINE REPLACEMENT THERAPY	
Intended Effects	› These nicotine replacements are pharmaceutical product substitutes for the nicotine in cigarettes or chewing tobacco. › The use of nicotine replacement therapy approximately doubles the rate of smoking cessation.
Nursing Interventions/ Client Education	› Clients should avoid using any nicotine products while pregnant or breastfeeding. › Nicotine gum (Nicorette) 　» Use of chewing gum is not recommended for longer than 6 months. 　» Advise clients to chew gum slowly and intermittently over 30 min. 　» Advise clients to avoid eating or drinking 15 min prior to and while chewing the gum. › Nicotine patch (Nicotrol) 　» Clients should apply a nicotine patch to an area of clean, dry skin each day. 　» Advise clients to avoid using any nicotine products while the patch is on. 　» Follow product directions for dosage times. 　» Advise clients to stop using patches and to notify the provider if local skin reactions occur. 　» Remove the patch prior to a magnetic resonance imaging scan, and replace after the scan. › Nicotine nasal spray (Nicotrol NS) 　» Provides pleasurable effects of smoking due to a rapid rise of nicotine level in the client's blood. 　» One spray in each nostril delivers the amount of nicotine in one cigarette. 　» Advise clients to follow product instructions for dosage frequency. 　» Not recommended for clients who have disorders affecting the upper respiratory system such as chronic sinus problems, allergies, or asthma.

VARENICLINE (CHANTIX)	
Intended Effects	› Varenicline is a nicotinic receptor agonist that promotes the release of dopamine to simulate the pleasurable effects of nicotine. › Reduces cravings for nicotine as well as the severity of withdrawal manifestations. › Reduces the incidence of relapse by blocking the desired effects of nicotine.
Nursing Interventions/ Client Education	› Instruct clients to take the medication after a meal. › Monitor BP during treatment. › Monitor clients who have diabetes mellitus for loss of glycemic control. › Follow instructions for titration to minimize adverse effects. › Advise clients to notify the provider if nausea, vomiting, insomnia, new-onset depression, or suicidal thoughts occur. › Chronic depression, serious mental illness, and suicidal ideation are contraindications for varenicline.

Nursing Evaluation of Medication Effectiveness

- Depending on therapeutic intent, clients demonstrate effectiveness by:
  - Absence of injury.
  - Abstinence from substances.
  - Regular attendance at a self-help group.

APPLICATION EXERCISES

1. A nurse is reinforcing teaching for a client who is withdrawing from alcohol and has a new prescription for propranolol (Inderal). Which of the following information is appropriate for the nurse to include?

    A. Increases the risk for seizure activity

    B. Provides a form of aversion therapy

    C. Decreases cravings

    D. Results in mild hypertension

2. A nurse is planning a staff education session to discuss medications appropriate during the care of a client undergoing alcohol detoxification. Which of the following should the nurse include? (Select all that apply.)

    _____ A. Lorazepam (Ativan)

    _____ B. Diazepam (Valium)

    _____ C. Disulfiram (Antabuse)

    _____ D. Naltrexone (Vivitrol)

    _____ E. Acamprosate (Campral)

3. A nurse is reinforcing teaching for a client who has a new prescription for clonidine (Catapres) to assist with maintenance of abstinence from opioids. The nurse should remind the client to watch for which of the following adverse effects?

    A. Diarrhea

    B. Dry mouth

    C. Insomnia

    D. Hypertension

4. A nurse is reinforcing teaching for a female client who has tobacco use disorder about nicotine replacement therapy. Which of the following statements by the client indicates understanding of the information?

    A. "I should avoid eating right before I chew a piece of nicotine gum."

    B. "I will need to stop using the nicotine gum after 1 year."

    C. "I know that nicotine gum is a safe alternative to smoking if I become pregnant."

    D. "I must chew the nicotine gum quickly for about 15 minutes."

5. A nurse in an acute mental health facility is caring for a client who is withdrawing from opioid use and has a new prescription for clonidine (Catapres). Which of the following is the priority nursing action?

    A. Administer the clonidine as prescribed.

    B. Provide ice chips at the client's bedside.

    C. Inform the client about the effects of clonidine.

    D. Measure the client's baseline vital signs.

6. A nurse is informing a client who has tobacco use disorder about a new prescription for varenicline (Chantix) to promote smoking cessation. Use the ATI Active Learning Template: Medication to complete this item to include the following:

    A. Expected Pharmacological Action

    B. Therapeutic Use

    C. Side and Adverse Effects: Identify at least three.

    D. Client Education: Identify at least two points.

    E. Evaluation of Medication Effectiveness: Identify a client outcome to indicate medication effectiveness.

APPLICATION EXERCISES KEY

1. A. INCORRECT: Seizure activity is a potential effect of alcohol withdrawal. However, propranolol does not increase this risk.

    B. INCORRECT: Disulfiram, rather than propranolol, provides a form of aversion therapy.

    C. **CORRECT:** Propranolol is an adjunct medication used during detoxification to decrease the client's craving for alcohol.

    D. INCORRECT: Propranolol is an antihypertensive medication that can result in hypotension rather than hypertension.

    Ⓝ NCLEX® Connection: Psychosocial Integrity, Chemical and Other Dependencies

2. A. **CORRECT:** Lorazepam is a benzodiazepine used during alcohol detoxification to decrease anxiety and reduce the risk for seizures.

    B. **CORRECT:** Diazepam is a benzodiazepine used during alcohol detoxification to decrease anxiety and reduce the risk for seizures.

    C. INCORRECT: Disulfiram assists the client in maintaining abstinence from alcohol following detoxification.

    D. INCORRECT: Naltrexone assists the client in maintaining abstinence from alcohol following detoxification.

    E. INCORRECT: Acamprosate decreases unpleasant effects, such as anxiety or restlessness, resulting from abstinence.

    Ⓝ NCLEX® Connection: Psychosocial Integrity, Chemical and Other Dependencies

3. A. INCORRECT: Constipation, rather than diarrhea, is a common adverse effect of clonidine use.

    B. **CORRECT:** Dry mouth is a common adverse effect of clonidine use.

    C. INCORRECT: Sedation, rather than insomnia, is a common adverse effect of clonidine use.

    D. INCORRECT: Clonidine is more likely to cause hypotension than hypertension.

    Ⓝ NCLEX® Connection: Pharmacological Therapies, Adverse Effects/Contraindications/ Side Effects/Interactions

4. A. **CORRECT:** The client should avoid eating or drinking 15 min prior to and while chewing the nicotine gum.

    B. INCORRECT: The client should not use nicotine gum for longer than 6 months.

    C. INCORRECT: The client should avoid all nicotine products, including nicotine gum, while pregnant or breastfeeding.

    D. INCORRECT: The client should chew the nicotine gum slowly and intermittently over 30 min.

    Ⓝ NCLEX® Connection: Psychosocial Integrity, Chemical and Other Dependencies

5. A. INCORRECT: Administering the clonidine as prescribed is an important nursing action. However, it is not the priority action according to the nursing process.

    B. INCORRECT: Providing ice chips is an important nursing action. However, it is not the priority action according to the nursing process.

    C. INCORRECT: Educating the client about the medication is an important nursing action. However, it is not the priority action according to the nursing process.

    D. **CORRECT:** Assessment is the initial step of the nursing process. Therefore, obtaining the client's baseline vital signs is the priority nursing action.

    Ⓝ NCLEX® Connection: Psychosocial Integrity, Chemical and Other Dependencies

6. *Using the ATI Active Learning Template: Medication*

   A. Expected Pharmacological Action
   - Varenicline is a nicotinic receptor agonist that promotes the release of dopamine to simulate the pleasurable effects of nicotine.

   B. Therapeutic Use
   - Varenicline is indicated to reduce nicotine cravings and block the desired effects of nicotine in clients who have tobacco use disorder.

   C. Side and Adverse Effects
   - New-onset hypertension
   - Loss of glycemic control in clients who have diabetes mellitus
   - Nausea
   - Vomiting
   - Insomnia
   - New-onset depression

   D. Client Education
   - Clients who have chronic depression, serious mental illness, or suicidal ideation should not take varenicline.
   - Take the medication after a meal.
   - Titrate as prescribed to minimize adverse effects.
   - Notify the provider if adverse effects occur.

   E. Evaluation of Medication Effectiveness
   - The client will maintain smoking cessation.
   - The client will report reduced cravings for nicotine.

   (N) NCLEX® Connection: Pharmacological Therapies, Expected Actions/Outcomes

chapter 12

Overview

- Medications administered for chronic neurologic disorders are used to manage symptoms and improve quality of life.
- Chronic neurologic disorders include myasthenia gravis, Parkinson's disease, and seizure disorder.

MEDICATION CLASSIFICATION: CHOLINESTERASE INHIBITORS

- Cholinesterase inhibitors are known as anticholinesterase agents and have two categories.
  - Reversible inhibitors – The effect is for a moderate duration used to treat myasthenia gravis, Alzheimer's disease, and Parkinson's disease.
  - Irreversible inhibitors, echothiophate (Phospholine Iodide) – The effect is for a long duration used to treat glaucoma.
    - Pralidoxime (2-PAM) is used to reverse the effect of echothiophate.
- Select Prototype Medication: neostigmine (Prostigmin)
- Other Medications
  - Ambenonium (Mytelase)
  - Pyridostigmine (Mestinon)
  - Edrophonium (Tensilon)

Purpose

- Expected Pharmacological Action
  - Cholinesterase inhibitors prevent the enzyme cholinesterase (ChE) from inactivating acetylcholine (ACh), thereby increasing the amount of ACh available at receptor sites. Transmission of nerve impulses is increased at all cholinergic junctions responding to ACh as a transmitter.
- Therapeutic Uses

THERAPEUTIC USES FOR CHOLINESTERASE INHIBITORS				
	Neostigmine	Ambenonium	Pyridostigmine	Edrophonium
Treatment of myasthenia gravis	✓	✓	✓	
Diagnosis of myasthenia gravis				✓
Reversal of nondepolarizing neuromuscular blocking agents	✓		✓	✓

Complications

ADVERSE EFFECTS	NURSING INTERVENTIONS/CLIENT EDUCATION
› Excessive muscarine stimulation as evidenced by increased gastrointestinal (GI) motility, increased GI secretions, bradycardia, and urinary urgency	› Advise the client of potential adverse effects. If effects become intolerable, instruct the client to notify the provider. › Adverse effects may be treated with atropine.
› Cholinergic crisis (excessive muscarinic stimulation and respiratory depression from neuromuscular blockade and CNS depression)	› Muscarinic effects (increased salivation, increased gastric secretions and GI motility, urinary urgency, eye spasms, and bradycardia) can be treated with atropine. › Provide respiratory support through mechanical ventilation and oxygen.

Contraindications/Precautions

- Pregnancy Risk Category C.
- Obstruction of GI and renal system.
- Use cautiously in clients who have seizure disorders, hyperthyroidism, peptic ulcer disease, asthma, bradycardia, and hypotension.

Interactions

MEDICATION/FOOD INTERACTIONS	NURSING INTERVENTIONS/CLIENT EDUCATION
› Atropine (Atropair) counteracts the effects of neostigmine.	› Atropine is used to treat neostigmine toxicity (increased muscarinic stimulation and respiratory depression). › Monitor the client closely, and provide mechanical ventilation until the client has regained full muscle function.
› Neostigmine reverses neuromuscular blockade caused by neuromuscular blocking agents after surgical procedures and overdose.	› Monitor the client for return of respiratory function. Support respiratory function as necessary. If used to treat overdose, provide mechanical ventilation until the client has regained full muscle function.
› Succinylcholine is a depolarizing short-acting neuromuscular blockade for surgical procedures.	› Avoid concurrent use. Cholinesterase inhibitors cannot counteract the effects of this medication and will intensify neuromuscular blockade caused by succinylcholine.

Nursing Considerations

- Neostigmine may be given PO, IM, IV, or subcutaneously.
- Instruct clients who have myasthenia gravis to take medications as prescribed.
- Advise clients that dosage is very individualized, starts at very low doses, and is titrated until desired muscle function is achieved.
- Instruct clients who have myasthenia gravis to take the oral medication at the same time each day to prevent weakness of respiratory and swallowing muscles.
- Encourage clients who have myasthenia gravis to participate in dosage self-adjustments of neostigmine medication. This can be accomplished by having the client do the following.
  - Keep records of medication administration and effects.
  - Recognize signs of inadequate dosing, such as difficulty swallowing, and signs of overmedication, such as urinary urgency.
  - Modify dosage based on response.
- Advise clients to wear a medical alert bracelet.

Nursing Evaluation of Medication Effectiveness

- Depending on therapeutic intent, effectiveness can be evidenced by:
  - Fewer episodes of fatigue.
  - Improvement in strength as demonstrated by chewing, swallowing, and performing activities of daily living (ADLs) such as bathing, walking, eating, and dressing.

MEDICATION CLASSIFICATION: ANTI-PARKINSON'S MEDICATIONS

Classifications

- Select Prototype Medications

  ○ Dopaminergic medications promote dopamine synthesis, activate dopamine receptors, prevent dopamine breakdown, promote dopamine release, or enhance the effect by blocking degradation of levodopa.

    ▪ Dopamine synthesis medication is prepared in combination with a dopamine agonist, carbidopa (Lodosyn), or listed as levodopa/carbidopa (Sinemet, Parcopa).

      □ Levodopa crosses the blood-brain barrier, whereas dopamine alone cannot cross this barrier and has a very short half-life. Levodopa is taken up by dopaminergic nerve terminals and converted to dopamine (DA). This newly synthesized DA is released into the synaptic space and causes stimulation of DA receptors.

      □ Carbidopa is used to augment levodopa by decreasing the amount of levodopa that is converted to DA in the intestine and periphery. This results in larger amounts of levodopa reaching the CNS.

  ○ Dopamine agonists activate dopamine receptors in the striatum: pramipexole (Mirapex); bromocriptine (Parlodel); ropinirole (Requip), a first-line supplement to levodopa; apomorphine (Apokyn), a rescue medication for "off" times.

    ▪ Catecholamine-O-methyltransferase (COMT) inhibitor enhances the effect of levodopa by blocking its breakdown: entacapone (Comtan), tolcapone (Tasmar). Entacapone is safer and more effective than tolcapone (preferred drug).

    ▪ Monoamine oxidase-B (MAO-B) prevents dopamine breakdown: selegiline (Carbex, Zelapar), rasagiline (Azilect).

    ▪ Dopamine releaser prevents dopamine reuptake: amantadine (Symmetrel).

    ▪ Anticholinergic medication blocks the muscarinic receptors, which assist in maintaining balance between dopamine and acetylcholine receptors in the brain.

    ▪ Dopamine agonists, COMT inhibitors, MAO-B inhibitors, dopamine releasers, and centrally acting anticholinergic antagonists can be used concurrently to increase the beneficial effects of levodopa/carbidopa.

Purpose

- Expected Pharmacological Action
  - These medications do not halt the progression of Parkinson's disease (PD). However, they do offer symptomatic relief from dyskinesias (bradykinesia, resting tremors, and muscle rigidity) and an increase in the ability to perform ADLs by maintaining the balance between dopamine and acetylcholine in the extrapyramidal nervous system.
- Therapeutic Uses
  - Levodopa/carbidopa is most effective for PD treatment, but the beneficial effects diminish by the end of year five.
    - "Wearing off" times occur at the end of the dose cycle or can occur at any time even at high dose levels, lasting minutes to several hours.

LEVODOPA/CARBIDOPA (SINEMET, PARCOPA) – USUALLY DOSE DEPENDENT	
Adverse Effects	Nursing Interventions/Client Education
› Nausea and vomiting, drowsiness	› Administer with food, in small doses, at the start of treatment. › Avoid administering with meals or with foods high in protein because adsorption is delayed and reduces the therapeutic effect, causing an "off" episode. › Advise clients to avoid vitamin preparations and foods containing pyridoxine (wheat germ, green vegetables, bananas, whole-grain cereals, liver, legumes), which reduce the therapeutic effects of levodopa/carbidopa. › Advise clients to eat protein in several small portions during the day. › Carbidopa administered as extra doses can reduce nausea and vomiting.
› Dyskinesias (head bobbing, tics, grimacing, tremors)	› Decrease the dosage. The decrease can result in resumption of PD symptoms. › Administer amantadine (releases and uptakes DA) to decrease dyskinesias. › Surgical or electrical stimulation.
› Orthostatic hypotension	› Monitor the client's blood pressure. › Instruct clients about signs of postural hypotension (lightheadedness, dizziness) and avoiding sudden changes of position.
› Cardiovascular effects from beta₁ stimulation (tachycardia, palpitations, irregular heartbeat)	› Monitor vital signs. › Monitor ECG. › Notify the provider if symptoms occur. › Use cautiously in clients who have cardiovascular disorders.
› Psychosis (visual hallucinations, nightmares, paranoia)	› Administer second-generation antipsychotic medications as prescribed to decrease psychotic symptoms without increasing the symptoms of Parkinson's disease. › Second-generation antipsychotic medications do not block dopamine receptors in the striatum. › Avoid concurrent use of conventional-antipsychotic agents, such as haloperidol (Haldol), which block dopamine receptors. › Check for the concurrent use of antipsychotic MAOI medications, which can result in hypertensive crisis. Do not use levodopa/carbidopa within 2 weeks of MAOI use.
› Discoloration of sweat and urine	› Advise the client that this is a harmless side effect.
› Activation of malignant melanoma	› Avoid use of medication in clients who have skin lesions that have not been diagnosed.

- Therapeutic Uses of Dopamine Agonist

  ○ Pramipexole, Ropinirole, Apomorphine

    ▪ Administered as monotherapy in early-stage PD and used in conjunction with levodopa/carbidopa in late-stage PD to allow for lower dosage of levodopa/carbidopa.

    ▪ Administered more often in younger clients who are better able to tolerate daytime drowsiness and postural hypotension.

    ▪ Bromocriptine, an ergot derivative, is poorly tolerated and has a high incidence of valvular heart injury. This medication is administered less frequently.

DOPAMINE AGONISTS: PRAMIPEXOLE, ROPINIROLE, APOMORPHINE, BROMOCRIPTINE	
Adverse Effects	Nursing Interventions/Client Education
› Sudden inability to stay awake	› Advise clients to notify the provider immediately if this occurs.
› Daytime sleepiness	› Advise clients of the potential for drowsiness and to avoid hazardous activities. › Advise clients to avoid other CNS depressants, such as alcohol.
› Orthostatic hypotension	› Instruct clients about the signs of postural hypotension (lightheadedness, dizziness) and to avoid sudden changes of position.
› Psychosis (visual hallucinations, nightmares)	› Administer second-generation antipsychotic medications, such as clozapine (Clozaril), if manifestations occur.
› Impulse control disorder (gambling, shopping, binge eating, and hypersexuality)	› Manifestations appear 9 months after initial dose. Manifestations subside when medication is discontinued. › Screen for compulsive behavior before initiating therapy.
› Dyskinesias (head bobbing, tics, grimacing, tremors)	› Decrease dosage of medication.
› Nausea	› Advise clients to take medication with food (slows absorption of medication).

- Therapeutic Uses of Dopamine Releaser

  ○ Releases dopamine where it is stored in the neurons, prevents dopamine reuptake and stimulation of dopamine release, and may block cholinergic and glutamate receptors: amantadine.

DOPAMINE RELEASER: AMANTADINE	
Adverse Effects	Nursing Interventions/Client Education
› CNS effects (confusion, dizziness, restlessness)	› Advise the client to avoid hazardous activities while taking the medication.
› Atropine-like effects (dry mouth, blurred vision, mydriasis, urinary hesitancy or retention, constipation)	› Advise the client to observe for symptoms and notify the provider. › Monitor I&O, and check the client for hesitancy or urinary retention. › Advise the client to chew sugarless gum, eat high-fiber foods, and increase fluid intake to 2 to 3 L/day from beverage and food.
› Discoloration of skin, also called livedo reticularis	› Advise the client that discoloration of the skin will subside when the medication is discontinued.

- Therapeutic Uses of COMT Inhibitors
  - COMT inhibitors are beneficial in combination with levodopa/carbidopa to inhibit the metabolism of levodopa in the intestines and peripheral tissues: entacapone, tolcapone.

COMT INHIBITORS: ENTACAPONE, TOLCAPONE

Adverse Effects	Nursing Interventions/Client Education
› Adverse effects are the same as for pramipexole when administered with levodopa/carbidopa. › Other common adverse effects: dyskinesias, orthostatic hypotension, hallucinations, sleep disturbances.	› Interventions are the same as for pramipexole when administered with levodopa/carbidopa.
› GI symptoms (vomiting, diarrhea, constipation)	› Treat GI adverse effects according to symptoms.
› Discoloration of urine to a yellow-orange	› Assure the client that the urine color is harmless.
› Use with caution if hepatic function is impaired.	› Monitor liver enzymes periodically.
	› Advise the client that the "wear off" effect is delayed and that the "on" times are extended.

- Therapeutic Uses of MAO-B Inhibitors
  - MAO-B is a first line medication in combination with levodopa/carbidopa to decrease the "wear-off" effect.
    - Selegiline can preserve dopamine produced from levodopa, and prolong the effects of levodopa but only up to 1 or 2 years.
    - Rasagiline preserves dopamine in the brain and is not converted into amphetamine or methamphetamine like selegiline does.

MAO-B INHIBITORS: SELEGILINE, RASAGILINE

Adverse Effects	Nursing Interventions/Client Education
› Insomnia (selegiline)	› Administer selegiline no later than noon.
› Hypertensive crisis triggered from foods containing tyramine	› Advise the client to avoid eating foods that contain tyramine (avocados, soybeans, figs, smoked meats, dried or cured fish, cheese, yeast products, beer, chianti wine, chocolate, caffeinated beverages).
› Hypertensive crisis and even death from certain medications	› Provide a list of medications to avoid (e.g., meperidine [Demerol], fluoxetine [Prozac], MAO inhibitors, antidepressants, sympathomimetics).

- Therapeutic Uses of Centrally Acting Anticholinergics
  - Centrally acting anticholinergic antagonists diminish cholinergic effect (neuron excitability) due to decreased dopamine: benztropine (Cogentin), trihexyphenidyl (Artane). They are considered second-line therapy for tremors, most appropriate for younger clients who have mild symptoms, and generally avoided in older adult clients because of CNS effects.

CENTRALLY ACTING ANTICHOLINERGICS: BENZTROPINE, TRIHEXYPHENIDYL	
Adverse Effects	Nursing Interventions/Client Education
› Nausea, vomiting	› Advise clients to take medication with food but to avoid high-protein snacks.
› Atropine-like effects (dry mouth, blurred vision, mydriasis, urinary retention, constipation)	› Advise clients to observe for symptoms and notify the provider if they occur. › Monitor I&O and for urinary retention. › Advise clients to chew sugarless gum, eat foods high in fiber, and increase fluid intake to 2 to 3 L/day from beverage and food sources. › Advise the client to schedule periodic eye exam to measure for increased intraocular pressure that can result in glaucoma.
› Antihistamine effects (sedation, drowsiness)	› Advise the client to avoid hazardous activities while taking the medication. › Avoid administering to older adult clients due to CNS adverse effects (sedation, confusion, delusions and hallucinations).

Client Education

- Instruct family members to assist clients with the medication at home.
- Instruct the client about the possible sudden loss of the effects of medication and to notify the provider if manifestations occur.
- Inform the client that effects might not be noticeable for several weeks to several months.
- Medication "holidays" may be indicated, but they must be monitored in a hospital setting.
- Advise clients to avoid high-protein meals and snacks.

- Advise client, if applicable, to avoid pregnancy when taking levodopa or pramipexole.

Nursing Evaluation of Medication Effectiveness

- Depending on therapeutic intent, effectiveness can be evidenced by:
  - Improvement of manifestations as demonstrated by absence of tremors, and reduction of irritability and stiffness.
  - Increase in ability to perform ADLs.

MEDICATION CLASSIFICATION: ANTIEPILEPTICS (AEDs)

TRADITIONAL ANTIEPILEPTIC MEDICATIONS

	Simple Partial, Complex Partial, Secondarily Generalized Seizures	Primary Generalized Seizures		
		Tonic-Clonic	Absence	Myoclonic
Phenobarbital (Luminal)	✓	✓		
Primidone (Mysoline)	✓	✓		
Phenytoin (Dilantin)	✓	✓		
Carbamazepine (Tegretol)	✓	✓		
Valproic Acid (Depakote)	✓	✓	✓	✓
Ethosuximide (Zarontin)			✓	

NEWER ANTIEPILEPTIC MEDICATIONS

	Simple Partial, Complex Partial, Secondarily Generalized Seizures	Primary Generalized Seizures		
		Tonic-Clonic	Absence	Myoclonic
Lamotrigine (Lamictal)	✓	✓	✓	✓
Levetiracetam (Keppra)	✓	✓		✓
Topiramate (Topamax)	✓	✓		✓
Oxcarbazepine (Trileptal)	✓			
Gabapentin (Neurontin)	✓			
Pregabalin (Lyrica)	✓			
Tiagabine (Gabitril Filmtabs)	✓			
Zonisamide (Zonegran)	✓			
Lacosamide (Vimpat)	✓			
Vigabatrin (Sabril)	✓			
Ezogabine (Potiga)	✓			

- Other Medications
  - Benzodiazepines used for status epilepticus (acute prolonged seizure)
    - Diazepam (Valium)
    - Lorazepam (Ativan)

Purpose

- Expected Pharmacological Action
  - AEDs control seizure disorders by various mechanisms.
    - Slowing the entrance of sodium and calcium back into the neuron, thus extending the time it takes for the nerve to return to its active state
    - Suppressing neuronal firing, which decreases seizure activity and prevents propagation of seizure activity into other areas of the brain
    - Decreasing seizure activity by enhancing the inhibitory effects of gamma butyric acid (GABA)

Traditional Antiepileptic Medication

BARBITURATES: PHENOBARBITAL, PRIMIDONE	
Adverse Effects	**Nursing Interventions/Client Education**
› CNS effects in adults manifest as drowsiness, sedation, and depression, and in the older adult can cause confusion and anxiety. In children, CNS effects manifest as irritability and hyperactivity.	› Advise the client to observe for symptoms and to notify the provider if they occur. › Advise the client to avoid hazardous activities, such as driving. › Never administer primidone with phenobarbital because phenobarbital is an active metabolic (stimulates drug metabolism cell porphyria). › Primidone is generally administered with phenytoin or carbamazepine. › Avoid administering other CNS depressants (alcohol, benzodiazepines, opioids).
› Toxicity (nystagmus, ataxia, respiratory depression, coma, pinpoint pupils, hypotension, death)	› Stop medication. Administer oxygen and maintain respiratory function with ventilatory support. › Monitor vital signs.
› Phenobarbital and primidone decrease synthesis of vitamins K and D and decrease the effectiveness of warfarin (Coumadin).	› Monitor laboratory values (INR, calcium, vitamin D).
› Phenobarbital is not recommended during pregnancy.	› Inform the client of the potential risk of pregnancy and to consult with the provider.
› Phenobarbital and primidone decrease the effectiveness of oral contraceptives.	› Advise the client to consider other forms of contraceptives.
› Phenobarbital can intensify CNS depression caused by other drugs (alcohol, opioids, benzodiazepines). Severe respiratory depression and coma can result.	› Monitor for manifestations, and notify the provider if they occur.

HYDANTOINS: PHENYTOIN

Adverse Effects	Nursing Interventions/Client Education
› CNS effects (nystagmus, sedation, ataxia, double vision, cognitive impairment)	› Monitor for manifestations of CNS effects, and notify the provider if symptoms occur.
› Gingival hyperplasia (softening and overgrowth of gum tissue, tenderness, and bleeding gums)	› Advise clients to maintain good oral hygiene (dental flossing, massaging gums).
› Skin rash	› Stop medication if rash develops.
› Teratogenic (cleft palate, heart defects)	› Avoid use in pregnancy. › Classified as Pregnancy Risk Category D. Administer only if the benefits outweigh the risks.
› Cardiovascular effects (dysrhythmias, hypotension)	› Administer at slow IV rate and in dilute solution to prevent adverse CV effects. › Administer IV route for status epilepticus. › Avoid administering to a client who has sinus bradycardia, sinoatrial block, or Stokes-Adams syndrome.
› Endocrine and other effects (coarsening of facial features, hirsutism, and interference with vitamin D metabolism)	› Instruct the client to report changes. › Encourage the client to consume adequate amounts of calcium and vitamin D.
› Interference with vitamin K-dependent clotting factors causing bleeding in newborns	› Administer prophylactic vitamin K to the mother for 1 month before the infant is delivered.
Interactions	Nursing Interventions/Client Education
› Phenytoin causes a decrease in the effects of oral contraceptives, warfarin (Coumadin), and glucocorticoids because of the stimulation of hepatic drug-metabolizing enzymes.	› Dose of oral contraceptives may need to be adjusted, or an alternative form of birth control used. › Monitor for therapeutic effects of warfarin and glucocorticoids (INR, blood glucose levels). Dosages may need to be adjusted.
› Alcohol, diazepam (Valium), cimetidine (Tagamet), valproic acid, and isoniazid increase phenytoin levels.	› Advise clients to avoid alcohol use. › Monitor serum levels.
› Carbamazepine (Tegretol), phenobarbital, and chronic alcohol use decrease phenytoin levels.	› Encourage the client to avoid use of alcohol.
› Additive CNS depressant effects can occur with concurrent use of CNS depressants (barbiturates, alcohol).	› Advise clients to avoid concurrent use of alcohol and other CNS depressants.

CARBAMAZEPINE

Adverse Effects	Nursing Interventions/Client Education
› Cognitive function is minimally affected, but CNS effects (nystagmus, double vision, vertigo, staggering gait, headache) can occur.	› Administer in low doses initially and then gradually increase dosage. › Administer dose at bedtime. › Administered also for bipolar disorder, and trigeminal and glossopharyngeal neuralgias.
› Teratogenic: associated with birth defects (spina bifida, neural tube defect)	› Classified as Pregnancy Risk Category D. Administer only if the benefits outweigh the risks.
› Blood dyscrasias (leukopenia, anemia, thrombocytopenia)	› Obtain baseline CBC and platelets. Perform ongoing monitoring of CBC and platelets. › Observe for manifestations of bruising and bleeding of gums, sore throat, fever, pallor, weakness, and infection. Instruct client to notify provider if these occur. › Avoid administering to a client who has bone marrow suppression or bleeding disorders.
› Hypo-osmolarity (carbamazepine promotes secretion of ADH, which inhibits water excretion by the kidneys and places clients who have heart failure at risk for fluid overload)	› Monitor serum sodium periodically. › Monitor the client for edema, decrease in urine output, and hypertension.
› Skin disorders (dermatitis, rash, Stevens-Johnson syndrome)	› Treat mild reactions with anti-inflammatory or antihistamine medications. › Medication should be discontinued if there is a severe reaction.

Interactions	Nursing Interventions/Client Education
› Carbamazepine causes a decrease in the effects of oral contraceptives and warfarin (Coumadin) because of the stimulation of hepatic drug-metabolizing enzymes.	› Dose of oral contraceptives may need to be adjusted or an alternative form of birth control used. › Monitor for therapeutic effects of warfarin with PT and INR. › Dosages may need to be adjusted.
› Grapefruit juice inhibits metabolism, and thus increases carbamazepine levels.	› Advise the client to avoid intake of grapefruit juice.
› Phenytoin and phenobarbital decrease the effects of carbamazepine.	› Concurrent use is not recommended.

VALPROIC ACID	
Adverse Effects	Nursing Interventions/Client Education
› Gastrointestinal effects (nausea, vomiting, indigestion)	› Advise the client to take medication with food. Enteric-coated formulation can decrease symptoms.
› Hepatotoxicity (anorexia, abdominal pain, jaundice)	› Obtain baseline liver function and monitor liver function periodically. › Advise the client to observe for manifestations of anorexia, nausea, vomiting, abdominal pain, and jaundice, and to notify the provider if they occur. › This medication should not be used for children younger than 2 years old. › Medication should be prescribed in lowest effective dose. › Avoid administering to a client who has liver disease.
› Pancreatitis as evidenced by nausea, vomiting, and abdominal pain	› Advise the client to observe for manifestations and to notify the provider immediately if they occur. › Monitor amylase levels. › Medication should be discontinued if pancreatitis develops.
› Thrombocytopenia	› Advise the client to observe for manifestations such as bruising, and to notify the provider if these occur. › Monitor the client's platelet counts and bleeding time.
› Teratogenic (cleft palate, heart defects)	› Avoid use in pregnancy. › Classified as Pregnancy Risk Category D. Administer only if the benefits outweigh the risks.
› CNS effects from hyperammonemia (vomiting, lethargy, impaired cognitive alertness)	› Monitor blood ammonia levels periodically. › Discontinue the medication.
Interactions	Nursing Interventions/Client Education
› Concurrent use of valproic acid increases the levels of phenytoin and phenobarbital.	› Monitor phenytoin and phenobarbital levels. › Adjust dosage of medications as prescribed.

ETHOSUXIMIDE	
Adverse Effects	Nursing Interventions/Client Education
› Gastrointestinal effects (nausea, vomiting)	› Administer with food.
› CNS effects (sleepiness, lightheadedness, fatigue)	› Administer low initial dosage. › Advise clients to avoid hazardous activities, such as driving.
› Note: Ethosuximide is indicated only for absence seizures.	

Newer Antiepileptic Medications

LAMOTRIGINE (LAMICTAL)

Adverse Effects	Nursing Interventions/Client Education
› CNS effects (dizziness, somnolence, aphasia, double or blurred vision, headache, nausea, vomiting, depression)	› Monitor for manifestations of aseptic meningitis (headache, fever, stiff neck, nausea, vomiting, rash, sensitivity to light). › Discontinue medication severe reaction develops. › Monitor for suicidal ideation.
› Skin disorders can include life-threatening rashes (Stevens-Johnson syndrome and toxic epidermal necrolysis).	› Treat mild reactions with anti-inflammatory or antihistamine medications. › Discontinue medication if there is a severe reaction.
› Teratogenic effects (cleft palate, cleft lip) are low risk.	› Classified as Pregnancy Risk Category C. Avoid use in pregnancy.

LEVETIRACETAM (KEPPRA)

Adverse Effects	Nursing Interventions/Client Education
› CNS effects (dizziness, asthenia [loss of strength, weakness] agitation, anxiety, depression, suicidal ideation)	› Discontinue medication if there is a severe reaction. › Monitor for suicidal ideation.

TOPIRAMATE (TOPAMAX)

Adverse Effects	Nursing Interventions/Client Education
› CNS effects (somnolence, dizziness, ataxia, nervousness, diplopia, confusion, impaired cognitive function)	› Discontinue medication if there is a severe reaction.
› Teratogenic (cleft palate, cleft lip)	› Avoid use in pregnancy. › Classified as Pregnancy Risk Category D. Administer only if the benefits outweigh the risks.
› Metabolic acidosis	› Monitor serum bicarbonate levels. › Advise the client to report signs of hyperventilation, fatigue, anorexia. › Discontinue medication or reduce the dosage as prescribed by the provider.
› Angle-closure glaucoma	› Inform the client of manifestations of glaucoma (ocular pain, redness, blurring of vision). › Advise the client to have periodic eye exams to measure intraocular pressure.
› Medication Interaction: phenytoin and carbamazepine can decrease topiramate level. Topiramate can increase phenytoin levels.	› Consult provider before administering phenytoin or carbamazepine with topiramate.
› Hypohidrosis (reduced sweating), increasing the risk for hyperthermia	› Avoid vigorous activity and elevated environmental temperatures.

OXCARBAZEPINE (TRILEPTAL)

Adverse Effects	Nursing Interventions/Client Education
› CNS effects (dizziness, drowsiness, double vision, nystagmus, headache, nausea, and vomiting)	› Administer low initial dosage. › Advise the client to avoid hazardous activities, such as driving. › Monitor serum sodium levels if having nausea and vomiting.
› Skin disorders, including life-threatening rashes (Stevens-Johnson syndrome and toxic epidermal necrolysis)	› Treat mild reactions with anti-inflammatory or antihistamine medications. › Discontinue medication if there is a severe reaction.
› Teratogenic (cleft palate, heart defects)	› Classified as Pregnancy Risk Category D. Administer only if the benefits outweigh the risks.
› Hyponatremia (nausea, drowsiness, headache, and confusion)	› Monitor serum sodium laboratory values. › Use caution when the client is administered diuretic medication.
Interactions	Nursing Interventions/Client Education
› Decreases oral contraceptive levels.	› Advise the client to use alternate form of contraception.
› Phenytoin levels increase when administered with oxcarbazepine.	› Consult provider before administering with phenytoin.
› Depresses CNS if alcohol is consumed.	› Advise the client to avoid alcohol.

GABAPENTIN (NEURONTIN)

Adverse Effects	Nursing Interventions/Client Education
› CNS effects (somnolence, dizziness, ataxia, fatigue, nystagmus, peripheral edema) diminish in time.	› Advise the client to avoid driving if experiencing a high degree of drowsiness.

PREGABALIN (LYRICA)

Adverse Effects	Nursing Interventions/Client Education
› CNS effects (somnolence, dizziness, adverse cognitive effect, headache)	› Advise the client to avoid driving if experiencing a high degree of drowsiness. › Discontinue medication if there is a severe reaction.
› Weight gain, peripheral edema, dry mouth	› Monitor daily weight, and report major increase to the provider. › Advise the client to chew gum or suck on hard candy to increase salivation.
› Can cause infant birth defects (skeletal and visceral malformations).	› Classified as Pregnancy Risk Category C. Avoid use in pregnancy.
Interactions	Nursing Interventions/Client Education
› Benzodiazepines, alcohol, and opioids intensify CNS effects.	› Advise the client to avoid medications that affect the CNS.

Client Education

- Inform the client that monitoring therapeutic plasma levels is recommended as prescribed by the provider.

- Monitor therapeutic plasma levels. Be aware of therapeutic levels for medications prescribed. Notify the provider of results.

- Advise the client taking antiepileptic medications that treatment provides for control of seizures, not cure of disorder.

- Encourage the client to keep a seizure frequency diary to monitor effectiveness of therapy.

- Advise the client to take medications as prescribed and not to stop medications without consulting the provider. Sudden cessation of medication may trigger seizures.

- Advise the client to avoid hazardous activities (driving, operating heavy machinery) until seizures are fully controlled.

- Advise the client who is traveling to carry extra medication to avoid interruption of treatment in locations where their medication is not available.

- Advise the client of childbearing age to avoid pregnancy, because medications can cause birth defects and congenital abnormalities.

- Advise the client that phenytoin doses must be individualized. Dosing usually starts twice a day and can be switched to once-a-day dosing with an extended-release form when maintenance dose has been established.

- Advise the client that phenytoin has a narrow therapeutic range, and strict adherence to the medication regimen is imperative to prevent toxicity or therapeutic failure.

Nursing Evaluation of Medication Effectiveness

- Depending on therapeutic intent, effectiveness can be evidenced by:
  - Absence or decreased occurrence of seizures.
  - Ability to perform ADLs.
  - Absence of injury.

APPLICATION EXERCISES

1. A nurse is reinforcing teaching of discharge instructions for a client who has a new diagnosis of myasthenia gravis. The client is prescribed neostigmine (Prostigmin). Which of the following information should the nurse reinforce in the discharge instructions? (Select all that apply.)

_____ A. Wear a medical alert bracelet.

_____ B. Initially start with a high dose of medication then decrease the dosage.

_____ C. Take medication at the same time each day.

_____ D. Monitor for manifestations of urinary urgency.

_____ E. Modify medication dose based on response.

2. A nurse is providing information about pramipexole (Mirapex) to a client who has early Parkinson's disease. Which of the following possible adverse effects should the nurse include in the information?

A. Hallucinations

B. Memory loss

C. Diarrhea

D. Discoloration of urine

3. A nurse is reviewing food interactions with a client who is taking levodopa/carbidopa (Sinemet) for Parkinson's disease. Which of the following instructions should the nurse include?

A. Eat large amounts of protein-rich foods with the medication.

B. Take the medication with whole-grain cereal.

C. Consider eating a banana with the medication.

D. Take the medication crushed in grapefruit juice.

4. A nurse is preparing to administer medication to a client who has absence seizures. Which of the following medications are appropriate for the nurse to administer? (Select all that apply.)

_____ A. Phenytoin (Dilantin)

_____ B. Ethosuximide (Zarontin)

_____ C. Gabapentin (Neurontin)

_____ D. Carbamazepine (Tegretol)

_____ E. Valproic acid (Depakote)

_____ F. Lamotrigine (Lamictal)

5. A nurse is reviewing a new prescription for oxcarbazepine (Trileptal) with a female client who has partial seizures. Which of the following statements by the nurse are appropriate? (Select all that apply.)

_____ A. "Use caution if given a prescription for a diuretic medication."

_____ B. "Consider using an alternate form of contraception."

_____ C. "Chew gum to increase saliva production."

_____ D. "Avoid driving until you see how the medication affects you."

_____ E. "Notify your provider if you develop a skin rash."

6. A nurse is contributing to the plan of care for a client who has tonic-clonic seizures and a new prescription for phenytoin (Dilantin). Considering the adverse effects and nursing interventions, what should the nurse contribute to the plan of care? Use the ATI Active Learning Template: Medication to complete this item to include the following:

A. Therapeutic Use: Describe.

B. Adverse Effects/Interactions: Describe two adverse effects and two medication interactions.

C. Nursing Interventions/Client Education: Include two interventions that relate to the two adverse effects, and two interventions that relate to the two medication interactions.

APPLICATION EXERCISES KEY

1. A. **CORRECT:** The nurse should recommend that the client wear a medical alert bracelet when prescribed neostigmine because episodes of difficulty swallowing and muscle weakness can occur until the dose is regulated.

    B. INCORRECT: The nurse should advise the client initially to start with a low dose of neostigmine and titrate the dosage up until desired muscle function is achieved.

    C. **CORRECT:** The nurse should encourage the client to take the medication at the same time each day to prevent weakness of respiratory and swallowing muscles.

    D. **CORRECT:** The nurse should inform the client to monitor for manifestations of urinary urgency because neostigmine increases the urge to void.

    E. **CORRECT:** The nurse should instruct the client to modify the medication dose according to individualized response to improving muscle weakness.

    Ⓝ NCLEX® Connection: Pharmacological Therapies, Adverse Effects/Contraindications/ Side Effects/Interactions

2. A. **CORRECT:** Pramipexole can cause hallucinations within 9 months of the initial dose and may need to be discontinued.

    B. INCORRECT: Memory loss is not an adverse effect of pramipexole.

    C. INCORRECT: Diarrhea is not an adverse effect of pramipexole.

    D. INCORRECT: Discoloration of urine is not an adverse effect of pramipexole.

    Ⓝ NCLEX® Connection: Pharmacological Therapies, Adverse Effects/Contraindications/ Side Effects/Interactions

3. A. INCORRECT: The client should avoid protein-rich foods, which contain pyridoxine and result in decreased therapeutic effects of levodopa.

    B. INCORRECT: The client should avoid whole-grain cereal, which contains pyridoxine and results in decreased therapeutic effects of levodopa.

    C. INCORRECT: The client should avoid bananas, which contain pyridoxine and result in decreased therapeutic effects of levodopa.

    D. **CORRECT:** The client may crush a tablet or empty a capsule of levodopa/carbidopa in any type of juice if having difficulty swallowing.

    Ⓝ NCLEX® Connection: Pharmacological Therapies, Medication Administration

4.   A. INCORRECT: Phenytoin is prescribed for partial seizures and tonic-clonic seizures and has no therapeutic effect for a client who has absence seizures.

    B. **CORRECT:** Ethosuximide's only mechanism of action is to treat a client who has absence seizures.

    C. INCORRECT: Gabapentin is prescribed for partial seizures and tonic-clonic seizures and has no therapeutic effect for a client who has absence seizures.

    D. INCORRECT: Carbamazepine is prescribed for partial seizures and tonic-clonic seizures and has no therapeutic effect for a client who has absence seizures.

    E. **CORRECT:** Valproic acid has a therapeutic effect when treating a client who has absence seizures and all other forms of seizures.

    F. **CORRECT:** Lamotrigine has a therapeutic effect when treating a client who has absence seizures and all other forms of seizures.

    Ⓝ NCLEX® Connection: Pharmacological Therapies, Expected Actions/Outcomes

5.   A. **CORRECT:** Diuretic medication is administered with caution because of the high risk for hyponatremia when taking oxcarbazepine.

    B. **CORRECT:** An alternate form of contraception is recommended because oxcarbazepine decreases oral contraceptive levels.

    C. INCORRECT: Chewing gum to increase salivation is not indicated because the medication does not cause dry mouth.

    D. **CORRECT:** The client should avoid driving if CNS effects of dizziness, drowsiness, and double vision develop.

    E. **CORRECT:** The client should notify the provider if a skin rash occurs because life-threatening skin disorders can develop.

    Ⓝ NCLEX® Connection: Pharmacological Therapies, Adverse Effects/Contraindications/ Side Effects/Interactions

6. *Using the ATI Active Learning Template: Medication*

    A. Therapeutic Use
        -   Phenytoin (Dilantin) is a hydantoin medication that suppresses partial seizure and primary generalized seizure activity in the affected neurons.

    B. Adverse Effects/Interactions
        -   CNS effects
        -   Gingival hyperplasia
        -   Teratogenic birth defects
        -   Decreases effectiveness of oral contraceptives
        -   Causes stimulation of hepatic drug-metabolizing enzymes

    C. Nursing Interventions/Client Education
        -   Instruct the client to refrain from alcohol and other medications that cause CNS depression (e.g., barbiturates).
        -   Encourage the client to use dental floss and massage gums daily.
        -   Instruct the client to avoid pregnancy and use an alternate form of contraception.
        -   Monitor INR if on warfarin (Coumadin) and blood glucose levels if taking a glucocorticoid.
        -   Monitor therapeutic effects of warfarin and glucocorticoids.
        -   Never abruptly discontinue antiepileptic medications.

        Ⓝ NCLEX® Connection: Pharmacological Therapies, Adverse Effects/Contraindications/
        Side Effects/Interactions

chapter **13**

Overview

- Eye Disorders

    - Glaucoma is the leading cause of blindness in the U.S. Damage to the optic nerve occurs when aqueous humor does not exit from the anterior chamber of the eye. This results in the buildup of aqueous humor, increased intraocular pressure (IOP), and loss of vision.

        - Types of glaucoma

            - Primary open-angle glaucoma (POAG)

                - POAG occurs in about 90% of people who have glaucoma.

                - Peripheral vision is lost gradually, with central visual field loss occurring if damage to the optic nerve continues.

                - Clients typically do not experience clinical manifestations until there is widespread damage. IOP greater than 21 mm Hg is the highest risk factor for POAG.

                - Treatment includes medication therapy to reduce IOP. Surgical intervention is indicated if IOP cannot be reduced by medications.

                - POAG is treated with the following medications.

                    - Beta-adrenergic blockers

                    - Alpha$_2$-adrenergic agonists

                    - Prostaglandin analogs

                    - Cholinergic agonists

                    - Carbonic anhydrase inhibitors

                    - Nonselective adrenergic agonists

            - Angle-closure glaucoma (narrow-angle glaucoma)

                - This is an acute disorder with a sudden onset, resulting in irreversible blindness within 1 to 2 days without emergency treatment.

                - Clinical findings include acute onset of ocular pain, seeing halos around lights, blurred vision, and photophobia. The optic nerve is damaged when the aqueous humor builds up as a result of displacement of the iris.

- Ear disorders

    - Acute otitis media

        - This condition occurs most often in young children.

        - A bacterial or a viral infection causes a buildup of fluid in the middle ear (middle ear effusion).

        - The major indication is acute onset of pain. Objective findings include erythema, bulging of the tympanic membrane, and fever.

- Treatment for bacterial infection, especially in infants and young children, is an antibiotic. Treatment for viral infection is symptomatic.
  - □ Because of the increase in antibiotic-resistant bacteria, the current trend is to observe children over age 2 years and prescribe antibiotics only if the condition does not resolve or worsens over several days.
- Medications for treating otitis media
  - □ Oral penicillins
  - □ Other antimicrobials, oral or parenteral
- ○ Otitis externa
  - This condition, also known as "swimmer's ear," is caused by a bacterial infection of the external auditory canal.
  - Any object that abrades or leaves moisture in the canal facilitates colonization of bacteria and the onset of otitis externa.
  - Treatment usually resolves infection within 10 days.
- ○ Otitis externa is usually treated by topical antimicrobial/anti-inflammatory combination.
  - Incidence of acute otitis media in infants and children can be reduced by yearly influenza vaccination and vaccination with pneumococcal conjugate vaccine (PCV).

MEDICATIONS FOR EYE DISORDERS

MEDICATION CLASSIFICATION: BETA ADRENERGIC BLOCKERS

- Nonselective beta blockers (have both beta$_1$ and beta$_2$ properties)
  - ○ Timolol (Timoptic, Betimol)
  - ○ Carteolol (Ocupress)
  - ○ Metipranolol (OptiPranolol)
  - ○ Levobunolol (Betagan Liquifilm, AK-Beta)
- Cardioselective beta$_1$ blockers
  - ○ Betaxolol (Betoptic)
  - ○ Levobetaxolol (Betaxon)

Purpose

- Expected Pharmacological Action
  - ○ Beta blockers decrease IOP by decreasing the amount of aqueous humor produced.
- Therapeutic Uses
  - ○ Topical beta blockers are used primarily to treat POAG. They also may be prescribed in combination with other topical medications to lower IOP.
  - ○ These medications occasionally are used to treat closed-angle glaucoma on an emergency basis.

Complications

ADVERSE EFFECTS	NURSING INTERVENTIONS/CLIENT EDUCATION
› Temporary stinging discomfort in the eye immediately after drop is instilled	› Instruct clients that this effect is transient.
› Occasional conjunctivitis, blurred vision, photophobia, dry eyes	› Instruct clients to report these effects to the provider.
› Systemic effects of beta blockade on heart and lungs	› Warn clients that overdose could cause or increase the chance of systemic effects. › When taking beta$_1$ blockers, clients should monitor pulse rate for bradycardia. › Use beta$_1$ blockers for clients who have chronic respiratory disease.

Contraindications/Precautions

- Betaxolol is contraindicated for clients who have bradycardia and AV heart block and should be used carefully in clients who have heart failure.

Interactions

MEDICATION/FOOD INTERACTIONS	NURSING INTERVENTIONS/CLIENT EDUCATION
› Oral beta blockers or a calcium channel blocker can increase cardiovascular and respiratory effects.	› Instruct clients to inform the provider if they are taking any of these medications.
› Beta blockers can interfere with some effects of insulin.	› Advise clients who have diabetes to monitor their blood glucose.

Nursing Administration

- Instill one drop in the affected eye once or twice daily.
- Review the proper method of instilling eye drops, and provide instruction to a family member if indicated.
- Use sterile technique when handling the applicator portion of the container. Avoid touching any part of the applicator, and keep the lid in place when not in use.
- Hold gentle pressure on the nasolacrimal duct for 30 to 60 seconds immediately after instilling the drop(s) to prevent or minimize any expected systemic effect.

- Monitor pulse rate/rhythm as indicated for beta blocker.

MEDICATION CLASSIFICATION: ALPHA$_2$-ADRENERGIC AGONISTS

- Select Prototype Medication: brimonidine (Alphagan)
- Other Medication: apraclonidine (Iopidine)

Purpose

- Expected Pharmacological Action
  - Brimonidine decreases production and can increase outflow of aqueous humor to lower IOP.
- Therapeutic Uses
  - Brimonidine is used as a first-line medication for long-term topical treatment of POAG.
  - Apraclonidine is a short-term therapy for POAG only and is used preoperatively for laser eye surgeries.

Complications

ADVERSE EFFECTS	NURSING INTERVENTIONS/CLIENT EDUCATION
› Localized stinging discomfort and pruritus of conjunctiva; sensation that a foreign body is in the eye	› Advise clients not to rub their eyes.
› Blurred vision, headache, dry mouth	› Instruct clients to report these effects.
› Reddened sclera caused by blood-vessel engorgement	› Inform clients of the possibility of this effect.
› Hypotension, drowsiness (brimonidine crosses the blood-brain barrier)	› Advise clients to use caution with driving and other tasks, and to inform the provider if dizziness or weakness occur.

Contraindications/Precautions

- Advise clients who wear soft contact lenses that brimonidine should be administered with lenses removed. Delay insertion of the lens at least 15 min after administration to prevent absorption of medication into the lens.

Interactions

MEDICATION/FOOD INTERACTIONS	NURSING INTERVENTIONS/CLIENT EDUCATION
› Antihypertensive medications can intensify hypotension caused by brimonidine.	› Instruct clients to inform the provider if they are taking any antihypertensive medications.

Nursing Administration

- Review proper method of administering eye drops and minimizing systemic effects.
- Monitor blood pressure for hypotension.

MEDICATION CLASSIFICATION: PROSTAGLANDIN ANALOGS

- Select Prototype Medication: latanoprost (Xalatan)
- Other Medications
  - Travoprost (Travatan)
  - Bimatoprost (Lumigan)

Purpose

- Expected Pharmacological Action
  - Latanoprost increases aqueous humor outflow through relaxation of ciliary muscle.
- Therapeutic Uses
  - These agents are topical first-line medications for clients who have POAG and ocular hypertension.

Complications

ADVERSE EFFECTS	NURSING INTERVENTIONS/CLIENT EDUCATION
› Permanent increased brown pigmentation, usually occurring in individuals with brown-colored iris (also can cause pigmentation of lids, lashes)	› Inform clients about the possibility of this effect.
› Stinging, burning, reddened conjunctiva	› Instruct clients not to rub their eyes.
› Blurred vision	› Instruct clients to report to the provider.
› Migraine (rare adverse effect)	› Instruct clients to report to the provider.

Second-line Topical Medications for Glaucoma

CLASSIFICATION: DIRECT-ACTING CHOLINERGIC AGONIST	
Prototype	› Pilocarpine (Isopto Carpine, Pilocar)
Purpose	› Second-line treatment for POAG; lowers IOP indirectly through ciliary contraction. › Also used to treat closed-angle glaucoma.
Adverse Effects	› Retinal detachment › Parasympathetic effects, such as bradycardia › Decreased visual acuity
CLASSIFICATION: CARBONIC ANHYDRASE INHIBITOR	
Prototype	› Dorzolamide (Trusopt) › Available in combination with timolol (called Cosopt)
Purpose	› Second-line treatment for POAG, which decreases aqueous humor production. › Timolol/dorzolamide combination produces increased effect of both medications.
Adverse Effects	› Localized allergic reactions in up to 15% › Blurred vision, dryness, photophobia

MEDICATION CLASSIFICATION: OSMOTIC AGENTS

- Select Prototype Medication: mannitol (Osmitrol)

Purpose

- Expected Pharmacological Action
    - Osmotic agents decrease intraocular pressure by making the plasma hypertonic, thus drawing fluid from the anterior chamber of the eye.
- Therapeutic Uses
    - These agents treat the rapid progression of closed-angle glaucoma to prevent blindness.

MEDICATION CLASSIFICATION: CARBONIC ANHYDRASE INHIBITORS (SYSTEMIC)

- Select Prototype Medication: acetazolamide (Diamox Sequels)
- Other Medications: methazolamide

Purpose

- Expected Pharmacological Action
    - Reduces production of aqueous humor by causing diuresis through renal effects.
- Therapeutic Uses
    - These medications are used to quickly lower IOP in clients for whom other medications have been ineffective.
    - Acetazolamide, a non-antimicrobial sulfonamide, can be used as an emergency medication prior to surgery for acute angle-closure glaucoma and as a second-line medication for treatment of POAG.
    - Acetazolamide may be used to treat acute mountain sickness, seizures, and heart failure (as a diuretic).

Complications

ADVERSE EFFECTS	NURSING INTERVENTIONS/CLIENT EDUCATION
› Severe allergic reactions (anaphylaxis) › Possible cross-sensitivity with sulfonamides	› Educate clients about effects and to notify provider. › Ask about sulfonamide allergy.
› Rare serious blood disorders, such as bone marrow depression	› Educate clients to recognize and immediately report effects.
› Gastrointestinal (GI) effects (nausea and diarrhea)	› Report GI adverse effects and weight loss to provider.

ADVERSE EFFECTS	NURSING INTERVENTIONS/CLIENT EDUCATION
› Electrolyte depletion (sodium and potassium), altered liver function	› Prepare clients for the need to obtain regular laboratory testing.
› Generalized influenza-like symptoms (headache, fever, body aches)	› Educate clients about possible reactions.
› Central nervous system disturbances (paresthesias of extremities, fatigue, sleepiness, rarely seizures)	› Educate clients about possible reactions. › Medication may be discontinued.
› Glucose disturbances in clients who have diabetes mellitus	› Instruct clients who have diabetes to closely monitor blood glucose and watch for indications of hypo- or hyperglycemia.

Contraindications/Precautions

- Acetazolamide is Pregnancy Risk Category C (teratogenic).
- Use during lactation only after evaluation by the provider.

Interactions

MEDICATION/FOOD INTERACTIONS	NURSING INTERVENTIONS/CLIENT EDUCATION
› Serious effects, such as metabolic acidosis, can occur in clients using high-dose aspirin.	› Question clients about aspirin use, and notify the provider.
› Acetazolamide can increase the risk of toxic effects of quinidine.	› Instruct clients to notify the provider of concurrent use and to watch for indications of toxicity, such as decreased heart rate.
› Acetazolamide can decrease blood levels of lithium.	› Instruct clients taking lithium to watch for increased indications of mania. Lithium levels should be monitored regularly.
› Acetazolamide can increase osteomalacia, an adverse effect of phenytoin.	› Instruct clients taking phenytoin to watch for bone pain or weakness and report symptoms to the provider.
› Sodium bicarbonate increases the risk of kidney stones.	› Question clients about the use of sodium bicarbonate and other over-the-counter antacids.

Nursing Administration

- Acetazolamide may be administered orally as a tablet or a capsule. It is also available for parenteral administration.

Nursing Evaluation of Medication Effectiveness

- Depending on therapeutic intent, effectiveness can be evidenced by:
  - Reduced IOP.
  - Safe self-administration of medication.
  - Prevention or minimization of systemic effects.

MEDICATIONS FOR EAR DISORDERS
MEDICATION CLASSIFICATION: ANTIMICROBIALS

- Select Prototype Medication: amoxicillin (Amoxil)
- Other Medication: amoxicillin/clavulanate (Augmentin) PO
- The following antibiotics are used to treat acute otitis media in clients who have a penicillin allergy or penicillin-resistant otitis media.
  - Ceftriaxone (Rocephin) IM, IV (severe illness)
  - Cefdinir (Omnicef) PO
  - Cefuroxime (Ceftin) PO, IM, IV
  - Cefpodoxime (Vantin) PO
  - Azithromycin (Zithromax) PO, IV
  - Clindamycin (Cleocin), PO, IM, IV (a macrolide antibiotic)

Purpose

- Expected Pharmacological Action
  - Eradication of infection
- Therapeutic Uses
  - Used to treat otitis media and various other bacterial infections throughout the body.

Complications

ADVERSE EFFECTS	NURSING INTERVENTIONS/CLIENT EDUCATION
› Possible allergic reaction is the most common risk when taking penicillin.	› Question the client and family regarding the presence of penicillin or other antibiotic allergy. › The client may need alternative medication. › A skin test may be used to test for sensitivity.
› GI upset (usually less with amoxicillin than with ampicillin)	› Educate family to inform the provider of severe diarrhea, especially in an infant or young child.
› Suprainfection with other microbes, such as oral candidiasis	› Report indications of new infection to the provider.

Contraindications/Precautions

- Amoxicillin is contraindicated for clients who have a severe allergy to penicillin or cephalosporins.
- Use cautiously in infants younger than 3 months of age because of immature renal system and increased risk for toxicity.

Nursing Administration

- Amoxicillin is prescribed usually 3 times daily PO.
- Amoxicillin may be taken with meals.
- As with all antibiotics, instruct the client to take the full course of medication.

Nursing Evaluation of Medication Effectiveness

- Depending on therapeutic intent, effectiveness may be evidenced by:
  - Reduction of manifestations (e.g., fever, earache).
  - Absence of infection.
  - Absence of recurrence of infection.

MEDICATION CLASSIFICATION:
FLUOROQUINOLONE ANTIBIOTIC PLUS STEROID MEDICATION

- Select Prototype Medication: ciprofloxacin plus hydrocortisone (Cipro HC) otic drops
- Other Medications
  - Acetic acid 2% solution otic drops (Vasolate)
  - Ciprofloxacin plus dexamethasone otic drops (Ciprodex)
  - Ofloxacin otic drops (Floxin)

Purpose

- Expected Pharmacological Action
  - The bactericidal effect of the ciprofloxacin and anti-inflammatory effect of the hydrocortisone should decrease pain, edema, and erythema in the ear canal.
- Therapeutic Uses
  - These topical medications are used to treat otitis externa.

Complications

ADVERSE EFFECTS	NURSING INTERVENTIONS/CLIENT EDUCATION
› CNS effects (dizziness, lightheadedness, tremors, restlessness, convulsions)	› Instruct clients to inform the provider if any of these occur.
› Rash	› Question the client/family about allergies to fluoroquinolone antibiotics or to steroids such as dexamethasone or cortisone.

Nursing Administration

- Review the method for instilling otic drops.
- Inform clients that movement of the tragus or pinna can be very painful when instilling otic drops.
- Warm the medication by gently rolling the container between hands before instilling drops. Cold drops can cause dizziness. Gently shake medication that is in suspension form.
- Place the client on the unaffected side.
- Keep clients in a side-lying position for 5 min with the affected ear up after instilling drops. Place a small piece of cotton in the ear. Avoid packing it tightly.

- Instruct client/family to prevent otic medications from being placed in the eye or ingested orally.
- Reinforce to client/family to prevent otitis externa by:
  - Keeping foreign bodies, such as cotton swabs, out of the ear canal, and avoiding the use of manual measures to remove cerumen.
  - Drying the ear canal after bathing or swimming, using a towel, and tilting the head to promote drainage.
  - Avoiding the use of earplugs except for swimming.

Nursing Evaluation of Medication Effectiveness

- Depending on therapeutic intent, effectiveness can be evidenced by:
  - Subsiding of clinical manifestations.
  - Use of measures to prevent reinfection.

APPLICATION EXERCISES

1. A nurse is reinforcing teaching to a client who has a new prescription for timolol (Timoptic) how to insert eye drops. The nurse should tell the client to press on which of the following to prevent systemic absorption of the medication?

    A. Bony orbit

    B. Nasolacrimal duct

    C. Conjunctival sac

    D. Outer canthus of the eye

2. A client has a new prescription for brimonidine (Alphagan) ophthalmic, one drop three times a day. He tells the nurse he also wears soft contact lenses and wants to know whether he can put the drops in his eyes with the lenses in place. Which of the following should the nurse tell this client?

    A. "Go ahead and put the drop in your eye with the contact lens in place."

    B. "Take the contact lens out of your eye, then instill the eye drop, and immediately reinsert the contact lens."

    C. "Take the contact lens out of your eye, then instill the eye drop, and wait at least 15 minutes before putting the contact lens back in place."

    D. "You will need to discontinue the use of contact lenses while using brimonidine eye drops."

3. A nurse in an emergency unit is reviewing the medical record of a client who is being evaluated for angle-closure glaucoma. Which of the following findings are indicative of this condition?

    A. Insidious onset of painless loss of vision

    B. Gradual reduction in peripheral vision

    C. Report of seeing halos around lights

    D. An intraocular pressure (IOP) of 12 mm Hg

4. A nurse is preparing to administer azithromycin (Zithromax) 500 mg to a client who has otitis media. Available is azithromycin oral suspension 40 mg/mL. How many mL should the nurse administer? (Round the answer to the nearest tenth.)

5. A nurse in a provider's office is reinforcing teaching to a parent how to administer ear drops. Which of the following instructions should the nurse include? (Select all that apply.)

_____ A. "Place the child on his unaffected side when you are ready to administer the medication."

_____ B. "Warm the medication by gently rolling it between your hands for a few minutes."

_____ C. "Gently shake medication that is in suspension form."

_____ D. "Keep the child on his side for 5 minutes after instillation of the ear drops."

_____ E. "Tightly pack the ear with cotton after instillation of the ear drops."

6. A nurse in a provider's office is reinforcing teaching to a client who has a prescription for ciprofloxacin/hydrocortisone (Cipro HC) about the medication and how to prevent otitis externa. Use the ATI Active Learning Template: Medication to complete this item to include the following sections:

A. Therapeutic Uses: Identify two therapeutic effects of the medication.

B. Nursing Administration: Identify two actions to prevent otitis externa.

APPLICATION EXERCISES KEY

1. A. INCORRECT: Pressing on the bony orbit will not prevent systemic absorption.

    B. **CORRECT:** Pressing on the nasolacrimal blocks the lacrimal punctum and prevents systemic absorption of the medication.

    C. INCORRECT: Pressing on the conjunctival sac will not prevent systemic absorption.

    D. INCORRECT: Pressing on the outer canthus will not prevent systemic absorption.

    Ⓝ NCLEX® Connection: Pharmacological Therapies, Medication Administration

2. A. INCORRECT: Contact lenses absorb brimonidine. Therefore, this response by the nurse is incorrect.

    B. INCORRECT: Contact lenses absorb brimonidine. Therefore, this response by the nurse is incorrect.

    C. **CORRECT:** The client can continue to wear his contacts. He should instill the medication and wait at least 15 min before putting in his contacts.

    D. INCORRECT: Although contact lenses absorb brimonidine, he can continue to wear his contacts by following proper procedure for installation.

    Ⓝ NCLEX® Connection: Pharmacological Therapies, Medication Administration

3. A. INCORRECT: Acute-angle glaucoma is painful and has a sudden onset.

    B. INCORRECT: Gradual loss of peripheral vision occurs in the presence of primary open-angle glaucoma.

    C. **CORRECT:** Halos around lights occurs in the presence of angle-closure glaucoma.

    D. INCORRECT: An IOP of 12 mm Hg is within the expected reference range. An elevated IOP is an expected finding in the presence of angle-closure glaucoma.

    Ⓝ NCLEX® Connection: Physiological Adaptations, Unexpected Response to Therapies

4. **12.5** mL

Using Ratio and Proportion

STEP 1: *What is the unit of measurement to calculate?*
mL

STEP 2: *What is the dose needed? Dose needed = Desired.*
500 mg

STEP 3: *What is the dose available? Dose available = Have.*
40 mg

STEP 4: *Should the nurse convert the units of measurement?*
No

STEP 5: *What is the quantity of the dose available?*
1 mL

STEP 6: *Set up an equation and solve for X.*

$$\frac{Have}{Quantity} = \frac{Desired}{X}$$

$$\frac{40\ mg}{1\ mL} = \frac{500\ mg}{X\ mL}$$

X = 12.5

STEP 7: *Round if necessary.*

STEP 8: *Reassess to determine whether the amount to administer makes sense.*
If there is 40 mg/mL and the prescribed amount is 500 mg, it makes sense to administer 12.5 mL. The nurse should administer azithromycin oral suspension 12.5 mL PO.

Using Desired Over Have

STEP 1: *What is the unit of measurement to calculate?*
mL

STEP 2: *What is the dose needed? Dose needed = Desired.*
500 mg

STEP 3: *What is the dose available? Dose available = Have.*
40 mg

STEP 4: *Should the nurse convert the units of measurement?*
No

STEP 5: *What is the quantity of the dose available?*
1 mL

STEP 6: *Set up an equation and solve for X.*

$$\frac{Desired \times Quantity}{Have} = X$$

$$\frac{500\ mg \times 1\ mL}{40\ mg} = X\ mL$$

12.5 = X

STEP 7: *Round if necessary.*

STEP 8: *Reassess to determine whether the amount to administer makes sense.*
If there is 40 mg/mL and the prescribed amount is 500 mg, it makes sense to administer 12.5 mL. The nurse should administer azithromycin oral suspension 12.5 mL PO.

Using Dimensional Analysis

STEP 1: *What is the unit of measurement to calculate?*
mL

STEP 2: *What quantity of the dose is available?*
1 mL

STEP 3: *What is the dose available? Dose available = Have.*
40 mg

STEP 4: *What is the dose needed? Dose needed = Desired.*
500 mg

STEP 5: *Should the nurse convert the units of measurement?*
No

STEP 6: *Set up an equation of factors and solve for X.*

$$X = \frac{Quantity}{Have} \times \frac{Conversion\ (Have)}{Conversion\ (Desired)} \times \frac{Desired}{}$$

$$\frac{1\ mL}{40\ mg} \times \frac{500\ mg}{}$$

X = 12.5

STEP 7: *Round if necessary.*

STEP 8: *Reassess to determine whether the amount to administer makes sense.*
If there is 40 mg/mL and the prescribed amount is 500 mg, it makes sense to administer 12.5 mL. The nurse should administer azithromycin oral suspension 12.5 mL PO.

 NCLEX® Connection: Pharmacological Therapies, Dosage Calculation

5. A. **CORRECT:** The parent should have the child on his unaffected side to allow access to the affected ear and to promote drainage of the medication by gravity into the ear.

   B. **CORRECT:** The parent should warm the medication by rolling it between her hands. Administering the medication cold can cause dizziness.

   C. **CORRECT:** The parent should gently shake medication that is in suspension form to evenly disperse the medication.

   D. **CORRECT:** The parent should keep the child on his side to promote drainage of the medication by gravity into the ear.

   E. INCORRECT: The parent should loosely pack the ear with cotton.

   Ⓝ NCLEX® Connection: Pharmacological Therapies, Medication Administration

6. *Using ATI Active Learning Template: Medication*

   A. Therapeutic Uses
   - The bactericidal effects of ciprofloxacin and the anti-inflammatory effect of hydrocortisone decreases the pain, edema, and erythremia in the ear.

   B. Nursing Administration
   - Preventing otitis externa
     ○ Keep foreign bodies out of ear canal.
     ○ Avoid manual measures to remove cerumen.
     ○ Dry ear canal after bathing or swimming using a towel.
     ○ Avoid use of ear plugs except for swimming.

   Ⓝ NCLEX® Connection: Pharmacological Therapies, Expected Actions/Outcomes

chapter 14

Overview

- Neuromuscular blocking agents have various uses, including assisting with sedation during general anesthesia, control of seizures during electroconvulsive therapy, and suppression of gag reflex during endotracheal intubation.
  - Medications include succinylcholine (Anectine) and vecuronium.
- Muscle relaxants and antispasmodic agents can affect both the central and peripheral nervous systems.
  - These agents are used for spasticity related to muscle injury, cerebral palsy, spinal cord injury, and multiple sclerosis.
  - Agents include diazepam (Valium), baclofen (Lioresal), and dantrolene (Dantrium).
  - Bethanechol (Urecholine), a muscarinic agonist, is used for urinary retention.
  - Oxybutynin (Ditropan), a muscarinic antagonist, is used for neurogenic bladder.

MEDICATION CLASSIFICATION: NEUROMUSCULAR BLOCKING AGENTS

- Select Prototype Medication
  - Depolarizing neuromuscular blockers: succinylcholine (Anectine)
  - Nondepolarizing neuromuscular blockers: pancuronium
- Other Medications
  - Nondepolarizing neuromuscular blockers: atracurium, vecuronium, doxacurium, mivacurium

Purpose

- Expected Pharmacological Action

  - Neuromuscular blocking agents block acetylcholine (ACh) at the neuromuscular junction, resulting in muscle relaxation and hypotension. They do not cross the blood-brain barrier and have no effect on the CNS. Consequently, complete paralysis can be achieved without loss of consciousness or decreased pain sensation.

MEDICATION ACTIONS
Succinylcholine
› Mimics ACh by binding with cholinergic receptors at the neuromuscular junction. This agent fills the cholinergic receptors, preventing ACh from binding with them, and causes sustained depolarization of the muscle, resulting in muscle paralysis.
› Short duration of action due to degradation by the plasma enzyme pseudocholinesterase causes plasma levels of succinylcholine to decline, thereby allowing repolarization of the end-plate.
Pancuronium, atracurium, vecuronium
› Block ACh from binding with cholinergic receptors at the motor end plate. Muscle paralysis occurs because of inhibited nerve depolarization and skeletal muscle contraction.
› Reversal agent: neostigmine (Prostigmin)

- Therapeutic Uses

  - Neuromuscular blocking agents are used as adjuncts to general anesthesia to promote muscle relaxation.

  - These agents are used to control spontaneous respiratory movements in clients receiving mechanical ventilation.

  - These agents are used as seizure control during electroconvulsive therapy.

  - Neuromuscular blocking agents are used during endotracheal intubation, endoscopy, and other short procedures.

Complications

ADVERSE EFFECTS	NURSING INTERVENTIONS/CLIENT EDUCATION
› Respiratory arrest from paralyzed respiratory muscles	› Maintain continuous cardiac and respiratory monitoring. › Have equipment ready for resuscitation and mechanical ventilation. › Monitor clients for return of respiratory function when medication is discontinued.
› Hypotension possible with atracurium	› Monitor for decreased blood pressure. Administer antihistamine if indicated.
Succinylcholine	
› Low pseudocholinesterase activity can lead to prolonged apnea.	› Test the client's blood or administer a small test dose for clients suspected of having low levels of pseudocholinesterase. › Withhold medication if pseudocholinesterase activity is low.
› Indications of malignant hyperthermia include muscle rigidity accompanied by increased temperature, reaching levels as high as 43° C (109.4° F).	› Monitor vital signs. › Stop succinylcholine and other anesthetics. › Administer oxygen at 100%. › Initiate cooling measures, including administration of iced 0.9% sodium chloride, applying a cooling blanket, and placing ice bags in groin and other areas. › Administer dantrolene to decrease metabolic activity of skeletal muscle.
› After 12 to 24 hr postoperative, clients can experience muscle pain in the upper body and back.	› Advise clients that this response is not unusual and eventually will subside. › Notify the provider to consider short-term use of muscle relaxant.
› Hyperkalemia	› Monitor potassium levels. › Observe for signs of hyperkalemia.

Contraindications/Precautions

- Pregnancy Risk Category C.
- Succinylcholine is contraindicated in clients who have a risk of hyperkalemia (clients who have major trauma, severe burns).
- Use cautiously in clients who have myasthenia gravis, respiratory dysfunction, and fluid and electrolyte imbalances.
- Note that neuromuscular blocker medications are not anesthetics and therefore have no effect on a client's hearing, thinking, or ability to feel pain.
- Contraindicated in patients who have low pseudocholinesterase activity.

Interactions

MEDICATION/FOOD INTERACTIONS	NURSING INTERVENTIONS/CLIENT EDUCATION
› General anesthetics often are used concurrently in surgery.	› Dosage of tubocurarine should be reduced to prevent extreme neuromuscular blockade.
› Aminoglycosides and tetracyclines can increase the effects of neuromuscular blockade.	› Take complete medication history of clients who are to receive neuromuscular blockade.
› Neostigmine and other cholinesterase inhibitors increase the effects of depolarizing neuromuscular blockers, such as succinylcholine.	› Monitor clients during neuromuscular blockade reversal after surgery.

Nursing Administration

- Clients must receive continuous cardiac and respiratory monitoring during therapy.
- Monitor clients following administration of a neuromuscular blocker for respiratory depression and have life support equipment available.
- Continue to carefully monitor clients for return of respiratory function.

Nursing Evaluation of Medication Effectiveness

- Depending on therapeutic intent, effectiveness can be evidenced by:
  - Muscle relaxation during surgery.
  - No spontaneous respiratory movements in clients receiving mechanical ventilation.
  - Absence of seizures in clients receiving electroconvulsive therapy.
  - Successful endotracheal intubation.

MEDICATION CLASSIFICATION: MUSCLE RELAXANTS AND ANTISPASMODICS

- Select Prototype Medications
  - Centrally acting muscle relaxant: diazepam (Valium)
  - Peripherally acting muscle relaxant: dantrolene (Dantrium)
- Other Medications
  - Centrally acting muscle relaxants
    - Baclofen (Lioresal)
    - Cyclobenzaprine
    - Tizanidine (Zanaflex)

Purpose

EXPECTED PHARMACOLOGICAL ACTION	THERAPEUTIC USES
Diazepam	

› Diazepam acts in the CNS to suppress spasticity by mimicking the actions of GABA, produce sedative effects, and depress spasticity of muscles.	› Relief of
	  » Muscle spasm related to muscle injury and spasticity
	  » Anxiety and panic disorders
	  » Insomnia
	  » Status epilepticus
	  » Alcohol withdrawal
	› Anesthesia induction

Cyclobenzaprine, tizanidine	
› These medications act in the CNS to enhance GABA, produce sedative effects, and depress spasticity of muscles. They have no direct muscle-relaxant action and so do not decrease muscle strength.	› Relief of muscle spasm related to muscle injury
Baclofen	
› Baclofen acts within the spinal cord to suppress hyperactive reflexes, which regulate muscle movement › Baclofen is a structural analog of GABA (an inhibitory neurotransmitter) and acts by mimicking the actions of GABA.	› Relief of spasticity related to cerebral palsy, spinal cord injury, and multiple sclerosis
Dantrolene	
› Dantrolene is a peripherally acting muscle relaxant that acts directly on spastic muscles and inhibits muscle contraction by preventing release of calcium in skeletal muscles. Hence, the muscle is less able to contract.	› Relief of spasticity related to cerebral palsy, spinal cord injury, and multiple sclerosis › Treatment of malignant hyperthermia

Complications

ADVERSE EFFECTS	NURSING INTERVENTIONS/CLIENT EDUCATION
All muscle relaxants and antispasmodics	
› CNS depression (sleepiness, lightheadedness, fatigue)	› Start at low doses. › Inform clients of potential adverse effects. › Advise clients to avoid hazardous activities, such as driving and concurrent use of other CNS depressants, including alcohol.
Centrally acting agents: Diazepam, cyclobenzaprine, tizanidine	
› Hepatic toxicity with tizanidine (anorexia, nausea, vomiting, abdominal pain, jaundice)	› Obtain baseline liver function, and perform periodic follow-up liver function tests. › Observe for signs of toxicity, and notify the provider if they occur. › Start at a low dose.
› Physical dependence from chronic long-term use	› Advise clients not to discontinue the medication abruptly.
Baclofen	
› Nausea, constipation, urinary retention	› Advise clients of adverse effects and to notify the provider if they occur. › Monitor I&O. › Advise clients to increase intake of high-fiber foods.
Peripherally acting agent: Dantrolene	
› Hepatic toxicity (anorexia, nausea, vomiting, abdominal pain, jaundice)	› Obtain baseline liver function studies and perform periodic follow-up liver function tests. › Observe for indications of toxicity, and notify the provider if they occur. › Start at the lowest effective dosage and for the shortest time necessary.
› Muscle weakness	› Monitor effectiveness of the medication.

Contraindications/Precautions

- Baclofen and dantrolene
  - Pregnancy Risk Category C
- Diazepam
  - Controlled Substance (Schedule IV)
  - Pregnancy Risk Category D
- Use both of these medications cautiously in clients who have impaired liver or kidney function.

Interactions

MEDICATION/FOOD INTERACTIONS	NURSING INTERVENTIONS/CLIENT EDUCATION
› CNS depressants (alcohol, opioids, antihistamines) have additive CNS depressant effects.	› Advise clients to avoid concurrent use.

Nursing Administration

- Instruct clients to take medications as prescribed.
- Advise clients not to stop taking the medication abruptly to avoid withdrawal reaction.
- Advise clients to avoid CNS depressants while using these medications.
- Provide assistance as needed in self-administration of medication and performance of ADLs.
- Advise clients to not drive or handle heavy equipment.

Nursing Evaluation of Medication Effectiveness

- Depending on therapeutic intent, effectiveness can be evidenced by:
  - Absence of muscle rigidity and spasms, good range of motion.
  - Absence of pain.
  - Increased ability to perform ADLs.

MEDICATION CLASSIFICATION: MUSCARINIC AGONISTS

- Select Prototype Medication: bethanechol (Urecholine)

Purpose

- Expected Pharmacological Action
  - Stimulation of muscarine receptors of the GU tract, thereby causing relaxation of the trigone and sphincter muscles and contraction of the detrusor muscle, resulting in bladder emptying
- Therapeutic Uses
  - Nonobstructive urinary retention, usually postoperatively or postpartum
  - On an investigational basis to treat gastroesophageal reflux; can help treat disorders associated with GI paralysis

Complications

ADVERSE EFFECTS	NURSING INTERVENTIONS/CLIENT EDUCATION
› Extreme muscarinic stimulation can result in sweating, tearing, urinary urgency, bradycardia and hypotension.	› Instruct clients to report manifestations if they occur.

Contraindications/Precautions

- Contraindicated in clients who have urinary or gastrointestinal obstruction, peptic ulcer disease, coronary insufficiency, asthma, and hyperthyroidism

Nursing Administration

- Administer by oral route, 1 hr before or 2 hr after meals to minimize nausea and vomiting.
- Monitor I&O.

Nursing Evaluation of Medication Effectiveness

- Depending on therapeutic intent, effectiveness can be evidenced by relief of urinary retention.

MEDICATION CLASSIFICATION: MUSCARINIC ANTAGONISTS

- Select Prototype Medication
  - ○ M_3 receptor selective: oxybutynin (Ditropan)
- Other Medications
  - ○ M_3 receptor selective: darifenacin (Enablex)
  - ○ Nonselective: tolterodine (Detrol)

Purpose

- Expected Pharmacological Action
  - ○ Muscarinic antagonists inhibit muscarinic receptors of the detrusor muscle of the bladder, which prevents contractions of the bladder and the urge to void.
- Therapeutic Use
  - ○ Overactive bladder

Complications

ADVERSE EFFECTS	NURSING INTERVENTIONS/CLIENT EDUCATION
› Anticholinergic effects (constipation, dry mouth, blurred vision, photophobia, dry eyes, tachycardia, asthma)	› Instruct clients to increase dietary fiber, consume 2 to 3 L/day of fluid from beverage and food sources, sip fluids, and avoid hazardous activities if vision is impaired.
› CNS effects (hallucinations, confusion, insomnia, nervousness)	› Instruct clients to report manifestations to the provider. The medication may need to be discontinued.

Contraindications/Precautions

- These medications are contraindicated in clients who have glaucoma, myasthenia gravis, paralytic ileus, GI or GU obstruction, or urinary retention.
- Use cautiously in children and older adults.
- Use cautiously in clients who have gastroesophageal reflux disease (GERD), heart failure, or kidney or liver impairment.

Interactions

MEDICATION/FOOD INTERACTIONS	NURSING INTERVENTIONS/CLIENT EDUCATION
› Antihistamines, tricyclic antidepressants, or phenothiazines used concurrently can result in extreme muscarinic blockage.	› Concurrent use is not recommended.

Nursing Administration

- Oral formulations are available as syrup, immediate release (IR) tablets, and extended release (ER) tablets that minimize anticholinergic effects.
- Advise clients to swallow ER tablets whole and to avoid chewing or crushing the tablets.
- Instruct clients that the shell of ER tablets will be eliminated whole in the stool.
- The transdermal patch is administered two times per week. Instruct clients to apply to dry skin of the hip, abdomen, or buttock and to rotate sites.

Nursing Evaluation of Medication Effectiveness

- Depending on therapeutic intent, effectiveness can be evidenced by a decrease in urinary urgency and frequency, nocturia, and urge incontinence.

APPLICATION EXERCISES

1. A nurse is assisting with the care of a client who received a bolus dose of succinylcholine (Anectine) IV before an endoscopy procedure. During the procedure, the client suddenly develops rigidity, and his body temperature begins to rise. The nurse should anticipate a prescription for which of the following medications?

    A. A second dose of succinylcholine (Anectine)

    B. Naloxone as an antagonist at receptor sites

    C. Dantrolene (Dantrium) to slow metabolic activity of muscles

    D. Vecuronium (Norcuron) as an adjunct to muscle relaxation

2. A nurse is assisting with the development of a treatment plan for a client following surgery. The client has been administered dantrolene to treat malignant hyperthermia, and the administration of succinylcholine and other anesthetics has been discontinued. Which of the following additional actions should be included in the plan? (Select all that apply.)

_____ A. Place a cooling blanket on the client.

_____ B. Administer oxygen at 100%.

_____ C. Administer iced 0.9% sodium chloride.

_____ D. Administer potassium chloride IV.

_____ E. Monitor core body temperature.

3. A nurse is reinforcing teaching with a client who has begun taking oral baclofen (Lioresal) three times daily to treat muscle spasms caused by a spinal cord injury. Which of the following statements by the client indicates a need for further teaching?

    A. "I will stop taking this medication right away if I develop dizziness."

    B. "I know the doctor will gradually increase my dose of this medication for awhile."

    C. "I'll make sure that I empty my bladder completely while taking this medication."

    D. "I won't be able to drink alcohol while I'm taking this medication."

4. A nurse in a provider's office is reviewing the health care record of a client who reported urinary incontinence and asked about a prescription for oxybutynin (Ditropan). The nurse should recognize that oxybutynin is contraindicated in the presence of which of the following conditions?

   A. Bursitis

   B. Sinusitis

   C. Depression

   D. Glaucoma

5. A nurse is caring for a client who has a prescription for bethanechol (Urecholine) 50 mg PO three times a day. The nurse should recognize that which of the following findings is a clinical manifestation of extreme muscarinic stimulation?

   A. Tachycardia

   B. Hypertension

   C. Excessive perspiration

   D. Fecal impaction

6. A nurse in a surgical center is reviewing nursing responsibilities regarding assisting with the administration of succinylcholine. Use the ATI Active Learning Template: Medication to complete this item to include the following sections:

   A. Therapeutic Uses: Identify two common indications for its use.

   B. Nursing Administration: Identify two conditions that require the nurse to question the use of succinylcholine.

APPLICATION EXERCISES KEY

1. A. INCORRECT: Muscle rigidity and a sudden rise in temperature are indications of malignant hyperthermia. A second dose of succinylcholine would exacerbate the client's condition.

    B. INCORRECT: Muscle rigidity and a sudden rise in temperature are indications of malignant hyperthermia. Naloxone is used to reverse the effects of opioids. It is not used to treat malignant hyperthermia.

    C. **CORRECT:** Muscle rigidity and a sudden rise in temperature are indications of malignant hyperthermia. Dantrolene acts on skeletal muscles to reduce metabolic activity.

    D. INCORRECT: Muscle rigidity and a sudden rise in temperature are indications of malignant hyperthermia. Vecuronium is an intermediate-acting nondepolarizing neuromuscular blocker, but it is not useful in treating malignant hyperthermia.

    Ⓝ NCLEX® Connection: Pharmacological Therapies, Adverse Effects/Contraindications/ Side Effects/Interactions

2. A. **CORRECT:** The nurse should apply a cooling blanket and apply ice to the axilla and groin.

    B. **CORRECT:** The nurse should administer oxygen at 100% to treat the client's decreased oxygen saturation.

    C. **CORRECT:** The nurse should take action to decrease the client's body temperature by administering iced IV fluids.

    D. INCORRECT: A client who has malignant hyperthermia is at risk for hyperkalemia. Therefore, this action is not appropriate.

    E. **CORRECT:** The nurse should monitor the client's core body temperature to prevent hypothermia and to determine progress with measures taken to treat the client's condition.

    Ⓝ NCLEX® Connection: Pharmacological Therapies, Adverse Effects/Contraindications/ Side Effects/Interactions

3. A. **CORRECT:** Abrupt withdrawal from baclofen can result in a number of adverse effects, including visual hallucinations and seizures.

    B. INCORRECT: The provider starts the client on a low dose, and the dose is increased gradually to prevent CNS depression.

    C. INCORRECT: Urinary retention is an adverse effect that can occur with baclofen. Therefore, the client is taught to empty the bladder when urinating.

    D. INCORRECT: The intake of alcohol and other CNS depressants can exacerbate the CNS depressant effects of baclofen. Therefore, the client is instructed to avoid CNS depressants while taking baclofen.

    Ⓝ NCLEX® Connection: Pharmacological Therapies, Adverse Effects/Contraindications/ Side Effects/Interactions

4. A. INCORRECT: Oxybutynin is not contraindicated for a client who has bursitis.

    B. INCORRECT: Oxybutynin is not contraindicated for a client who has sinusitis.

    C. INCORRECT: Oxybutynin is not contraindicated for a client who has depression.

    D. **CORRECT:** Oxybutynin is an anticholinergic and can increase intraocular pressure. Therefore, it is contraindicated for clients who have glaucoma.

    Ⓝ NCLEX® Connection: Pharmacological Therapies, Adverse Effects/Contraindications/
    Side Effects/Interactions

5. A. INCORRECT: Bradycardia is a clinical manifestation of extreme muscarinic stimulation.

    B. INCORRECT: Hypotension is a clinical manifestation of extreme muscarinic stimulation.

    C. **CORRECT:** Bethanechol is a muscarinic agonist. Extreme muscarinic stimulation can result in sweating.

    D. INCORRECT: Fecal impaction is an adverse effect of bethanechol, but it is not a clinical manifestation of extreme muscarinic stimulation.

    Ⓝ NCLEX® Connection: Pharmacological Therapies, Adverse Effects/Contraindications/
    Side Effects/Interactions

6. *Using the Active Learning Template: Medication*

    A. Therapeutic Uses
      • Endotracheal intubation
      • Electroconvulsive therapy
      • Endoscopy
      • Adjunct to mechanical ventilation
      • Muscle relaxation during surgery

    B. Nursing Administration
      • Clients must receive continuous cardiac and respiratory monitoring during therapy.
      • Monitor clients following administration of a neuromuscular blocker for respiratory depression, and have life support equipment available.
      • Continue to carefully monitor clients for return of respiratory function.
      • Succinylcholine is contraindicated for clients at risk for hyperkalemia (trauma, severe burns).

    Ⓝ NCLEX® Connection: Safety and Infection Control, Accident/Error/Injury Prevention

chapter 15

Overview

- Sedatives are CNS depressants that induce a sense of calm and decrease anxiety. Hypnotics are CNS depressants that induce sleep.

- The three types of sedative-hypnotics are benzodiazepines, barbiturates, and benzodiazepine-like medications. The most commonly used are benzodiazepines and benzodiazepine-like medications because barbiturates cause tolerance and dependence, have multiple interactions, and are powerful respiratory depressants.

- IV anesthetics usually are administered during induction of general anesthesia. Most have a quick onset of action and short duration. These medications can be nonopioids or opioids.

MEDICATION CLASSIFICATION: BENZODIAZEPINES

- Select Prototype Medication: triazolam (Halcion)
- Other Medications
  - Alprazolam (Xanax)
  - Lorazepam (Ativan)
  - Midazolam (Versed)
  - Temazepam (Restoril)

Purpose

- Expected Pharmacological Action
  - These medications enhance the action of gamma-aminobutyric acid (GABA) in the CNS.
- Therapeutic Uses
  - Anxiety disorders
  - Seizure disorders
  - Insomnia
  - Muscle spasm
  - Alcohol withdrawal
  - Panic disorder
  - Induction of anesthesia

Complications

ADVERSE EFFECTS	NURSING INTERVENTIONS/CLIENT EDUCATION
› CNS depression (lightheadedness, drowsiness, incoordination)	› Advise clients to observe for symptoms and notify the provider if they occur. › Advise clients to avoid hazardous activities, such as driving or operating heavy equipment/machinery.
› Anterograde amnesia	› Advise clients to observe for symptoms and notify the provider if they occur.
› Paradoxical response, such as insomnia, excitation, euphoria, anxiety, rage	› Advise clients to observe for symptoms. If symptoms occur, instruct clients to notify the provider and stop the medication.
› Respiratory depression, especially with IV administration	› Monitor vital signs. › Have resuscitation equipment available.

› Physical dependence
  » Withdrawal following short-term therapy manifests as anxiety, insomnia, tremors and dizziness.
  » Withdrawal following long-term therapy manifests as delirium, paranoia, panic, hypertension, and seizures.
	› Discontinue medication slowly by tapering dose over weeks to months.

› Acute toxicity; oral toxicity (drowsiness, lethargy, confusion); IV toxicity (respiratory depression)	› For oral toxicity, gastric lavage can be used, followed by the administration of activated charcoal or saline cathartics. › For IV toxicity, administer flumazenil to counteract sedation and reverse side effects. › Monitor vital signs, maintain patent airway, and provide fluids to maintain blood pressure. › Have resuscitation equipment available.

Contraindications/Precautions

- These medications are Pregnancy Risk Category D; estazolam, flurazepam, quazepam, triazolam, and temazepam are Pregnancy Risk Category X.
- These medications are contraindicated in clients who have sleep apnea, respiratory depression, organic brain disease, or who are breastfeeding.
- Use cautiously in clients who have a history of substance use disorder, liver dysfunction, and kidney failure. Older adults may need decreased dosages.

Interactions

MEDICATION/FOOD INTERACTIONS	NURSING INTERVENTIONS/CLIENT EDUCATION
› CNS depressants, such as alcohol, barbiturates, and opioids, cause additive CNS depressant effects with concurrent use.	› Take complete medication history to identify concurrent use of other CNS depressants. › Advise clients to avoid alcohol and other CNS depressants.

Nursing Administration

- Ensure proper route of administration.
  - All agents may be given by oral route.
  - IV administration is acceptable with diazepam, midazolam, and lorazepam.
  - Lorazepam is the agent of choice for IM injection.
- Advise clients to take the medication as prescribed and to avoid abrupt discontinuation of treatment to prevent withdrawal manifestations.
- When discontinuing benzodiazepines, taper dose over several weeks.
- Administer medication with meals. Advise clients to swallow sustained-release tablets and to avoid chewing or crushing the tablet.
- Inform clients about possible development of dependency during and after treatment, and to notify the provider if manifestations occur.

Nursing Evaluation of Medication Effectiveness

- Depending on therapeutic intent, effectiveness can be evidenced by improvement of well-being as evidenced by absence of panic attacks, decrease or absence of anxiety, normal sleep pattern, absence of seizures, absence of withdrawal symptoms from alcohol, and relaxation of muscles.

MEDICATION CLASSIFICATION: NONBENZODIAZEPINES

- Select Prototype Medication: zolpidem (Ambien)
- Other Medications
    - Zaleplon (Sonata)
    - Eszopiclone (Lunesta)
    - Trazodone (Oleptro)

Purpose

- Expected Pharmacological Action
    - These medications enhance the action of gamma-aminobutyric acid (GABA) in the CNS. This results in prolonged sleep duration and decreased awakenings. These medications do not function as antianxiety, muscle relaxant, or antiepileptic agents. There is a low risk of tolerance, substance use disorder, and dependence.
- Therapeutic Uses
    - Management of insomnia

Complications

ADVERSE EFFECTS	NURSING INTERVENTIONS/CLIENT EDUCATION
› Daytime sleepiness and lightheadedness	› Administer medication at bedtime.
	› Advise clients to take medication allowing for at least 8 hr of sleep.
	› Advise clients that more rapid absorption occurs when the medication is taken when the stomach is empty.

Contraindications/Precautions

- Pregnancy Risk Category C.
- Contraindicated in clients who are breastfeeding.

 - Use cautiously in older adult clients and in clients who have impaired kidney, liver, or respiratory function.

Interactions

MEDICATION/FOOD INTERACTIONS	NURSING INTERVENTIONS/CLIENT EDUCATION
› CNS depressants, such as alcohol, barbiturates, and opioids, cause additive CNS depression.	› Advise clients to avoid alcohol and other CNS depressants.

Nursing Administration

- Advise clients to take the medication just before bedtime.
- Administer all agents by oral or sublingual route.

Nursing Evaluation of Medication Effectiveness

- Depending on therapeutic intent, effectiveness can be evidenced by an effective sleep pattern.

MEDICATION CLASSIFICATION: MELATONIN AGONIST

- Select Prototype Medication: ramelteon (Rozerem)

Purpose

- Expected Pharmacological Action
  - Activation of melatonin receptors
- Therapeutic Use
  - Management of insomnia

Complications

ADVERSE EFFECTS	NURSING INTERVENTIONS/CLIENT EDUCATION
› Sleepiness, dizziness, fatigue	› Ramelteon is generally well tolerated. Instruct clients to notify the provider if manifestations occur. › Advise clients to avoid activities such as driving if manifestations occur.
› Hormonal effects (amenorrhea, decreased libido, infertility, galactorrhea)	› Instruct clients to notify the provider if manifestations occur. Medication may be discontinued.

Contraindications/Precautions

- Contraindicated in pregnancy and lactation, in severe forms of liver disease, depression, apnea, and COPD.
- Use cautiously in older adults and clients who have moderate liver disease.

Interactions

MEDICATION/FOOD INTERACTIONS	NURSING INTERVENTIONS/CLIENT EDUCATION
› High-fat meals and grapefruit juice increase absorption.	› Take medication on an empty stomach.
› Concurrent use of fluvoxamine (Luvox) can increase levels of ramelteon.	› Avoid concurrent use.
› CNS depressants, such as opioids and alcohol, can cause additive CNS depression.	› Avoid concurrent use.

Nursing Administration

- Administer by oral route.
- Instruct clients to take medication 30 min prior to bedtime.
- Instruct clients to take medication on an empty stomach.

Nursing Evaluation of Medication Effectiveness

- Depending on therapeutic intent, effectiveness can be evidenced by improvement in sleep patterns.

MEDICATION CLASSIFICATION: INTRAVENOUS ANESTHETICS

- Intravenous nonopioid agents
  - ○ Select Prototype Medications
    - ▪ Barbiturates: pentobarbital sodium (Nembutal Sodium), thiopental (Pentothal)
    - ▪ Benzodiazepines: midazolam, diazepam (Valium)
  - ○ Other Medications: propofol (Diprivan), ketamine (Ketalar)
- Intravenous opioid agents
  - ○ Select Prototype Medication: fentanyl (Sublimaze)
  - ○ Other Medications: alfentanil (Alfenta), sufentanil (Sufenta)

Purpose

- Expected Pharmacological Action
  - ○ These medications produce loss of consciousness and elimination of response to painful stimuli.
- Therapeutic Uses
  - ○ Induction and maintenance of anesthesia
  - ○ Moderate (conscious) sedation (usually an IV nonopioid agent combined with an opioid agent)
  - ○ Intubation and mechanical ventilation
  - ○ Painful procedures (i.e., burn dressing changes)

Complications

ADVERSE EFFECTS	NURSING INTERVENTIONS/CLIENT EDUCATION
› Respiratory and cardiovascular depression with high risk for hypotension	› Provide continuous monitoring of vital signs and ECG. › Maintain mechanical ventilation during procedure. › Have equipment ready for resuscitation.
› Bacterial infection (with propofol)	› Use opened vials within 6 hr. › Monitor for indications of infection, such as fever or malaise after surgery.

› Psychologic reactions (with ketamine)
  » Hallucinations, mental confusion
  » Children less than 15 years of age and adults older than 65 years of age at lower risk
	› Avoid use in clients who have a history of mental illness.
	› Maintain a quiet, low-stimulus environment during recovery.
	› Give diazepam prior to ketamine.

Contraindications/Precautions

- Avoid use in clients who have a history of mental illness.
- Use cautiously in clients who have respiratory and cardiovascular disease.
- Midazolam is contraindicated in clients who have glaucoma, status asthmaticus, and acute alcohol intoxication.
- Pentobarbital and midazolam are Pregnancy Risk Category D.

Interactions

MEDICATION/FOOD INTERACTIONS	NURSING INTERVENTIONS/CLIENT EDUCATION
› CNS depressants (alcohol, barbiturates, opioids) create additive CNS depression.	› Clients may require lower doses. › Provide continuous monitoring of vital signs and ECG. › Have equipment ready for resuscitation.
› CNS stimulants (amphetamines, cocaine) create additive CNS stimulation.	› Clients may require higher doses. › Provide continuous monitoring of vital signs and ECG. › Have equipment ready for resuscitation.
› Opioid analgesics (fentanyl) provide analgesia and cough suppression.	› Monitor bladder and bowel function. › Encourage early ambulation, and assist clients to void.

Nursing Administration

- For moderate (conscious) sedation or for neonatal anesthesia, administer slowly over 2 min.
- Monitor carefully during and after moderate sedation or anesthesia for respiratory arrest or hypotension.
- Inject propofol into large vein to decrease pain at injection site.
- Instruct clients to arrange for a ride home following outpatient procedure.

Nursing Evaluation of Medication Effectiveness

- Depending on therapeutic intent, effectiveness can be evidenced by the following.
  - Surgical procedure occurs with loss of consciousness and elimination of pain.
  - Postoperative recovery as demonstrated by the following.
    - Vital signs return to baseline.
    - Client is oriented to time, place, and person.
    - Bowel sounds return.
    - Voiding occurs within 8 hr.
    - Nausea and vomiting are controlled.

APPLICATION EXERCISES

1. A nurse in a provider's office is reinforcing teaching to a client who has a new prescription for lorazepam (Ativan). The nurse should inform the client that which of the following are adverse effects of lorazepam? (Select all that apply.)

_____ A. Incoordination

_____ B. Euphoria

_____ C. Pruritus

_____ D. Flatus

_____ E. Amnesia

2. A nurse is assisting with the care of a client who is receiving moderate sedation with diazepam (Valium) IV. The client is oversedated. Which of the following medications should the nurse anticipate being administered to this client?

A. Ketamine (Ketalar)

B. Naltrexone (ReVia)

C. Flumazenil

D. Fluvoxamine (Luvox)

3. A nurse is reinforcing teaching with a client who has a new prescription for ramelteon (Rozerem). The nurse should instruct the client to avoid which of the following foods while taking this medication?

A. Eggs

B. Grapefruit juice

C. Whole-grain bread

D. Chicken

4. A client is admitted to undergo a surgical procedure. The nurse should be aware that which of the following preexisting conditions can be a contraindication for the use of ketamine (Ketalar) as an intravenous anesthetic for this client?

A. Peptic ulcer disease

B. Breast cancer

C. Diabetes mellitus

D. Schizophrenia

5. A nurse is reinforcing teaching with a female client who has a new prescription for zolpidem (Ambien). Which of the following instructions should the nurse include?

    A. Notify the provider if you plan to become pregnant.

    B. Take the medication 1 hr before you plan to go to sleep.

    C. Allow at least 6 hr for sleep when taking zolpidem.

    D. To increase the effectiveness of zolpidem, take it with a bedtime snack.

6. A nurse is assisting with an educational session to review client use of benzodiazepines for the nurses on her unit. Use the ATI Active Learning Template: Medication to complete this item to include the following sections:

    A. Therapeutic Uses: Identify five therapeutic uses for the benzodiazepines.

    B. Nursing Administration: Identify four contraindications for taking benzodiazepines.

APPLICATION EXERCISES KEY

1. A. **CORRECT:** Due to central nervous system depression, incoordination is an adverse effect of lorazepam.

    B. **CORRECT:** Euphoria can occur as a paradoxical adverse effect of lorazepam.

    C. INCORRECT: Pruritus is not an adverse effect of lorazepam.

    D. INCORRECT: Flatus is not an adverse effect of lorazepam.

    E. **CORRECT:** Retrograde amnesia, the inability to remember the events that occurred after taking the medication, can occur as an adverse effect of lorazepam.

    (N) NCLEX® Connection: Pharmacological Therapies, Adverse Effects/Contraindications/ Side Effects/Interactions

2. A. INCORRECT: Ketamine is an anesthetic agent.

    B. INCORRECT: Naltrexone is an opioid antagonist used to treat opioid overdose and alcohol use disorders.

    C. **CORRECT:** Flumazenil is a competitive benzodiazepine antagonist used to reverse the sedation and other effects of benzodiazepines.

    D. INCORRECT: Fluvoxamine is a selective serotonin reuptake inhibitor used to treat depression.

    (N) NCLEX® Connection: Pharmacological Therapies, Adverse Effects/Contraindications/ Side Effects/Interactions

3. A. INCORRECT: Eggs are not contraindicated for a client who is taking ramelteon.

    B. **CORRECT:** Grapefruit juice and high-fat foods increase ramelteon absorption.

    C. INCORRECT: Whole-grain breads are not contraindicated for a client who is taking ramelteon.

    D. INCORRECT: Chicken is not contraindicated for a client who is taking ramelteon.

    (N) NCLEX® Connection: Pharmacological Therapies, Adverse Effects/Contraindications/ Side Effects/Interactions

4. A. INCORRECT: Peptic ulcer disease is not a contraindication for the use of ketamine.

   B. INCORRECT: Breast cancer is not a contraindication for the use of ketamine.

   C. INCORRECT: Diabetes mellitus is not a contraindication for the use of ketamine.

   D. **CORRECT:** Ketamine can produce psychological effects such as hallucinations. Therefore, schizophrenia can be a contraindication for the use of ketamine.

   (N) NCLEX® Connection: Pharmacological Therapies, Adverse Effects/Contraindications/ Side Effects/Interactions

5. A. **CORRECT:** Zolpidem is Pregnancy Risk Category C. Therefore, the client should notify the provider if she plans to become pregnant.

   B. INCORRECT: Zolpidem should be taken at bedtime.

   C. INCORRECT: The client should allow at least 8 hr for sleep when taking zolpidem.

   D. INCORRECT: Zolpidem is absorbed best on an empty stomach.

   (N) NCLEX® Connection: Pharmacological Therapies, Medication Administration

6. *Using the ATI Active Learning Template: Medication*

   A. Therapeutic Uses
   - Anxiety disorders
   - Seizure disorders
   - Insomnia
   - Muscle spasms
   - Alcohol withdrawal
   - Panic disorder
   - Induction of anesthesia

   B. Nursing Administration: Contraindications
   - Pregnancy – benzodiazepines are Pregnancy Risk Category D (a high risk to the fetus)
   - Sleep apnea
   - Respiratory depression
   - Organic brain disease
   - Lactation
   - Cautious use in clients who have a history of substance use disorders, liver dysfunction, and kidney failure

   (N) NCLEX® Connection: Pharmacological Therapies, Expected Actions/Outcomes

UNIT 3 Medications Affecting the Respiratory System

CHAPTERS

› Airflow Disorders
› Upper Respiratory Disorders

NCLEX® CONNECTIONS

When reviewing the chapters in this unit, keep in mind the relevant sections of the NCLEX® outline, in particular:

Client Needs: Pharmacological Therapies

› Relevant topics/tasks include:

» Adverse Effects/Contraindications/Side Effects/Interactions

› Reinforce client teaching on possible effects of medications (common side effects or adverse effects, when to notify the primary health care provider).

» Expected Actions/Outcomes

› Apply knowledge of pathophysiology when addressing the client's pharmacological agents.

» Medication Administration

› Reinforce client teaching on client self-administration of medications (insulin, subcutaneous insulin pump).

| UNIT 3 | MEDICATIONS AFFECTING THE RESPIRATORY SYSTEM |
| CHAPTER 16 | Airflow Disorders |

Overview

- Asthma is a chronic inflammatory disorder of the airways. It is an intermittent and reversible airflow obstruction that affects the bronchioles. The obstruction occurs either by inflammation or airway hyper-responsiveness leading to bronchoconstriction.
- Medication management usually addresses both inflammation and bronchoconstriction. These same medications may be used in symptomatic treatment of chronic obstructive pulmonary disease (COPD).
- Medications include bronchodilator agents, such as beta$_2$-adrenergic agonists; methylxanthines; inhaled anticholinergics; and anti-inflammatory agents, such as glucocorticoids, mast cell stabilizers, and leukotriene modifiers.

 View Animation: Bronchoconstriction

MEDICATION CLASSIFICATION: BETA$_2$-ADRENERGIC AGONISTS

- Select Prototype Medication: albuterol (Proventil, Ventolin)
- Other Medications
  - Formoterol (Foradil Aerolizer)
  - Salmeterol (Serevent)
  - Terbutaline (Brethine)

Purpose

- Expected Pharmacological Action
  - Beta$_2$-adrenergic agonists act by selectively activating the beta$_2$-receptors in the bronchial smooth muscle, resulting in bronchodilation. As a result of this:
    - Bronchospasm is relieved.
    - Histamine release is inhibited.
    - Ciliary motility is increased.

- Therapeutic Uses

MEDICATION	ROUTE	THERAPEUTIC USES
Albuterol (Proventil, Ventolin)	› Inhaled, short-acting › Oral, long-acting	› Prevention of asthma episode (exercise-induced) › Inhaled, short-acting, used for prevention of asthma › Treatment for bronchospasm › Long-term control of asthma
Formoterol (Foradil Aerolizer) Salmeterol (Serevent)	› Inhaled, long-acting	› Long-term control of asthma
Terbutaline (Brethine)	› Oral, long-acting	› Long-term control of asthma

Complications

ADVERSE EFFECTS	NURSING INTERVENTIONS/CLIENT EDUCATION
› Oral agents can cause tachycardia and angina because of activation of alpha$_1$ receptors in the heart.	› Advise clients to observe for chest, jaw, or arm pain or palpitations and to notify the provider if they occur. › Instruct clients to check pulse and to report an increase of greater than 20 to 30/min. › Advise clients to avoid caffeine. › Dosage may need to be reduced.
› Tremors caused by activation of beta$_2$ receptors in skeletal muscle.	› Tremors usually resolve with continued medication use. › Dosage may need to be reduced.

Contraindications/Precautions

- Pregnancy Risk Category C.
- Contraindicated in clients who have tachydysrhythmia.
- Use cautiously in clients who have diabetes, hyperthyroidism, heart disease, hypertension, or angina.

Interactions

MEDICATION/FOOD INTERACTIONS	NURSING INTERVENTIONS/CLIENT EDUCATION
› Use of beta-adrenergic blockers (propranolol) can negate effects of both medications.	› Beta-adrenergic blockers should not be used concurrently.
› MAOIs and tricyclic antidepressants can increase the risk of tachycardia and angina.	› Instruct clients to report changes in heart rate and chest pain.

Nursing Administration

- Instruct clients to follow manufacturer's instructions for use of metered-dose inhaler (MDI), dry-powder inhaler (DPI), and nebulizer.

 View Image: Metered-Dose Inhaler

- When a client has a prescription for an inhaled beta$_2$-agonist and an inhaled glucocorticoid, advise the client to inhale the beta$_2$-agonist before inhaling the glucocorticoid. The beta$_2$-agonist promotes bronchodilation and enhances absorption of the glucocorticoid.

- Advise clients not to exceed prescribed dosages.

- Ensure that clients know the appropriate dosage schedule (if the medication is to be taken on a fixed or a as-needed schedule).

- Formoterol and salmeterol are long-acting beta$_2$-agonist inhalers. These inhalers are used every 12 hr for long-term control and are not used to abort an asthma attack, or exacerbation. They should always be taken on a fixed schedule and never PRN. These long-acting agents are not used alone but are prescribed in combination with an inhaled corticosteroid.

- A short-acting beta$_2$-agonist is used to treat an acute episode. Short-acting also can be used PRN for prophylaxis of exercise-induced bronchospasm (EIB).

- Advise clients to observe for indications of an impending asthma episode and to keep a log of the frequency and intensity of exacerbations.

- Instruct clients to notify the provider if there is an increase in the frequency and intensity of asthma exacerbations.

Nursing Evaluation of Medication Effectiveness

- Depending on therapeutic intent, effectiveness can be evidenced by:
  - Long-term control of asthma.
  - Prevention of exercise-induced asthma.
  - Resolution of asthma exacerbations as evidenced by absence of shortness of breath, clear breath sounds, absence of wheezing, and return of respiratory rate to baseline.

MEDICATION CLASSIFICATION: METHYLXANTHINES

- Select Prototype Medication: theophylline (Theolair, Theo-24)

Purpose

- Expected Pharmacological Action
  - Theophylline causes relaxation of bronchial smooth muscle, resulting in bronchodilation.
  - Theophylline, once the first-line medication for asthma, is now used infrequently because newer medications are safer and more effective.

- Therapeutic Uses
  - ○ Oral theophylline is used for long-term control of chronic stable asthma.
  - ○ Route of administration: oral or IV (emergency use only).

Complications

ADVERSE EFFECTS	NURSING INTERVENTIONS/CLIENT EDUCATION
› Mild toxicity reaction can include GI distress and restlessness. › More severe reactions can occur with higher therapeutic levels and can include dysrhythmias and seizures. › Death can result from cardiorespiratory collapse.	› Monitor theophylline serum levels to keep within therapeutic range (5 to 15 mcg/mL). Adverse effects are unlikely to occur at levels less than 20 mcg/mL. › If manifestations occur, stop the medication. Activated charcoal is used to decrease absorption, lidocaine is used to treat dysrhythmias, and diazepam is used to control seizures. › Inform the client that periodic blood levels are needed. Advise the client to report nausea, diarrhea, or restlessness, which are indicative of toxicity.

Contraindications/Precautions

- Pregnancy Risk Category C
- Use cautiously in clients who have heart disease, hypertension, liver and kidney dysfunction, and diabetes.

- Use cautiously in children and older adults.

Interactions

MEDICATION/FOOD INTERACTIONS	NURSING INTERVENTIONS/CLIENT EDUCATION
› Caffeine increases CNS and cardiac adverse effects of theophylline. › Caffeine can increase theophylline levels.	› Advise clients to avoid consuming caffeinated beverages (coffee, caffeinated colas).
› Phenobarbital, phenytoin, and rifampin decrease theophylline levels.	› When theophylline is used concurrently with these medications, increase the dosage of theophylline.
› Cimetidine (Tagamet), ciprofloxacin (Cipro), and other fluoroquinolone antibiotics increase theophylline levels.	› When theophylline is used concurrently with these medications, decrease the dosage of theophylline.

Nursing Administration

- Advise clients to take the medication as prescribed. If a dose is missed, the following dose should not be doubled.
- Instruct clients not to chew or crush sustained-release preparations. These medications should be swallowed whole.

Nursing Evaluation of Medication Effectiveness

- Depending on therapeutic intent, effectiveness can be evidenced by long-term control of asthma and COPD.

MEDICATION CLASSIFICATION: INHALED ANTICHOLINERGICS

- Select Prototype Medication: ipratropium (Atrovent)
- Other Medications: tiotropium (Spiriva)

Purpose

- Expected Pharmacological Action
  - Block muscarinic receptors of the bronchi, resulting in bronchodilation.
- Therapeutic Uses
  - Relieve bronchospasm associated with COPD. The drug is approved only for COPD, but is used for asthma also.
  - Allergen-induced and exercise-induced asthma.
  - Route of administration: inhalation

Complications

ADVERSE EFFECTS	NURSING INTERVENTIONS/CLIENT EDUCATION
› Local anticholinergic effects (dry mouth, hoarseness)	› Advise clients to sip fluids and suck on hard candies to control dry mouth.

Contraindications/Precautions

- Pregnancy Risk Category B.
- Contraindicated in clients who have an allergy to peanuts because the medication preparations can contain soy lecithin.
- Use cautiously in clients who have narrow-angle glaucoma and benign prostatic hyperplasia (due to anticholinergic effects).

Nursing Administration

- Advise clients to rinse the mouth after inhalation to decrease unpleasant taste.
- Usual adult dosage is two puffs. Instruct clients to wait the length of time directed between puffs.
- If two inhaled medications are prescribed, instruct clients to wait at least 5 min between medications.

Nursing Evaluation of Medication Effectiveness

- Depending on therapeutic intent, effectiveness may be evidenced by:
    - ○ Control of bronchospasm in clients who have COPD.
    - ○ Prevention of allergen- and exercise-induced asthma.

MEDICATION CLASSIFICATION: GLUCOCORTICOIDS

- Select Prototype Medications
    - ○ Inhalation: beclomethasone (QVAR)
    - ○ Oral: prednisone
- Other Medications
    - ○ Inhalation
        - ▪ Budesonide (Pulmicort Flexhaler)
        - ▪ Budesonide and formoterol (Symbicort)
        - ▪ Fluticasone and salmeterol (Advair)
        - ▪ Fluticasone (Flovent)
        - ▪ Mometasone furoate and formoterol fumarate dihydrate (Dulera)
    - ○ Oral: prednisolone (Prelone)
    - ○ IV
        - ▪ Hydrocortisone sodium succinate (Solu-Cortef)
        - ▪ Methylprednisolone sodium succinate (Solu-Medrol)

Purpose

- Expected Pharmacological Action
    - ○ These medications prevent inflammation, suppress airway mucus production, and promote responsiveness of beta$_2$ receptors in the bronchial tree.
    - ○ The use of glucocorticoids does not provide immediate effects, but rather promotes decreased frequency and severity of exacerbations and acute attacks.
- Therapeutic Uses
    - ○ Short-term IV agents are used for status asthmaticus.
    - ○ Inhaled agents are used for long-term prophylaxis of asthma.
    - ○ Short-term oral therapy is used to treat manifestations following an acute asthma episode.
    - ○ Long-term oral therapy is used to treat chronic asthma.
    - ○ Promote lung maturity and decrease respiratory distress in fetuses at risk for preterm birth.

Complications

ADVERSE EFFECTS	NURSING INTERVENTIONS/CLIENT EDUCATION
Beclomethasone	
› Difficulty speaking, hoarseness, and candidiasis	› Advise clients to rinse mouth or gargle with water or salt water after use.
	› Advise clients to monitor for redness, sores, or white patches and to report them to the provider if they occur. Candidiasis may be treated with nystatin oral suspension.
	› In children, glucocorticoids can suppress or slow growth.
Prednisone when used for 10 days or more can result in:	
› Suppression of adrenal gland function, such as a decrease in the ability of the adrenal cortex to produce glucocorticoids, can occur with inhaled agents and oral agents.	› Administer oral glucocorticoid on an alternate-day dosing schedule.
	› Monitor blood glucose levels.
	› Taper the dose. Do not stop abruptly.
› Bone loss (can occur with inhaled agents and oral agents)	› Advise clients to perform weight-bearing exercises.
	› Advise clients to consume a diet with sufficient calcium and vitamin D intake.
	› Use the lowest dose possible to control manifestations.
	› Oral medications should be given on an alternate-day dosing schedule.
› Hyperglycemia and glucosuria	› Clients who have diabetes should have their blood glucose monitored.
	› Clients may need an increase in insulin dosage.
› Myopathy as evidenced by muscle weakness	› Instruct clients to report signs of muscle weakness.
	› Medication dosage should be decreased.
› Peptic ulcer disease	› Advise clients to avoid NSAIDs.
	› Advise clients to report black, tarry stools. Check stool for occult blood periodically.
	› Administer with food or meals.
› Infection	› Advise clients to notify the provider if early signs of infection occur (sore throat, weakness, malaise).
› Disturbances of fluid and electrolytes (fluid retention as evidenced by weight gain, and edema and hypokalemia as evidenced by muscle weakness)	› Instruct clients to observe for symptoms and report to the provider.

Contraindications/Precautions

- Pregnancy Risk Category C.

- Contraindicated in clients who have received a live virus vaccine and those with systemic fungal infections.

- Use cautiously in children, and in clients who have diabetes, hypertension, peptic ulcer disease, or kidney dysfunction.

- Use cautiously in clients taking NSAIDs.

Interactions

MEDICATION/FOOD INTERACTIONS	NURSING INTERVENTIONS/CLIENT EDUCATION
Prednisone	
› Concurrent use of potassium-depleting diuretics increases the risk of hypokalemia.	› Monitor potassium level and administer supplements as needed.
› Concurrent use of NSAIDs increases the risk of GI ulceration.	› Advise clients to avoid use of NSAIDs. Instruct clients to notify the provider if GI distress occurs.
› Concurrent use of glucocorticoids and hypoglycemic agents (oral and insulin) counteract the effects.	› Clients should notify the provider if hyperglycemia occurs. The client may need increased dosage of insulin or oral hypoglycemics.

Nursing Administration

- Instruct clients to use glucocorticoid inhalers on a regular, fixed schedule for long-term therapy of asthma. Glucocorticoids are not to be used to treat an acute episode.

- Administer using an MDI device, DPI, or nebulizer.

- Glucocorticoid MDIs using chlorofluorocarbons (CFCs) as a propellant are being withdrawn from the market. The new devices using HFA no longer require a spacer to increase drug delivery.

- When a client is prescribed an inhaled beta$_2$-agonist and an inhaled glucocorticoid, advise the client to inhale the beta$_2$-agonist before inhaling the glucocorticoid. The beta$_2$-agonist promotes bronchodilation and enhances absorption of the glucocorticoid.

- Oral glucocorticoids are used short-term, 3 to 10 days following an acute asthma exacerbation.

- If client is on long-term oral therapy, additional dosages of oral glucocorticoids are required in times of stress (infection, trauma).

- Clients who discontinue oral glucocorticoid medications or switch from oral to inhaled agents require additional doses of glucocorticoids during periods of stress.

Nursing Evaluation of Medication Effectiveness

- Depending on therapeutic intent, effectiveness may be evidenced by:
  - Long-term control of asthma.
  - Resolution of acute exacerbation as demonstrated by absence of shortness of breath, clear breath sounds, absence of wheezing, and return of respiratory rate to baseline.

MEDICATION CLASSIFICATION: LEUKOTRIENE MODIFIERS

- Select Prototype Medication: montelukast (Singulair)
- Other Medication: zileuton (Zyflo), zafirlukast (Accolate)

Purpose

- Expected Pharmacological Action
  - Leukotriene modifiers prevent the effects of leukotrienes, thereby suppressing inflammation, bronchoconstriction, airway edema, and mucus production.
- Therapeutic Uses
  - Leukotriene modifiers are used for long-term therapy of asthma in adults and children, and to prevent exercise-induced bronchospasm. Current guidelines recommend using these agents as second-line therapy, and as add-on therapy when an inhaled glucocorticoid alone is inadequate.
    - Singulair can be used in children as young as 12 months of age.
    - Accolate can be used in children age 5 years and up.
    - Zyflo can be used in adolescents and adults.
  - Route of administration: oral

Complications

ADVERSE EFFECTS	NURSING INTERVENTIONS/CLIENT EDUCATION
› Liver injury with use of zileuton (Zyflo) and zafirlukast (Accolate)	› Obtain baseline liver function tests and monitor periodically. › Advise clients to monitor for signs of liver damage (nausea, anorexia, abdominal pain). › Instruct clients to notify the provider if symptoms occur.

Contraindications/Precautions

- Singulair and Accolate are Pregnancy Category B. Zyflo is Pregnancy Category C.
- Use cautiously in clients who have liver dysfunction.

Interactions

MEDICATION/FOOD INTERACTIONS	NURSING INTERVENTIONS/CLIENT EDUCATION
› Zileuton and zafirlukast inhibit metabolism of warfarin (Coumadin), leading to increased warfarin levels.	› Advise clients to observe for signs of bleeding and to notify the provider if they occur. › Monitor prothrombin time (PT) and INR levels.
› Zileuton and Zafirlukast inhibit metabolism of theophylline, leading to increased theophylline levels.	› Monitor theophylline levels. › Advise clients to observe for signs of theophylline toxicity (nausea, vomiting, seizures), and to notify the provider.

Nursing Administration

- Advise clients to take zileuton as prescribed. Zileuton can be given with or without food.
- Advise clients to avoid taking zafirlukast with food, and to take it 1 hr before or 2 hr after meals.
- Advise clients to take montelukast once daily at bedtime.

Nursing Evaluation of Medication Effectiveness

- Depending on therapeutic intent, effectiveness can be evidenced by long-term control of asthma.

APPLICATION EXERCISES

1. A nurse is providing instructions to a young adult female client who has a new prescription for beclomethasone (QVAR). Which of the following should the nurse include in the teaching?

    A. "Rinse your mouth after each use."

    B. "Limit fluid intake while taking this medication."

    C. "Increase your intake of vitamin B_{12} while taking this medication."

    D. "You can take the medication as needed."

2. A nurse is providing instructions to a client who has been prescribed albuterol (Proventil) and beclomethasone (QVAR) inhalers for the control of asthma. Which of the following instructions should the nurse include?

    A. Alternate which inhaler is used so that both are not taken the same time of day.

    B. Use the albuterol inhaler prior to using the beclomethasone inhaler.

    C. Only use beclomethasone if experiencing an acute episode.

    D. Use the beclomethasone inhaler first and immediately follow with the albuterol inhaler.

3. A nurse is providing instructions to the parent of an adolescent client who has a new prescription for albuterol (Proventil) PO. Which of the following instructions should the nurse include?

    A. "You can take this medication to abort an acute asthma attack."

    B. "Tremors are an adverse effect of this medication."

    C. "Prolonged use of this medication can cause hyperglycemia."

    D. "This medication can slow skeletal growth rate."

4. A client has a prescription for long-term use of oral prednisone for treatment of chronic asthma. The nurse should instruct the client to watch for which of the following?

    A. Weight gain and fluid retention

    B. Nervousness and insomnia

    C. Chest pain and tachycardia

    D. Dry mouth and constipation

5. A nurse is instructing a client who has a new prescription for albuterol PO. What should the nurse include in the teaching? Use the ATI Active Learning Template: Medication to complete this item to include the following.

    A. Therapeutic Effect

    B. Adverse Effects: List two.

APPLICATION EXERCISES KEY

1. A. **CORRECT:** The client should rinse her mouth after each use to reduce the risk of oral fungal infections.

    B. INCORRECT: A client who has asthma should have a liberal intake of fluids to liquefy secretions, unless contraindicated by another condition.

    C. INCORRECT: Glucoroticoids place the client at risk for bone loss. There is no need for the client to increase her intake of vitamin B_{12}. The client should ensure an adequate intake of calcium and vitamin D.

    D. INCORRECT: Beclomethasone is an inhaled glucocorticoid and should be taken on a fixed schedule.

    Ⓝ NCLEX® Connection: Pharmacological Therapies, Medication Administration

2. A. INCORRECT: This is not the proper use of a combined albuterol beclomethasone regimen.

    B. **CORRECT:** When a client is prescribed an inhaled beta$_2$-agonist, such as albuterol, and an inhaled glucocorticoid, such as beclomethasone, the beta$_2$-agonist should be administered first. The beta$_2$-agonist promotes bronchodilation and enhances absorption of the glucocorticoid.

    C. INCORRECT: Beclomethasone is administered on a fixed schedule. It is not used to treat an acute attack.

    D. INCORRECT: The client should use the albuterol inhaler first.

    Ⓝ NCLEX® Connection: Pharmacological Therapies, Medication Administration

3. A. INCORRECT: Inhaled albuterol is used to abort an acute asthma episode.

    B. **CORRECT:** Tremors can occur due to excessive stimulation of beta$_2$ receptors of skeletal muscles.

    C. INCORRECT: Prolonged use of glucocorticoids can cause hyperglycemia.

    D. INCORRECT: Glucocorticoids slow skeletal growth rate in children and adolescents. However, height when the child reaches adulthood is not reduced.

    Ⓝ NCLEX® Connection: Pharmacological Therapies, Adverse Effects/Contraindications/ Side Effects/Interactions

4. A. **CORRECT:** Weight gain and fluid retention are adverse effects of oral prednisone due to the effect of sodium and water retention.

    B. INCORRECT: Nervousness and insomnia are adverse effects of beta agonists, not glucocorticoids.

    C. INCORRECT: Angina and tachycardia are adverse effects of beta agonists.

    D. INCORRECT: Dry mouth and constipation are adverse effects of tiotropium (Spiriva).

    Ⓝ NCLEX® Connection: Pharmacological Therapies, Adverse Effects/Contraindications/ Side Effects/Interactions

5. *Using the ATI Active Learning Template: Medication*

    A. Therapeutic Effect

    - Beta$_2$-adrenergic agonists act by selectively activating the beta$_2$-receptors in the bronchial smooth muscle, resulting in bronchodilation. They also suppress histamine release and promote ciliary motility.

    B. Adverse Effects

    - Oral agents can cause tachycardia and angina due to activation of alpha$_1$ receptors in the heart.
    - Activation of beta$_2$ receptors in skeletal muscle causes tremors.

    Ⓝ NCLEX® Connection: Pharmacological Therapies, Expected Actions/Outcomes

chapter 17

Overview

- The medications in this section work on the CNS, nasal passages, or other parts of the respiratory system to treat the effects of allergic or nonallergic rhinitis or coughs from the common cold, influenza, and other disorders.
  - Antihistamines, often prescribed for allergic rhinitis, also may be used to treat nausea, motion sickness, allergic reactions, and insomnia.
- This section includes opioid and nonopioid antitussives, nasal glucocorticoids to treat allergic rhinitis, expectorants, mucolytics, decongestants, and antihistamine medications.
- Medications in this section frequently are combined for increased effectiveness. For example, an antitussive may be combined with an expectorant to better control a cough.

MEDICATION CLASSIFICATION: ANTITUSSIVES – OPIOIDS

- Select Prototype Medication: codeine
- Other Medication: hydrocodone

Purpose

- Expected Pharmacological Action
  - Codeine suppresses cough through its action on the central nervous system.
- Therapeutic Uses
  - Codeine is used for chronic nonproductive cough.

Complications

ADVERSE EFFECTS	NURSING INTERVENTIONS/CLIENT EDUCATION
› CNS effects (dizziness, lightheadedness, drowsiness, respiratory depression)	› Obtain baseline vital signs. › Monitor clients when ambulating. › Advise clients to lie down if feeling lightheaded. › Observe for manifestations of respiratory depression, such as respiratory rate less than 12/min. Stimulate the client to breathe if respiratory depression occurs. It can be necessary to stop the medication and administer naloxone. › Advise clients to avoid driving while taking codeine.
› GI distress (nausea, vomiting, constipation)	› Instruct clients to take oral codeine with food. › Advise clients to increase fluids and dietary fiber.
› Potential for abuse	› Advise clients of the potential for abuse. › Use for short duration.

Contraindications/Precautions

- Codeine is a Pregnancy Category Risk C medication.
- This medication is contraindicated in clients who have acute asthma, head trauma, liver and kidney dysfunction, and acute alcohol use disorder.

- Use cautiously in children, older adults, and clients who have a history of substance use disorder.

Nursing Interventions

- Advise clients to avoid hazardous activities, such as driving while taking codeine.
- Advise clients to change positions slowly and to lie down if feeling dizzy.
- Advise clients to avoid alcohol and other CNS depressants while taking codeine.

MEDICATION CLASSIFICATION: ANTITUSSIVES – NONOPIOIDS

- Select Prototype Medication: dextromethorphan (found in many different products for cough, such as Robitussin)
- Other Medications: benzonatate (Tessalon), diphenhydramine

Purpose

- Expected Pharmacological Action
  - Dextromethorphan suppresses cough through its action on the CNS. Although not an opioid, it is derived from opioids.
- Therapeutic Use
  - Cough suppression

Complications

- This medication has few adverse effects.
- Some mild nausea, dizziness, and sedation can occur.
- Can cause euphoria when taken in high doses. This medication can be abused for this effect.

Contraindications/Precautions

- Pregnancy Category Risk C

Interactions

- Can cause high fever when used within 2 weeks of MAOI antidepressants

Nursing Interventions

- Some formulations can contain alcohol or sucrose.
- Available forms include capsules, lozenges (for clients older than 12 years), liquids, and syrups.

Nursing Evaluation of Medication Effectiveness

- Depending on therapeutic intent, effectiveness can be evidenced by absence or decreased episodes of coughing.

MEDICATION CLASSIFICATION: EXPECTORANTS

- Select Prototype Medication: guaifenesin (Mucinex)

Purpose

- Expected Pharmacological Action
  - Guaifenesin promotes increased cough production through increasing mucous secretion. These actions allow clients to decrease chest congestion by coughing out secretions.
- Therapeutic Uses
  - Although guaifenesin is available as an expectorant alone, it most often is combined with antitussives (either opioid or nonopioid), or a decongestant for treating symptoms of colds, allergic or nonallergic rhinitis, or for cough caused by lower respiratory disorders.

Complications

ADVERSE EFFECTS	NURSING INTERVENTIONS/CLIENT EDUCATION
› GI upset	› Take with food if GI upset occurs.
› Drowsiness, dizziness	› Do not take prior to driving or activities if these reactions occur.
› Allergic reaction (rash)	› Stop taking guaifenesin and obtain medical care if rash or other manifestations of allergy occur.

Contraindications/Precautions

- Guaifenesin is a Pregnancy Risk Category C medication.
- Advise clients who are breastfeeding to talk to the provider before taking medications containing guaifenesin.
- Depending on the formulation and medication combinations, preparations containing guaifenesin may not be recommended for children.

Nursing Interventions

- Advise clients to increase fluid intake when taking guaifenesin, in order to promote liquefying secretions.
- This medication is available in tablets (which should not be crushed) and capsules (which may be opened to sprinkle on foods).
- Advise clients to read over-the-counter labels carefully to discover what medications have been combined in the preparation used. Guaifenesin frequently is combined with other medications (antitussives, decongestants) as a liquid or syrup (for example, Mucinex D combines guaifenesin with the sympathomimetic decongestant, pseudoephedrine).
- Any cough lasting longer than 1 week should be reported to the provider.

Nursing Evaluation of Medication Effectiveness

- Depending on therapeutic intent, effectiveness can be evidenced by the following.
  - Cough is more productive, and mucous is easier to expectorate.
  - Chest congestion is decreased.

MEDICATION CLASSIFICATION: MUCOLYTICS

- Select Prototype Medication: acetylcysteine (Mucomyst, Acetadote)
- Other Medication: hypertonic saline

Purpose

- Expected Pharmacological Action
  - Mucolytics enhance the flow of secretions in the respiratory passages. They react directly with mucus to make it more watery.
- Therapeutic uses
  - Mucolytics are used in clients who have acute and chronic pulmonary disorders exacerbated by large amounts of secretions.
  - Mucolytics are used in clients who have cystic fibrosis.
  - Acetylcysteine is the antidote for acetaminophen poisoning.

Complications

ADVERSE EFFECTS	NURSING INTERVENTIONS/CLIENT EDUCATION
› Aspiration and bronchospasm when administered orally	› Monitor clients for manifestations of aspiration and bronchospasm. Stop medication immediately and notify the provider.

Contraindications/Precautions

- Acetylcysteine is a Pregnancy Risk Category B medication.
- This medication should not be used in clients at risk for GI hemorrhage.
- Use cautiously in clients who have peptic ulcer disease, esophageal varices, and severe liver disease.
- Due to the potential for bronchospasm, acetylcysteine should be used cautiously in clients who have asthma.

Nursing Administration

- Advise clients that acetylcysteine has an odor like rotten eggs.
- Acetylcysteine is administered by inhalation to liquefy nasal and bronchial secretions and facilitate coughing.
- The medication is administered orally or IV for acetaminophen overdose.
- Be prepared to suction clients if aspiration occurs with oral administration.

Nursing Evaluation of Medication Effectiveness

- Depending on therapeutic intent, effectiveness can be evidenced by improvement of manifestations as demonstrated by regular respiratory rate, clear lung sounds, and increased ease of expectoration

---

MEDICATION CLASSIFICATION: DECONGESTANTS

- Select Prototype Medication: phenylephrine (Neo-Synephrine)
- Other Medications
  - Ephedrine
  - Naphazoline (Privine)
  - Pseudoephedrine (Sudafed)

Purpose

- Expected Pharmacological Action
  - Sympathomimetic decongestants stimulate alpha$_1$-adrenergic receptors on nasal blood vessels, causing vasoconstriction and reduction in the inflammation of the nasal membranes.
- Therapeutic Uses
  - Treat allergic or nonallergic rhinitis by relieving nasal stuffiness
  - Decongestant for clients who have sinusitis and the common cold

Complications

ADVERSE EFFECTS	NURSING INTERVENTIONS/CLIENT EDUCATION
› Rebound congestion secondary to prolonged use of topical agents	› Advise clients to use for short-term therapy, no more than 3 to 5 days. › Taper use and discontinue medication using one nostril at a time.
› CNS stimulation (agitation, nervousness, uneasiness)	› CNS stimulation is rare with the use of topical agents. › Advise clients to observe for manifestations of CNS stimulation, and to notify the provider if they occur. › Stop medication.
› Vasoconstriction	› Advise clients who have hypertension and coronary artery disease to avoid using these medications.

Contraindications/Precautions

- These medications are contraindicated in clients who have chronic rhinitis.
- Use cautiously in clients who have coronary artery disease and hypertension.

Nursing Administration

- When administering nasal drops, instruct clients to be in the lateral, head-low position to increase the desired effect and to prevent swallowing the medication.
- Drops are preferred for children because they can be administered precisely and toxicity can be prevented.
- When nasal spray preparations are prescribed, teach clients their proper use.
- Instruct clients in the differences between topical and oral agents.
  - Topical agents are usually more effective and work faster.
  - Topical agents have a shorter duration.
  - Vasoconstriction and CNS stimulation are uncommon with topical agents, but are a concern with oral agents.
  - Oral agents do not lead to rebound congestion.
- Advise clients to use topical decongestants for no longer than 3 to 5 days to avoid rebound congestion.
- Instruct clients not to exceed recommended doses.

Nursing Evaluation of Medication Effectiveness

- Depending on therapeutic intent, effectiveness can be evidenced by improvement of manifestations (relief of congestion, increased ease of breathing, ability to sleep comfortably).

MEDICATION CLASSIFICATION: ANTIHISTAMINES

- Select Prototype Medications
  - 1st generation H_1 antagonists
    - Diphenhydramine
    - Chlorpheniramine (Chlor-Trimeton)
  - 2nd generation H_1 antagonists
    - Loratadine (Claritin)
    - Cetirizine (Zyrtec)
    - Fexofenadine (Allegra)
    - Desloratadine (Clarinex)
  - Intranasal antihistamines
    - Azelastine (Astelin, Astepro)
    - Olopatadine (Patanase)

Purpose

- Expected Pharmacological Action
  - Antihistamine action is on the H_1 receptors, which results in the blocking of histamine release in the small blood vessels, capillaries, and nerves during allergic reactions. When used for upper respiratory infections, antihistamines relieve manifestations by suppressing mucous secretion because of their anticholinergic effect.
- Therapeutic Uses
  - Mild allergic reactions (seasonal allergic rhinitis, urticaria, mild transfusion reaction)
  - Anaphylaxis (hypotension, acute laryngeal edema, bronchospasm)
  - Motion sickness
  - Insomnia
  - Often used in combination with sympathomimetics to provide a nasal decongestive effect

Complications

ADVERSE EFFECTS	NURSING INTERVENTIONS/CLIENT EDUCATION
› Sedation (common with 1st generation H_1 antagonists)	› Advise clients to take the medication at night to minimize daytime sedative effect.
	› Avoid driving, hazardous activities, consumption of alcohol, and other CNS depressant medications (barbiturates, benzodiazepines, opioids).
› Anticholinergic effects (dry mouth, constipation) – more common with 1st generation agents	› Advise clients to take sips of water, suck on sugarless candies, and maintain 2 to 3 L of water each day from food and beverage sources.

ADVERSE EFFECTS	NURSING INTERVENTIONS/CLIENT EDUCATION
› Gastrointestinal discomfort (nausea, vomiting, constipation)	› Advise clients to take antihistamine with meals.
› Acute toxicity (flushed face, high fever, tachycardia, dry mouth, urinary retention, pupil dilation) › Excitation, hallucinations, incoordination, and seizures in children	› Advise clients to notify the provider if effects occur. › Induce vomiting to remove the antihistamine. › Administer activated charcoal and cathartic to decrease absorption of antihistamine. › Administer acetaminophen for fever. › Apply ice packs or sponge baths.

Contraindications/Precautions

- Antihistamines are contraindicated during the third trimester of pregnancy, for mothers who are breastfeeding, and for newborns. Newborns are sensitive to the adverse effects, such as sedation, of these medications.
- Promethazine is a Pregnancy Category C medication. It is contraindicated in clients who have cardiac dysrhythmias and hepatic diseases, and those on MAOI therapy.
- Use cautiously in children and older adults (adverse effects, especially respiratory depression).
- Use cautiously in clients who have asthma, urinary retention, open-angle glaucoma, hypertension, and prostate hypertrophy (effect of anticholinergic medications).

Interactions

MEDICATION/FOOD INTERACTIONS	NURSING INTERVENTIONS/CLIENT EDUCATION
› CNS depressants, including alcohol, cause additive CNS depression.	› Advise clients to avoid alcohol and medications causing CNS depression (opioids, barbiturates, and benzodiazepines).

Nursing Interventions

- Advise clients taking 1st generation medications to be aware of sedating effects.

Nursing Evaluation of Medication Effectiveness

- Depending on therapeutic intent, effectiveness can be evidenced by:
  - Improvement of allergic reaction (absence of rhinitis, urticaria).
  - Relief of manifestations of motion sickness (decreased nausea and vomiting).

MEDICATION CLASSIFICATION: NASAL GLUCOCORTICOIDS

- Select Prototype Medication: mometasone (Nasonex)
- Other Medications
  - Fluticasone (Veramyst)
  - Budesonide (Rhinocort Aqua)

Purpose

- Expected Pharmacological Action
  - Nasal glucocorticoids decrease inflammation associated with allergic rhinitis. They are the first line of treatment for nasal congestion.
- Therapeutic Use
  - Reduce the effects of allergic rhinitis, including congestion, erythema, sneezing, nasal itching, runny nose.

Complications

- Adverse Effects
  - Sore throat, nosebleed, headache, burning in the nose
- Nursing Intervention and Client Education
  - Contact the provider if adverse effects occur.

Contraindications/Precautions

- Pregnancy Risk Category C.
- Nursing Interventions
  - Full doses are given initially. Dose is tapered to minimal effective dose once symptoms are under control.
  - Advise the client that a metered-dose spray devise is used to administer the medication.
  - Advise the client to administer dose daily, not just when manifestations occur.
  - Advise clients who have seasonal allergic rhinitis that it can take 7 days or more to get the maximum relief.
  - Advise clients who have perennial allergic rhinitis that it can take as long as 21 days to get the maximum relief.

APPLICATION EXERCISES

1. A nurse is caring for a client who states she has been taking phenylephrine (Neo-Synephrine) nasal drops for the past 10 days for her upper respiratory symptoms. For which of the following adverse effects should the nurse monitor?

    A. Sedation

    B. Nasal congestion

    C. Productive cough

    D. Constipation

2. A nurse is reinforcing teaching with a client to self-administer nasal drops for allergic rhinitis manifestations. The nurse should instruct the client to lie in which of the following positions to obtain the best effect of the medication?

    A. Supine with head flexed

    B. Sitting with head in neutral position

    C. Lateral with head in low position

    D. Prone with head extended

3. A nurse is caring for a preschool child who has a new diagnosis of cystic fibrosis and a new prescription for acetylcysteine (Mucomyst). The nurse should instruct the client and her family that the purpose of this medication is to do which of the following?

    A. Suppress cough

    B. Decrease pain

    C. Minimize nasal congestion

    D. Loosen secretions

4. An adult client is taking diphenhydramine for manifestations of allergic rhinitis. For which of the following adverse reactions should the nurse instruct the client to watch? (Select all that apply.)

    _____ A. Dry mouth

    _____ B. Nonproductive cough

    _____ C. Skin rash

    _____ D. Diarrhea

    _____ E. Urinary hesitation

5. A nurse is evaluating a client's understanding of the instructions about the use of fluticasone (Flonase) to treat perennial rhinitis. Which of the following statements by the client indicate he understands the instructions?

    A. "I should use the spray every 4 hours while I am awake."

    B. "It may take as long as 3 weeks before the medication takes a maximum effect."

    C. "This medication can also be used to treat motion sickness."

    D. "I can use this medication when my nasal passages are blocked."

6. A nurse in a provider's office is reinforcing teaching with a client who has a new prescription for guaifenesin (Mucinex). Use the ATI Active Learning Template: Medication to complete this item to include the following:

    A. Adverse Effects: Identify two adverse effects of this medication.

    B. Medication Effectiveness: Identify two findings that indicate that the medication is effective.

APPLICATION EXERCISES KEY

1. A. INCORRECT: Insomnia, rather than sedation, is a possible adverse effect of this medication.

    B. **CORRECT:** When used for more than 5 days, rebound nasal congestion can occur when taking topical sympathomimetic medications, such as phenylephrine.

    C. INCORRECT: A productive cough is not an expected adverse effect.

    D. INCORRECT: Constipation, an anticholinergic adverse effect, is not caused by sympathomimetic medications such as phenylephrine.

    Ⓝ NCLEX® Connection: Pharmacological Therapies, Adverse Effects/Contraindications/ Side Effects/Interactions

2. A. INCORRECT: Supine with the head flexed does not allow the medication to best spread to affected areas.

    B. INCORRECT: Sitting with the head in a neutral position does not allow the medication to best spread to affected areas.

    C. **CORRECT:** Lying on the side with the head in a low position helps spread the nasal drops, allows the medication to be more effective, and prevents swallowing the medication.

    D. INCORRECT: Prone with head extended does not allow the medication to best spread to affected areas.

    Ⓝ NCLEX® Connection: Pharmacological Therapies, Medication Administration

3. A. INCORRECT: Acetylcysteine does not suppress cough.

    B. INCORRECT: Acetylcysteine does not decrease pain.

    C. INCORRECT: Acetylcysteine does not minimize nasal congestion.

    D. **CORRECT:** Acetylcysteine, when administered by inhalation, is a mucolytic medication that liquefies secretions and allows them to be expectorated more easily.

    Ⓝ NCLEX® Connection: Pharmacological Therapies, Expected Actions/Outcomes

4. A. **CORRECT:** Dry mouth is an anticholinergic effect that can occur when a client takes diphenhydramine.

    B. INCORRECT: Cough is not an expected adverse reaction to this medication. Diphenhydramine is sometimes prescribed to treat nonproductive cough.

    C. INCORRECT: Skin rash is not an expected adverse reaction to this medication. Diphenhydramine sometimes is prescribed for skin rash caused by allergies.

    D. INCORRECT: Constipation, rather than diarrhea, is an adverse reaction of this medication.

    E. **CORRECT:** Urinary hesitation is an anticholinergic effect that can occur when a client takes diphenhydramine.

    (N) NCLEX® Connection: Pharmacological Therapies, Medication Administration

5. A. INCORRECT: The client should use the medication once a day.

    B. **CORRECT:** The client might see some benefits of the medication within a few hours, but the maximum benefits might not be seen for as long as 3 weeks.

    C. INCORRECT: Diphenhydramine can be used to treat motion sickness, but this medication is not used for that purpose.

    D. INCORRECT: The client should blow his nose to clear the nasal passages prior to use of the medication.

    (N) NCLEX® Connection: Pharmacological Therapies, Medication Administration

6. Using the ATI Active Learning Template: Medication

    A. Adverse Effects
    - GI upset
    - Drowsiness
    - Dizziness
    - Rash

    B. Medication Effectiveness
    - Cough is more productive, and mucous is easier to expectorate.
    - Chest congestion is decreased.

    (N) NCLEX® Connection: Pharmacological Therapies, Adverse Effects/Contraindications/ Side Effects/Interactions

UNIT 4 ## Medications Affecting the Cardiovascular System

CHAPTERS

› Medications Affecting Urinary Output
› Medications Affecting Blood Pressure
› Cardiac Glycosides and Heart Failure
› Angina and Antilipemic Agents

chapter 18

Overview

- Indications for medications that affect urinary output include management of blood pressure; excretion of edematous fluid related to heart failure and kidney and liver disease; and prevention of kidney failure.
- Medications include high-ceiling loop diuretics, thiazide diuretics, potassium-sparing diuretics, and osmotic diuretics.

MEDICATION CLASSIFICATION: HIGH-CEILING LOOP DIURETICS

- Select Prototype Medication: furosemide (Lasix)
- Other Medications
  - Ethacrynic acid (Edecrin)
  - Bumetanide (Bumex)
  - Torsemide (Demadex)

Purpose

- Expected Pharmacological Action
  - High-ceiling loop diuretics work in the ascending limb of loop of Henle.
    - Blocks reabsorption of sodium and chloride and to prevent reabsorption of water
    - Causes extensive diuresis even with severe renal impairment
- Therapeutic Uses
  - High-ceiling loop diuretics are used when there is an emergent need for rapid mobilization of fluid.
    - Pulmonary edema caused by heart failure
    - Conditions not responsive to other diuretics, such as edema caused by liver, cardiac, or kidney disease; or hypertension
    - Can promote diuresis in patients who have severe renal impairment
  - These medications may be used to treat hypercalcemia related to kidney stone formation.
- Route of administration: oral, IV, IM

Complications

ADVERSE EFFECTS	NURSING INTERVENTIONS/CLIENT EDUCATION
› Dehydration, hyponatremia, hypochloremia	› Monitor for manifestations of dehydration: dry mouth, increased thirst, minimal urine output, and weight loss. › Monitor electrolytes. › Report urine output less than 30 mL/hr. Stop medication and notify the provider. › If signs of headache or chest, calf, or pelvic pain occur, notify the provider. This can be an indication of thrombosis or embolism. › Minimize the risk for dehydration by starting clients on low doses and monitoring daily weights.
› Hypotension	› Monitor blood pressure. › Instruct clients about signs of postural hypotension (lightheadedness, dizziness). If these occur, advise clients to sit or lie down. › Advise clients to avoid sudden changes of position and arise slowly from lying down or sitting.
› Ototoxicity (transient with furosemide and irreversible with ethacrynic acid)	› Advise clients to notify the provider of tinnitus, which can indicate ototoxicity. › Avoid use with other ototoxic medications, such as gentamicin.
› Hypokalemia (K^+ less than 3.5 mEq/L)	› Monitor cardiac status and potassium levels. › Report a decrease in potassium level (K^+ less than 3.5 mEq/L). › Instruct clients to consume high-potassium foods (e.g., bananas, potatoes, dried fruits, nuts, spinach, and citrus fruit). › Instruct clients about manifestations of hypokalemia, such as nausea, vomiting, and general weakness.
› Other adverse effects (hyperglycemia, hyperuricemia, decrease in calcium and magnesium levels)	› Monitor blood glucose, uric acid, and calcium and magnesium levels. › Report elevated levels.

Contraindications/Precautions

- Avoid using these medications during pregnancy unless absolutely required.
- Use cautiously in clients who have diabetes mellitus or gout.

Interactions

MEDICATION/FOOD INTERACTIONS	NURSING INTERVENTIONS/CLIENT EDUCATION
› Digoxin (Lanoxin) toxicity (ventricular dysrhythmias) can occur in the presence of hypokalemia.	› Monitor the client's cardiac status and potassium and digoxin levels. › Potassium-sparing diuretics often are used in conjunction with loop diuretics to reduce the risk of hypokalemia. › Administer potassium supplements as prescribed by the provider.
› Concurrent use of antihypertensives can have additive hypotensive effect.	› Monitor blood pressure.
› Lithium carbonate (Lithobid) serum levels can increase, which can lead to toxicity, if hyponatremia occurs due to the loop diuretic.	› Monitor lithium levels. Dosage may need to be adjusted.
› NSAIDs decrease blood flow to the kidneys, which reduces the diuretic effect.	› Watch for a decrease in the effectiveness of the diuretic, such as a decrease in urine output.

Nursing Considerations

- Obtain baseline data, including orthostatic blood pressure, weight, electrolytes, and location and extent of edema.

- Weigh the client at the same time each day with same amount of clothing and bed linen (if using a bed scale), usually upon awakening.

- Monitor blood pressure and I&O.

- Avoid administering the medication late in the day to prevent nocturia. Usual dosing time is 0800 and 1400.

- Administer furosemide orally, IV bolus dose, or continuous IV infusion. Infuse IV doses at 20 mg/min or slower to avoid abrupt hypotension and hypovolemia.

- If potassium level drops below 3.5 mEq/L, monitor the potassium level and notify the provider because the client may need to be placed on a potassium supplement.

- If the medication is used for hypertension, instruct clients to self-monitor blood pressure and weight by keeping a log.

- Advise clients to get up slowly to minimize postural hypotension and check orthostatic blood pressure to assess for hypovolemia. If faintness or dizziness occurs, instruct clients to sit or lie down.

- Instruct clients to report significant weight loss, lightheadedness, dizziness, GI distress, or general weakness to the provider, which can indicate hypokalemia or hypovolemia.

- Encourage clients to consume foods high in potassium.

- Instruct clients who have diabetes mellitus to monitor for elevated blood glucose levels.

- Instruct clients to observe for manifestations of low magnesium levels (e.g., weakness, muscle twitching, and tremors).

Nursing Evaluation of Medication Effectiveness

- Depending on therapeutic intent, effectiveness can be evidenced by the following.
  - Decrease in pulmonary or peripheral edema
  - Weight loss
  - Decrease in blood pressure
  - Increase in urine output

MEDICATION CLASSIFICATION: THIAZIDE DIURETICS

- Select Prototype Medication: hydrochlorothiazide (Microzide)
- Other Medications
  - Chlorothiazide (Diuril)
  - Methyclothiazide (Enduron)
  - Thiazide-type diuretics
    - Indapamide (Lozide, Lozol)
    - Chlorthalidone (Hygroton)
    - Metolazone (Zaroxolyn)

Purpose

- Expected Pharmacological Action
  - Thiazide diuretics work in the early distal convoluted tubule.
    - Blocks the reabsorption of sodium and chloride, and prevents the reabsorption of water at this site
    - Promotes diuresis when renal function is not impaired
- Therapeutic Uses
  - Thiazide diuretics are often the medication of first choice for essential hypertension.
  - These medications may be used for edema of mild-to-moderate heart failure and liver and kidney disease.
  - Thiazide diuretics often are used in combination with antihypertensive agents for blood pressure control.

Complications

ADVERSE EFFECTS	NURSING INTERVENTIONS/CLIENT EDUCATION
› Dehydration	› Monitor for manifestations of dehydration (dry mouth, increased thirst, minimal urine output, weight loss). › Monitor electrolytes and weight. › Report urine output less than 30 mL/hr. Stop medication and notify the provider.
› Hypokalemia (K⁺ less than 3.5 mEq/L)	› Monitor cardiac status and K⁺ levels, especially if taking digoxin. › Report a decrease in K⁺ level (less than 3.5 mEq/L). › Instruct clients to consume foods high in potassium. › Instruct clients to recognize manifestations of hypokalemia (nausea, vomiting, general weakness).
› Hyperglycemia	› Monitor for an increase in blood glucose levels.

Contraindications/Precautions

- Avoid administering thiazide diuretics during pregnancy because the medication decreases maternal blood volume and decreases placental perfusion, causing a compromise in the nutrients supplied to the fetus.

- If a thiazide diuretic is indicated during lactation, advise clients not to breastfeed because the diuretic enters the milk and is harmful to the infant.

Interactions

- Medication and food interactions are the same as for loop diuretic medications.

- Thiazide diuretics cause no risk of hearing loss and can be combined with ototoxic medications.

- NSAIDs can interfere with the diuretic effects of thiazides.

Nursing Considerations

- Chlorothiazide may be administered orally and IV. All others only can be given orally.

- Obtain baseline data, including orthostatic blood pressure, weight, electrolytes, and location and extent of edema.

- Monitor potassium levels.

- Instruct clients to take the medication first thing in the morning. If twice-a-day dosing is prescribed, be sure the second dose is taken by 1400 to prevent nocturia.

- Encourage clients to consume foods high in potassium and maintain adequate fluid intake (1,500 mL/day, unless contraindicated).

- If GI upset occurs, clients should take the medication with or after meals.

- Alternate-day dosing can decrease electrolyte imbalances.

Nursing Evaluation of Medication Effectiveness

- Depending on therapeutic intent, effectiveness may be evidenced by the following.

  - Decrease in blood pressure

  - Decrease in edema

  - Increase in urine output

MEDICATION CLASSIFICATION: POTASSIUM-SPARING DIURETICS

- Select Prototype Medication: spironolactone (Aldactone)
- Other Medications: triamterene (Dyrenium), amiloride (Midamor)

Purpose

- Expected Pharmacological Action

  - Potassium-sparing diuretics block the action of aldosterone (sodium and water retention), which results in potassium retention and the secretion of sodium and water.

- Therapeutic Uses

  - Potassium-sparing diuretics are combined with other diuretics (loop and thiazide diuretics) for potassium-sparing effects.

  - Potassium-sparing diuretics are administered for heart failure.

  - Potassium-sparing diuretics block actions of aldosterone in primary hyperaldosteronism by retaining potassium and increasing sodium excretion, causing an opposite effect of the action of aldosterone in the distal nephrons.

  - Therapeutic effects can take 12 to 48 hr.

- Route of administration: oral

Complications

ADVERSE EFFECTS	NURSING INTERVENTIONS/CLIENT EDUCATION
› Hyperkalemia (K⁺ greater than 5.0 mEq/L)	› Monitor potassium level. Initiate cardiac monitoring for serum potassium greater than 5 mEq/L.
	› Treat hyperkalemia by discontinuing medication, restricting potassium in the diet, and administering insulin injections to drive potassium back into the cell.
	› Potassium supplements or other potassium-sparing diuretics should never be administered in conjunction with spironolactone.
	› Caution is recommended when administered with ACE inhibitors, angiotensin receptor blockers, and direct renin inhibitors because these can cause elevated potassium levels.
› Endocrine effects (impotence in male clients; irregularities of menstrual cycle in female clients)	› Advise clients to observe for side effects.
	› Clients should notify the provider if these responses occur.

Contraindications/Precautions

- Do not administer to clients who have hyperkalemia.
- Do not administer to clients who have severe kidney failure and anuria.

Interactions

MEDICATION/FOOD INTERACTIONS	NURSING INTERVENTIONS/CLIENT EDUCATION
› Concurrent use of ACE inhibitors increases the risk of hyperkalemia.	› Monitor the client's K^+ levels. Notify the provider if K^+ is greater than 5.0 mEq/L.
› Concurrent use of potassium supplements increases the risk of hyperkalemia.	› Clients should not take this medication and a potassium supplement or salt substitute concurrently.

Nursing Considerations

- Obtain baseline data.
- Monitor potassium levels regularly.
- Instruct clients to avoid salt substitutes that contain potassium.
- Instruct clients to self-monitor blood pressure.
- Instruct clients to keep a log of blood pressure and weight.
- Warn clients that triamterene can turn urine a bluish color.

Nursing Evaluation of Medication Effectiveness

- Depending on therapeutic intent, effectiveness may be evidenced by the following.
  - Maintenance of normal potassium levels: between 3.5 mEq/L and 5.0 mEq/L
  - Weight loss
  - Decrease in blood pressure and edema

MEDICATION CLASSIFICATION: OSMOTIC DIURETICS

- Select Prototype Medication: mannitol (Osmitrol)

Purpose

- Expected Pharmacological Action
  - ○ Osmotic diuretics reduce intracranial pressure and intraocular pressure by raising serum osmolality and drawing fluid back into the vascular and extravascular space.
- Therapeutic Uses
  - ○ Osmotic diuretics prevent kidney failure in specific situations, such as hypovolemic shock and severe hypotension, because mannitol is not reabsorbed and remains in the nephron, drawing off water, thus preserving urine flow and preventing kidney failure.
  - ○ Decreases intracranial pressure (ICP) caused by cerebral edema by drawing off fluid from the brain into the bloodstream.
  - ○ Decreases intraocular pressure (IOP) by creating an osmotic force that draws ocular fluid into the bloodstream.
  - ○ Osmotic diuretics promote sodium retention and water excretion in clients who have hyponatremia and fluid volume excess.
  - ○ Administered for the oliguria phase of acute kidney injury.

Complications

ADVERSE EFFECTS	NURSING INTERVENTIONS/CLIENT EDUCATION
› Heart failure, pulmonary edema	› If indications of heart failure develop (dyspnea, weakness, fatigue, distended neck veins, or weight gain), stop the medication immediately and notify the provider.
› Kidney failure	› If indications of kidney failure develop (urine output less than 30 mL/hr, increased serum creatinine [greater than 1.2 mg/dL] and BUN [greater than 20 mg/dL]), stop the medication immediately and notify the provider.
› Fluid and electrolyte imbalances	› Monitor laboratory values.

Contraindications/Precautions

- Use extreme caution in clients who have heart failure because it can precipitate CHF and pulmonary edema.

Interactions

- Lithium excretion through the kidneys is increased. (Monitor lithium levels.)

Nursing Considerations

- Administer mannitol by continuous IV infusion.
- To prevent administering microscopic crystals, use a filter needle when drawing from the vial and a filter in the IV tubing.
- Monitor daily weight, I&O, and serum electrolytes.
- Monitor for signs of dehydration, acute kidney injury, and edema.

Nursing Evaluation of Medication Effectiveness

- Depending on therapeutic intent, effectiveness can be evidenced by:
  - Normal kidney function as demonstrated by:
    - Urine output of at least 30 mL/hr.
    - Serum creatinine between 0.6 to 1.2 mg/dL for men and 0.5 to 1.1 mg/dL for women.
    - BUN levels between 10 to 20 mg/dL.
  - Decrease in intracranial pressure.
  - Decrease in intraocular pressure.

APPLICATION EXERCISES

1. A nurse is contributing to the plan of care for a client who is receiving furosemide (Lasix) IV for peripheral edema. Which of the following should the nurse include in the plan? (Select all that apply.)

_____ A. Check for tinnitus.

_____ B. Report urine output of 50 mL/hr.

_____ C. Monitor serum potassium levels.

_____ D. Elevate the head of bed slowly before ambulation.

_____ E. Recommend eating a banana daily.

2. A nurse is reinforcing teaching with a client who has a new prescription for hydrochlorothiazide (Microzide). Which of the following information should the nurse include?

A. Take the medication with food.

B. Plan to take the medication at bedtime.

C. Expect increased swelling of the ankles.

D. Fluid intake should be limited in the morning.

3. A nurse is monitoring a client who is receiving spironolactone (Aldactone). Which of the following findings should the nurse report to the provider?

A. Serum sodium 148 mEq/L

B. Urine output of 120 mL in 4 hr

C. Serum potassium 5.2 mEq/L

D. Blood pressure 140/90 mm Hg

4. A nurse is monitoring a client who has increased intracranial pressure and is receiving mannitol (Osmitrol). Which of the following findings should the nurse report to the provider?

A. Blood glucose 150 mg/dL

B. Urine output 40 mL/hr

C. Dyspnea

D. Headache

5. A nurse is reviewing a client's medication history and notes that the client is taking digoxin (Lanoxin), an antihypertensive medication, and NSAIDs. The client has a new prescription for torsemide (Demadex). The nurse should plan to monitor for which of the following medication interactions? (Select all that apply.)

_____ A. Decrease in serum digoxin level

_____ B. Hypokalemia

_____ C. Hypotension

_____ D. Low urine output

_____ E. Ventricular dysrhythmias

6. A nurse is reviewing nursing considerations related to loop diuretics with a group of nurses. What are appropriate nursing interventions? Use the ATI Active Learning Template: Medication to complete this item to include the following:

A. Therapeutic Uses: Identify two.

B. Adverse Effects: Describe three.

C. Nursing Interventions/Client Education: Describe two interventions for each of the three adverse effects.

APPLICATION EXERCISES KEY

1. A. **CORRECT:** An adverse effect of furosemide is ototoxicity. Manifestations of tinnitus should be reported to the provider.

    B. INCORRECT: A urine output of 50 mL/hr is within the expected reference range.

    C. **CORRECT:** A decrease in serum potassium levels is an adverse effect of furosemide, and the provider should be notified.

    D. **CORRECT:** Slowly elevating the head of the bed will prevent the client from developing orthostatic hypotension, which is a sign of hypovolemia.

    E. **CORRECT:** A banana is high in potassium. The nurse should encourage the client to eat foods high in potassium to prevent hypokalemia.

    Ⓝ NCLEX® Connection: Pharmacological Therapies, Medication Administration

2. A. **CORRECT:** The client should take hydrochlorothiazide with or after meals to prevent gastrointestinal upset.

    B. INCORRECT: The client should take hydrochlorothiazide in the morning or no later than 1400, and not at bedtime, to prevent nocturia.

    C. INCORRECT: The client should expect decreased swelling of the ankles.

    D. INCORRECT: The client should maintain a normal fluid intake (1,500 mL) throughout the day unless contraindicated because of heart failure.

    Ⓝ NCLEX® Connection: Pharmacological Therapies, Medication Administration

3. A. INCORRECT: Serum sodium of 148 mEq/L is in the expected reference range and does not need to be reported to the provider.

    B. INCORRECT: Urine output of 30 mL/hr or 120 mL in 4 hr is in the expected reference range and does not need to be reported to the provider.

    C. **CORRECT:** Serum potassium of 5.2 mEq/L indicates hyperkalemia. Because spironolactone causes potassium retention, the nurse should withhold the medication and notify the provider.

    D. INCORRECT: A blood pressure of 140/90 mm Hg is within the expected reference range and does not need to be reported to the provider.

    Ⓝ NCLEX® Connection: Pharmacological Therapies, Adverse Effects/Contraindications/ Side Effects/Interactions

4. A. INCORRECT: Blood glucose of 150 mg/dL is not an adverse effect of mannitol.

    B. INCORRECT: Urine output of 40 mL/hr indicates adequate urine output. However, kidney failure is an adverse effect of mannitol for which the nurse should continue to monitor.

    C. **CORRECT:** Dyspnea can indicate heart failure, an adverse effect of mannitol. The nurse should stop the medication and notify the provider.

    D. INCORRECT: A headache is a manifestation of increased intracranial pressure. Mannitol is administered to draw fluid back into the vascular and extravascular space, which can relieve the headache.

    (N) NCLEX® Connection: Pharmacological Therapies, Adverse Effects/Contraindications/ Side Effects/Interactions

5. A. INCORRECT: The nurse should plan to monitor for digoxin toxicity, which is an increase in serum digoxin levels that can occur in a client receiving torsemide, if the client has hypokalemia.

    B. **CORRECT:** The nurse should plan to monitor for hypokalemia, which is an adverse effect of a loop diuretic and can place the client at risk for digoxin toxicity.

    C. **CORRECT:** The nurse should plan to monitor for hypotension when other antihypertensive medications are being administered, which can cause a decrease in blood pressure.

    D. **CORRECT:** The nurse should plan to monitor for low urine output when NSAIDs are administered with a loop diuretic. NSAIDs decrease blood flow to the kidneys, which reduces the diuretic effect.

    E. **CORRECT:** The nurse should plan to monitor for ventricular dysrhythmias, which can occur with digoxin toxicity when torsemide is administered with digoxin.

    (N) NCLEX® Connection: Pharmacological Therapies, Adverse Effects/Contraindications/ Side Effects/Interactions

6. *Using the ATI Active Learning Template: Medication*

    A. Therapeutic Uses
       - Used when there is an emergent need for rapid mobilization of fluid
       - Pulmonary edema caused by heart failure
       - Liver, cardiac, or kidney disease
       - Hypertension
       - Kidney stone formation

    B. Adverse Effects
       - Dehydration
       - Hypotension
       - Ototoxicity
       - Hypokalemia

    C. Nursing Interventions/Client Education
       - Dehydration – Check for dry mouth, increased thirst, low urine output, and weight loss.
       - Hypotension – Monitor orthostatic blood pressure and pulse. Monitor for signs of postural hypotension.
       - Ototoxicity – Check for tinnitus. Avoid administering ototoxic medications.
       - Hypokalemia – Monitor laboratory values. Offer potassium-rich foods. Monitor for general weakness, nausea, and vomiting.

    (N) NCLEX® Connection: Pharmacological Therapies, Expected Actions/Outcomes

chapter 19

Overview

- Blood pressure may be controlled in a variety of ways with many agents that can be used alone or in combination. Guidelines for pharmacological management of hypertension can be found in The Eighth Report of the Joint National Committee on Prevention, Detection, Evaluation, and Treatment of High Blood Pressure (JNC 8) released in 2013 by the U.S. Department of Health and Human Services.

- The classifications of medications used to control blood pressure include the following.

  - Thiazide diuretics (often the first medication given for hypertension)

  - Angiotensin-converting enzyme (ACE) inhibitors

  - Angiotensin II receptor blockers (ARBs)

  - Aldosterone antagonists

  - Direct renin inhibitors

  - Calcium channel blockers (CCB)

  - Alpha adrenergic blockers

  - Centrally acting alpha$_2$ agonists

  - Beta adrenergic blockers

  - Vasodilators

MEDICATION CLASSIFICATION: ANGIOTENSIN-CONVERTING ENZYME (ACE) INHIBITORS

- Select Prototype Medication: captopril (Capoten)
- Other Medications
  - Enalapril (Vasotec)
  - Enalaprilat (Vasotec intravenous)
  - Fosinopril (Monopril)
  - Lisinopril (Prinivil)
  - Ramipril (Altace)
  - Moexipril (Univasc)

Purpose

- Expected Pharmacological Action
  - ACE inhibitors produce their effects by blocking the conversion of angiotensin I to angiotensin II, leading to:
    - Vasodilation (mostly arteriole).
    - Excretion of sodium and water, and retention of potassium by actions in the kidneys.
    - Reduction in pathological changes in the blood vessels and heart that result from the presence of angiotensin II and aldosterone.
- Therapeutic Uses
  - Hypertension
  - Heart failure
  - Myocardial infarction (to decrease mortality and to decrease risk of heart failure and left ventricular dysfunction)
  - Diabetic and nondiabetic nephropathy
  - For clients at high risk for a cardiovascular event, ramipril can be used to prevent MI, stroke, or death.

Complications

ADVERSE EFFECTS	NURSING INTERVENTIONS/CLIENT EDUCATION
› First-dose orthostatic hypotension	› If the client is already taking a diuretic, the medication should be stopped temporarily for 2 to 3 days prior to the start of an ACE inhibitor. › Taking another type of antihypertensive medication increases the hypotensive effects of an ACE inhibitor. › Start treatment with a low dosage of the medication. › Monitor blood pressure for 2 hr after initiation of treatment. › Instruct clients to change positions slowly and to lie down if feeling dizzy, lightheaded, or faint.
› Cough related to inhibition of kinase II (alternative name for ACE), which results in increase in bradykinin	› Inform clients of the possibility of experiencing a dry cough and to notify the provider. The medication should be discontinued.
› Hyperkalemia	› Monitor potassium levels to maintain a level within the expected reference range of 3.5 to 5 mEq/L. › Advise clients to avoid the use of salt substitutes containing potassium.
› Rash and dysgeusia (altered taste), primarily with captopril	› Clients should inform the provider if these effects occur. › Manifestations will stop with discontinuation of the medication.
› Angioedema (swelling of the tongue and oral pharynx)	› Treat severe effects with subcutaneous injection of epinephrine. › Medication should be discontinued.
› Neutropenia (rare but serious complication of captopril)	› Monitor WBC counts every 2 weeks for 3 months, then periodically. › This condition is reversible when detected early. › Inform clients to notify the provider at the first indications of infection (fever, sore throat) because medication should be discontinued.

Contraindications/Precautions

- Pregnancy Risk Category D during the second and third trimester, related to fetal injury.
- Contraindicated in clients who have history of allergy/angioedema to ACE inhibitors, in bilateral renal artery stenosis, or in clients who have a single kidney.
- Use cautiously in clients who have renal impairment and collagen vascular disease because they are at greater risk for developing neutropenia. Closely monitor these clients for indications of infection.

Interactions

MEDICATION/FOOD INTERACTIONS	NURSING INTERVENTIONS/CLIENT EDUCATION
› Diuretics can contribute to first-dose hypotension.	› Advise clients to temporarily stop taking diuretics 2 to 3 days before the start of therapy with an ACE inhibitor.
› Antihypertensive medications can have an additive hypotensive effect.	› Advise clients that dosage of medication may need to be adjusted if ACE inhibitors are added to the treatment regimen.
› Potassium supplements and potassium-sparing diuretics increase the risk of hyperkalemia.	› Clients should only take potassium supplements if prescribed by the provider. Clients should avoid salt substitutes that contain potassium.
› ACE inhibitors can increase levels of lithium carbonate (Lithobid).	› Monitor lithium levels to avoid toxicity.
› Use of NSAIDs can decrease the antihypertensive effect of ACE inhibitors.	› Avoid concurrent use.

Nursing Administration

- Administer ACE inhibitors orally, except enalaprilat, which is the only ACE inhibitor for IV use.
- Advise clients that the medication may be prescribed as a single formulation or in combination with hydrochlorothiazide.
- Advise clients that blood pressure has to be monitored after the first dose for at least 2 hr to detect hypotension.
- Instruct clients that captopril and moexipril should be taken at least 1 hr before meals. Other ACE inhibitors can be taken with or without food.
- Advise clients to notify the provider if cough, rash, dysgeusia (lack of taste), or indications of infection occur.

MEDICATION CLASSIFICATION: ANGIOTENSIN II RECEPTOR BLOCKERS (ARBs)

- Select Prototype Medication: losartan (Cozaar)
- Other Medications
  - Valsartan (Diovan)
  - Irbesartan (Avapro)
  - Candesartan (Atacand)
  - Olmesartan (Benicar)

Purpose

- Expected Pharmacological Action
  - These medications block the action of angiotensin II in the body. This results in:
    - Vasodilation (mostly arteriole).
    - Excretion of sodium and water, and retention of potassium (through effects on the kidney).
- Therapeutic Uses
  - Hypertension
  - Heart failure and prevention of mortality following MI
  - Stroke prevention
  - Delay progression of diabetic nephropathy

Complications

- The major difference between ARBs and ACE inhibitors is that cough and hyperkalemia are not adverse effects of ARBs.

ADVERSE EFFECTS	NURSING INTERVENTIONS/CLIENT EDUCATION
› Angioedema	› Advise clients to observe for indications (skin wheals, swelling of tongue) and to notify provider.
	› Treat severe effects with subcutaneous injection of epinephrine.
	› Medication should be discontinued.
› Fetal injury	› Advise women of risk during the second and third trimester of pregnancy.

Contraindications/Precautions

- Pregnancy Risk Category D. ARBs cause fetal damage in the second and third trimesters and should be discontinued as early in pregnancy as possible.

- These medications are contraindicated in clients who have renal stenosis when present bilaterally or in a single remaining kidney

- Use cautiously in clients who experienced angioedema with ACE inhibitor (not an absolute contraindication).

Interactions

MEDICATION/FOOD INTERACTIONS	NURSING INTERVENTIONS/CLIENT EDUCATION
› Antihypertensive medications can have an additive effect when used with ARBs.	› Advise clients that dosage of medication may need to be adjusted if ACE inhibitors are added to the treatment regimen.

Nursing Administration

- Administer medications by oral route.
- Advise clients that medication may be prescribed as a single formulation or in combination with hydrochlorothiazide.
- Advise clients that ARBs can be taken with or without food.

MEDICATION CLASSIFICATION: ALDOSTERONE ANTAGONISTS

- Select Prototype Medication: eplerenone (Inspra)
- Other Medication: spironolactone (Aldactone)

Purpose

- Expected Pharmacological Action
  - Aldosterone antagonists reduce blood volume by blocking aldosterone receptors in the kidney, thus promoting excretion of sodium and water.
- Therapeutic Uses
  - Hypertension
  - Heart failure

Complications

ADVERSE EFFECTS	NURSING INTERVENTIONS/CLIENT EDUCATION
› Hyperkalemia, hyponatremia	› Monitor serum potassium and sodium levels periodically. › Advise client not to use potassium supplements, salt substitutes containing potassium, or other potassium-sparing diuretics.
› Flulike manifestations, fatigue, headache, mild GI manifestations	› Advise the client to report severe manifestations to provider.
› Dizziness	› Instruct the client to not operate machinery or drive until reaction is known.

Contraindications/Precautions

- Contraindicated in clients who have high potassium levels, kidney impairment, and type 2 diabetes mellitus with albuminuria.
- Use cautiously in clients who have liver impairment.

Interactions

MEDICATION/FOOD INTERACTIONS	NURSING INTERVENTIONS/CLIENT EDUCATION
› Verapamil, ACE inhibitors, ARBs, erythromycin, and ketoconazole can increase risk of hyperkalemia.	› Monitor serum potassium more frequently if client must take these medication concurrently. › Instruct the client about manifestations of hyperkalemia.
› Lithium toxicity can occur if it is taken concurrently.	› Monitor clients on lithium more frequently for lithium toxicity.

Nursing Administration

- Administer orally with or without food.
- Do not administer with potassium supplements or potassium-sparing diuretics.

MEDICATION CLASSIFICATION: DIRECT RENIN INHIBITORS

- Select Prototype Medication: aliskiren (Tekturna)

Purpose

- Expected Pharmacological Action
  - Binds with renin to inhibit production of angiotensin I, thus decreasing production of both angiotensin II and aldosterone.
- Therapeutic Use
  - Relieves hypertension when used alone or with another antihypertensive medication.

Complications

ADVERSE EFFECTS	NURSING INTERVENTIONS/CLIENT EDUCATION
› Allergic reaction: angioedema (swelling of the pharynx, tongue, glottis) and rash	› Instruct client to monitor for rash and angioedema. Stop medication and notify provider, or call 911 for severe manifestations.
› Hyperkalemia	› Monitor serum potassium periodically during treatment. › Advise the client not to use potassium supplements or salt substitutes containing potassium.
› Diarrhea – dose-related, seen most often in females and older adult clients	› Instruct client to notify provider for severe diarrhea. › Monitor for dehydration, especially in older adults.

Contraindications/Precautions

- Pregnancy Risk Category C in first trimester, Category D in second and third trimesters.
- Contraindicated with previous allergy to aliskiren or in clients who have hyperkalemia
- Use cautiously in clients who have asthma or other respiratory disorders, history of angioedema, or diabetes mellitus, and in older adults.

MEDICATION/FOOD INTERACTIONS	NURSING INTERVENTIONS/CLIENT EDUCATION
› Decreases serum levels of furosemide (Lasix).	› Furosemide dosage may need to be increased.
› Increases effect of other antihypertensive medications.	› Monitor for hypotension when combinations are used.
› Atorvastatin (Lipitor) and ketoconazole increase levels of aliskiren.	› Monitor for hypotension if used concurrently.

Nursing Administration

- High-fat meals interfere with absorption. Instruct client to take at the same time daily away from foods high in fat.
- Available alone or in combination tablets with a variety of other antihypertensives (e.g., hydrochlorothiazide, a diuretic; valsartan, an ARB).

MEDICATION CLASSIFICATION: CALCIUM CHANNEL BLOCKERS

- Select Prototype Medications
  - Nifedipine (Adalat, Procardia)
  - Verapamil (Calan)
  - Diltiazem (Cardizem)
- Other Medications
  - Amlodipine (Norvasc)
  - Felodipine (Plendil)
  - Nicardipine (Cardene, Cleviprex)

Purpose

- Expected Pharmacological Action

EXPECTED PHARMACOLOGICAL ACTION	SITE OF ACTION AT THERAPEUTIC DOSES
Nifedipine	
› Blocking of calcium channels in blood vessels leads to vasodilation of peripheral arterioles and arteries/arterioles of the heart.	› Nifedipine acts primarily on arterioles. › Veins are not significantly affected.
Verapamil, diltiazem	
› Blocking of calcium channels in blood vessels leads to vasodilation of peripheral arterioles and arteries/arterioles of the heart. › Blocking of calcium channels in the myocardium, SA node, and AV node leads to a decreased force of contraction, decreased heart rate, and slowing of the rate of conduction through the AV node.	› These medications act on arterioles and the heart at therapeutic doses. › Veins are not significantly affected.

- Therapeutic Uses

MEDICATION	ANGINA PECTORIS	HYPERTENSION	CARDIAC DYSRHYTHMIAS (ATRIAL FIBRILLATION, ATRIAL FLUTTER, SVT)
Nifedipine	✓	✓	
Amlodipine	✓	✓	
Nicardipine	✓	✓	
Felodipine		✓	
Verapamil, diltiazem	✓	✓	✓

Complications

ADVERSE EFFECTS	NURSING INTERVENTIONS/CLIENT EDUCATION
Nifedipine	
› Reflex tachycardia	› Monitor for an increased heart rate. › A beta-blocker (metoprolol [Lopressor]) can be administered to counteract tachycardia.
› Peripheral edema	› Inform clients to observe for swelling in lower extremities and notify the provider if this occurs. › A diuretic may be prescribed to control edema.
› Acute toxicity	› With excessive doses, the heart, in addition to blood vessels, is affected. › Monitor vital signs and ECG. Gastric lavage and cathartic may be indicated. › Administer medications (norepinephrine, calcium, isoproterenol, lidocaine, and IV fluids). › Have equipment for cardioversion and cardiac pacer available.
Verapamil, diltiazem	
› Orthostatic hypotension and peripheral edema	› Monitor blood pressure, edema, and weight daily. › Instruct clients to observe for swelling in the lower extremities, and notify the provider if it occurs. › A diuretic may be prescribed to control edema. › Instruct clients about the manifestations of postural hypotension (lightheadedness, dizziness). If these occur, advise clients to sit or lie down. Effects can be minimized by getting up slowly.
› Constipation (primarily verapamil)	› Advise clients to increase intake of high fiber food and oral fluids, if not restricted.
› Suppression of cardiac function (bradycardia, heart failure)	› Monitor ECG, pulse rate, and rhythm. › Advise clients to observe for suppression of cardiac function (slow pulse, activity intolerance), and to notify provider if these occur. Medication may be discontinued.
› Dysrhythmias (QRS complex is widened and QT interval is prolonged)	› Monitor vital signs and ECG.
› Acute toxicity resulting in hypotension, bradycardia, AV block, and ventricular tachydysrhythmias	› Monitor vital signs and ECG. Gastric lavage and cathartic may be indicated. › Administer medications (norepinephrine, calcium, isoproterenol, lidocaine, and IV fluids). › Have equipment for cardioversion and cardiac pacer available.

Contraindications/Precautions

- Pregnancy Risk Category C.
- Nifedipine is contraindicated in acute MI, unstable angina, aortic stenosis, shock, and intestinal obstruction.
- Verapamil is contraindicated in heart block, digoxin toxicity, severe heart failure, and during lactation.
- Use cautiously in older adults and clients who have kidney disorders, liver disorders, mild to moderate heart failure, or GERD.

Interactions

MEDICATION/FOOD INTERACTIONS	NURSING INTERVENTIONS/CLIENT EDUCATION
Nifedipine	
› Beta-blockers, such as metoprolol (Lopressor), are used to decrease reflex tachycardia.	› Monitor for excessive slowing of heart rate.
› Consuming grapefruit juice and nifedipine can lead to toxicity.	› Monitor for indications of decrease in blood pressure, increase in heart rate, and flushing. › Advise clients to avoid drinking grapefruit juice.
Verapamil, diltiazem	
› Verapamil can increase digoxin (Lanoxin) levels, increasing the risk of digoxin toxicity. Digoxin can cause an additive effect and intensify AV conduction suppression.	› Monitor digoxin levels to maintain therapeutic range. › Monitor vital signs for bradycardia and for manifestations of AV block, such as a reduced ventricular rate.
› Concurrent use of beta-blockers can lead to heart failure, AV block, and bradycardia.	› Allow several hours between administration of IV verapamil (Calan) and beta-blockers.
› Consuming grapefruit juice and verapamil or diltiazem can lead to toxicity.	› Monitor clients for indications of constipation, decrease in blood pressure, decrease in heart rate, and AV block. › Advise clients to avoid drinking grapefruit juice.

Nursing Administration

- Advise clients not to chew or crush sustained-release tablets.
- For IV administration of verapamil, administer injections slowly over a period of 2 to 3 min.
- Advise clients who have angina to record pain frequency, intensity, duration, and location. Notify the provider if attacks increase in frequency, intensity, and/or duration.
- Instruct clients to monitor blood pressure and heart rate, as well as keep a blood pressure record.

MEDICATION CLASSIFICATION:
ALPHA-ADRENERGIC BLOCKERS (SYMPATHOLYTICS)

- Select Prototype Medication: prazosin (Minipress)
- Other Medications: doxazosin mesylate (Cardura), terazosin

Purpose

- Expected Pharmacological Action
  - Selective alpha$_1$ blockade prevents stimulation of alpha receptors on arterioles and veins, resulting in:
    - Venous and arterial dilation.
    - Smooth muscle relaxation of the prostatic capsule and bladder neck.
- Therapeutic uses
  - Primary hypertension.
  - Doxazosin and terazosin can be used to decrease manifestations of benign prostatic hyperplasia (BPH), which include urgency, frequency, and dysuria.

Complications

ADVERSE EFFECTS	NURSING INTERVENTIONS/CLIENT EDUCATION
› First-dose orthostatic hypotension	› Start treatment with low dosage of medication. › First dose often is given at night. › Monitor blood pressure for 2 hr after the initiation of treatment. › Instruct clients to avoid activities requiring mental alertness for the first 12 to 24 hr. › Instruct clients to change positions slowly and to lie down if feeling dizzy, lightheaded, or faint.

Contraindications/Precautions

- Pregnancy Risk Category C.
- Contraindicated in clients who have hypotension.
- Use cautiously clients who have angina pectoris or renal insufficiency, and in older adults.

Interactions

MEDICATION/FOOD INTERACTIONS	NURSING INTERVENTIONS/CLIENT EDUCATION
› Antihypertensive medications can have an additive hypotensive effect.	› Instruct clients to observe for indications of hypotension (dizziness, lightheadedness, faintness). › Instruct clients to lie down if these manifestations occur, and to change positions slowly.

Nursing Administration

- Instruct clients that the medication can be taken with food.
- Recommend that clients take the initial dose at bedtime to decrease "first-dose" hypotensive effect.
- Advise client about safety measures to minimize results of orthostatic hypotension/dizziness.

MEDICATION CLASSIFICATION: CENTRALLY ACTING ALPHA$_2$ AGONISTS

- Select Prototype Medication: clonidine (Catapres)
- Other Medications: guanfacine HCl (Tenex), methyldopa (Aldomet)

Purpose

- Expected Pharmacological Action
  - These medications act within the CNS to decrease sympathetic outflow, resulting in decreased stimulation of the adrenergic receptors (both alpha and beta receptors) of the heart and peripheral vascular system.
    - Decrease in sympathetic outflow to the myocardium results in bradycardia and decreased cardiac output (CO).
    - Decrease in sympathetic outflow to the peripheral vasculature results in vasodilation, which leads to decreased blood pressure.
- Therapeutic Uses
  - Primary hypertension (administered alone, with a diuretic, or with another antihypertensive agent)
  - Severe cancer pain (administered parenterally by epidural infusion)
  - Investigational use
    - Migraine headache
    - Flushing from menopause
    - Management of ADHD and Tourette syndrome
    - Management of withdrawal symptoms from alcohol, tobacco, and opioids

Complications

ADVERSE EFFECTS	NURSING INTERVENTIONS/CLIENT EDUCATION
› Drowsiness and sedation	› Drowsiness will diminish as use of medication continues. › Advise clients to avoid activities that require mental alertness until manifestations subside.
› Dry mouth	› Advise clients to be compliant with medication regimen. › Reassure clients that manifestations usually resolve in 2 to 4 weeks. › Encourage clients to chew gum or suck on hard candy, and to take small amounts of water or ice chips.
› Rebound hypertension if abruptly discontinued	› Advise clients not to discontinue treatment without consulting the provider. › Clonidine should be discontinued gradually over the course of 2 to 4 days.

Contraindications/Precautions

- Clonidine is Pregnancy Risk Category C. Methyldopa and guanfacine are Pregnancy Risk Category B.
- Avoid use during lactation.
- Avoid use of transdermal patch on affected skin in scleroderma and systemic lupus erythematosus (SLE).
- Use cautiously in clients who have had a stroke, recent MI, diabetes mellitus, major depressive disorder, or chronic renal failure.

Interactions

MEDICATION/FOOD INTERACTIONS	NURSING INTERVENTIONS/CLIENT EDUCATION
› Antihypertensive medications can have an additive hypotensive effect.	› Instruct clients to observe for manifestations of hypotension (dizziness, lightheadedness, faintness). › Instruct clients to lie down if feeling dizzy, lightheaded, or faint, and change positions slowly.
› Concurrent use of prazosin (Minipress), MAOIs, and tricyclic antidepressants can counteract the antihypertensive effect of clonidine.	› Monitor clients for therapeutic effect. Monitor blood pressure. Do not use concurrently.
› Additive CNS depression can occur with concurrent use of other CNS depressants, such as alcohol.	› Advise clients of additive CNS depression with alcohol, and encourage clients to avoid use.

Nursing Administration

- Administer medication by oral, epidural, and transdermal routes.
- Medication is usually administered twice a day in divided doses. Take larger dose at bedtime to decrease the occurrence of daytime sleepiness.
- Transdermal patches are applied every 7 days. Advise clients to apply patch on hairless, intact skin on the torso or upper arm.

MEDICATION CLASSIFICATION: BETA-ADRENERGIC BLOCKERS (SYMPATHOLYTICS)

- Select Prototype Medications
  - Cardioselective: beta₁ (affects only the heart)
    - Metoprolol (Lopressor)
    - Atenolol (Tenormin)
    - Metoprolol succinate (Toprol XL)
    - Esmolol HCl (Brevibloc)
  - Nonselective: beta₁ and beta₂ (affect both the heart and lungs)
    - Propranolol (Inderal)
    - Nadolol (Corgard)
  - Alpha- and beta-blockers
    - Carvedilol (Coreg)
    - Labetalol (Trandate)

Purpose

- Expected Pharmacological Action
  - In cardiac conditions, the primary effects of beta-adrenergic blockers are a result of beta₁-adrenergic blockade in the myocardium and in the electrical conduction system of the heart.
    - Decreased heart rate (negative chronotropic [rate] action).
    - Decreased myocardial contractility (negative inotropic [force] action).
    - Decreased rate of conduction through the AV node (negative dromotropic action).
    - Alpha blockade adds vasodilation in medications such as carvedilol and labetalol.
- Therapeutic Uses
  - Primary hypertension (exact mechanism unknown; might be related to long-term use causing reduction in peripheral vascular resistance).
  - Angina, tachydysrhythmias, heart failure, and myocardial infarction.
  - Other uses may include treatment of hyperthyroidism, migraine headache, stage fright, pheochromocytoma, and glaucoma.

Complications

ADVERSE EFFECTS	NURSING INTERVENTIONS/CLIENT EDUCATION
Beta₁ Blockade – metoprolol, propranolol	
› Bradycardia	› Monitor pulse. If below 60/min, hold medication and notify the provider.
	› Use cautiously in clients who have diabetes mellitus. This medication can mask tachycardia, an early sign of low blood glucose in clients who have diabetes. Advise clients to monitor blood glucose to detect hypoglycemia.
› Decreased cardiac output	› Use cautiously with clients in heart failure. Doses are started very low and titrated to the desired level.
	› Advise clients to observe for indications of worsening heart failure (shortness of breath, edema, fatigue).
	› The provider should be notified if symptoms occur.
› AV block	› Obtain a baseline ECG and monitor.
› Orthostatic hypotension	› Advise clients to sit or lie down if experiencing dizziness or faintness.
	› Advise clients to avoid sudden changes of position and rise slowly.
› Rebound myocardium excitation	› The myocardium becomes sensitized to catecholamines with long-term use of beta-blockers.
	› Advise clients not to stop taking beta-blockers abruptly, but to follow the provider's instructions.
	› Use of beta-blockers should be discontinued over 1 to 2 weeks.
Beta₂ Blockade – propranolol	
› Bronchoconstriction	› Avoid in clients who have asthma.
	› Clients who have asthma should be administered a beta₁ selective agent.
› Inhibited glycogenolysis	› Clients who have diabetes mellitus rely on the breakdown of glycogen into glucose to manage low blood glucose (can happen with insulin overdose).
	› In addition, a decreased heart rate can further mask manifestations of impending low blood glucose level. Clients who have diabetes should be administered a beta₁ selective agent.

Contraindications/Precautions

Q
S

- Contraindicated in clients who have AV block and sinus bradycardia.
- Nonselective beta-adrenergic blockers are contraindicated in clients who have asthma, bronchospasm, and heart failure.
- Use cardioselective beta-adrenergic blockers cautiously in clients who have asthma.

G

- In general, use beta-adrenergic blockers cautiously in clients who have myasthenia gravis, diabetes mellitus, depression, and in older adults and those with a history of severe allergies.

Interactions

MEDICATION/FOOD INTERACTIONS	NURSING INTERVENTIONS/CLIENT EDUCATION
Beta₁ Blockade – metoprolol, propranolol	
› Calcium channel blockers (CCB): verapamil (Calan) and diltiazem (Cardizem) intensify the effects of beta-blockers. » Decreased heart rate » Decreased myocardial contractility » Decreased rate of conduction through the AV node	› Monitor ECG and blood pressure. › Monitor clients closely if taking a CCB and beta-blocker concurrently. Reduce dose if needed.
› Concurrent use of antihypertensive medications with beta-blockers can intensify the hypotensive effect of both medications.	› Monitor for a drop in blood pressure.
Beta₂ Blockade – propranolol	
› Propranolol use can mask the hypoglycemic effect of insulin and prevent the breakdown of fat in response to hypoglycemia.	› Monitor blood glucose levels.

Nursing Administration

- Administer medications orally, usually once or twice a day.
- The following medications may be administered by the IV route: atenolol, metoprolol, labetalol, propranolol.
- Advise clients not to discontinue medication without consulting the provider.
- Advise clients to avoid sudden changes in position to prevent occurrence of orthostatic hypotension.
- Instruct clients not to crush or chew extended-release tablets.
- Instruct clients to self-monitor heart rate and blood pressure at home on a daily basis.

Nursing Evaluation of Medication Effectiveness

- Depending on therapeutic intent, effectiveness can be evidenced by:
  - Absence of chest pain.
  - Absence of cardiac dysrhythmias.
  - Normotensive blood pressure readings.
  - Control of heart failure manifestations.

MEDICATIONS FOR HYPERTENSIVE CRISIS

- Select Prototype Medication: nitroprusside (Nitropress), a centrally-acting vasodilator
- Other Medications
  - Nitroglycerin (Nitrostat IV), a vasodilator
  - Nicardipine (Cardene), a calcium channel blocker
  - Clevidipine (Cleviprex), a calcium channel blocker
  - Enalaprilat (Vasotec IV), an ACE inhibitor
  - Esmolol (Brevibloc), an ACE inhibitor

Purpose

- Expected Pharmacological Action
  - Direct vasodilation of arteries and veins resulting in rapid reduction of blood pressure (decreased preload and afterload)
- Therapeutic Use
  - Hypertensive crisis

Complications

ADVERSE EFFECTS	NURSING INTERVENTIONS/CLIENT EDUCATION
› Excessive hypotension	› Administer medication slowly because rapid administration will cause blood pressure to go down rapidly. › Monitor blood pressure and ECG. › Keep client supine during administration.
› Cyanide poisoning (headache and drowsiness, and may lead to cardiac arrest) – nitroprusside only	› Clients who have liver dysfunction are at increased risk. › Risk of cyanide poisoning can be reduced by administering medication at a rate of 5 mcg/kg/min or less, and giving thiosulfate concurrently. Medication should be discontinued if cyanide toxicity occurs.
› Thiocyanate toxicity (CNS findings, including delirium, psychosis) – accumulates when nitroprusside is given over several days	› Avoid prolonged use of nitroprusside. Monitor plasma levels if used for more than 3 days. Level should be maintained at less than 10 mg/dL.

Contraindications/Precautions

- Pregnancy Risk Category C.
- Use cautiously in clients who have liver and kidney disease or fluid and electrolyte imbalances, and in older adults.

Interactions

- Nitroprusside should not be administered in the same infusion as any other medication.

Nursing Administration

- Prepare medication by adding to diluent for IV infusion.
- Note color of solution, which can be light brown in color. Discard solution of any other color.
- Protect IV container and tubing from light.
- Discard medication after 24 hr.
- Monitor vital signs and ECG continuously.

Nursing Evaluation of Medication Effectiveness

- Depending on therapeutic intent, effectiveness can be evidenced by:
  - Decrease in blood pressure and maintenance of normotensive blood pressure.
  - Improvement of heart failure ,such as ability to perform activities of daily living, improved breath sounds, and absence of edema.
  - Improvement in renal function and delay of further progression of renal disease.

APPLICATION EXERCISES

1. A nurse is reviewing the health record of a client who is starting propranolol (Inderal) to treat hypertension. Which of the following conditions is a contraindication for taking propranolol?

    A. Asthma

    B. Diabetes

    C. Angina

    D. Tachycardia

2. A nurse is reinforcing teaching with a client who is starting verapamil (Calan) to control hypertension. Which of the following should the nurse include in the instructions?

    A   Increase the amount of dietary fiber in the diet.

    B. Drink grapefruit juice daily to increase vitamin C intake.

    C. Decrease the amount of calcium in the diet.

    D. Withhold food for 1 hr after the medication is taken.

3. A nurse is caring for a client who is starting captopril (Capoten) for hypertension. For which of the following adverse effects should the nurse monitor the client?

    A. Hypokalemia

    B. Hypernatremia

    C. Neutropenia

    D. Anemia

4. A nurse in an acute care facility is assisting with the infusion of IV nitroprusside for a client who is in hypertensive crisis. For which of the following adverse reactions should the nurse monitor this client?

    A. Intestinal ileus

    B. Neutropenia

    C. Delirium

    D. Hyperthermia

5. A nurse is planning to administer a first dose of captopril (Capoten) to a hospitalized client who has hypertension. Which of the following medications can intensify early adverse effects of captopril? (Select all that apply.)

_____ A. Simvastatin (Zocor)

_____ B. Hydrochlorothiazide (Microzide)

_____ C. Phenytoin (Dilantin)

_____ D. Clonidine (Catapres)

_____ E. Aliskiren (Tekturna)

6. A nurse in an outpatient facility is reinforcing teaching with a client who is starting aliskiren (Tekturna) to treat hypertension. What should the nurse instruct the client about this medication? Use the ATI Active Learning Template: Medication to complete this item to include the following:

A. Therapeutic Use: Identify the therapeutic use for aliskiren.

B. Adverse Effects: List two adverse effects of this medication.

C. Diagnostic Tests: Describe one to monitor.

D. Client Teaching: Identify two teaching points.

APPLICATION EXERCISES KEY

1. A. **CORRECT:** Propranolol is a nonselective beta-adrenergic blocker that blocks both beta$_1$ and beta$_2$ receptors. Blockade of beta$_2$ receptors in the lungs causes bronchoconstriction, so it is contraindicated in clients who have asthma.

    B. INCORRECT: Propranolol should be used cautiously in clients who have diabetes mellitus because it can mask signs of hypoglycemia, but it is not contraindicated for these clients.

    C. INCORRECT: Propranolol is prescribed to treat angina pectoris. It is not contraindicated for clients who have this disorder.

    D. INCORRECT: Propranolol is prescribed to treat tachydysrhythmias, such as tachycardia. It is contraindicated in clients who have bradycardia and heart block.

    ⓝ NCLEX® Connection: Pharmacological Therapies, Adverse Effects/Contraindications/ Side Effects/Interactions

2. A. **CORRECT:** Increasing dietary fiber intake can help prevent constipation, an adverse effect of verapamil.

    B. INCORRECT: Clients should be instructed to avoid drinking grapefruit juice when taking verapamil because concurrent use can lead to toxicity. In addition, it is not necessary to take extra vitamin C when taking verapamil.

    C. INCORRECT: There is no restriction on dietary calcium intake for clients taking verapamil.

    D. INCORRECT: There is no restriction regarding food when taking verapamil. Clients can take verapamil with food to prevent GI upset.

    ⓝ NCLEX® Connection: Pharmacological Therapies, Medication Administration

3. A. INCORRECT: Hyperkalemia, rather than hypokalemia, is a risk for clients taking ACE inhibitors.

    B. INCORRECT: ACE inhibitors cause excretion of sodium and water. Hypernatremia is not a risk for the client taking an ACE inhibitor.

    C. **CORRECT:** Neutropenia is a serious adverse effect that can occur in clients taking an ACE inhibitor. The nurse should monitor CBC and instruct the client to report manifestations of infection to the provider.

    D. INCORRECT: Anemia is not an adverse effect of an ACE inhibitor.

    ⓝ NCLEX® Connection: Pharmacological Therapies, Adverse Effects/Contraindications/ Side Effects/Interactions

4. A. INCORRECT: Intestinal ileus is not an adverse effect caused by nitroprusside infusion.

    B. INCORRECT: Neutropenia is not an adverse effect caused by nitroprusside infusion.

    C. **CORRECT:** Delirium and other mental status changes can occur in thiocyanate toxicity when IV nitroprusside is infused at a high dosage in clients who have kidney dysfunction. The thiocyanate level may be monitored during therapy and should remain below 10 mg/dL.

    D. INCORRECT: Hyperthermia is not an adverse effect caused by nitroprusside infusion.

    (N) NCLEX® Connection: Pharmacological Therapies, Adverse Effects/Contraindications/ Side Effects/Interactions

5. A. INCORRECT: Simvastatin, an antilipemic medication that lowers cholesterol, does not interact with captopril and does not intensify early adverse effects of captopril.

    B. **CORRECT:** Hydrochlorothiazide, a thiazide diuretic, often is used to treat hypertension. Diuretics can intensify first-dose orthostatic hypotension caused by captopril and can continue to interact with antihypertensive medications to cause hypotension. The nurse should monitor carefully for hypotension, especially after the first dose of captopril, and keep the client safe from injury.

    C. INCORRECT: Phenytoin, an antiseizure medication, does not interact with captopril and does not intensify early adverse effects of captopril.

    D. **CORRECT:** Clonidine, a centrally acting alpha2 agonist, is an antihypertensive medication that can interact with captopril to intensify first-dose orthostatic hypotension. The nurse should monitor carefully for hypotension, especially after the first dose of captopril, and keep the client safe from injury.

    E. **CORRECT:** Aliskiren, a direct renin inhibitor, is an antihypertensive medication that can interact with captopril to intensify its first-dose orthostatic hypotension. The nurse should monitor carefully for hypotension, especially after the first dose of captopril, and keep the client safe from injury.

    (N) NCLEX® Connection: Pharmacological Therapies, Adverse Effects/Contraindications/ Side Effects/Interactions

6. *Using the ATI Active Learning Template: Medication*

A. Therapeutic Use

- Aliskiren binds with renin to inhibit production of angiotensin I, thus decreasing production of both angiotensin II and aldosterone. Aliskiren is used solely for treating hypertension alone or in combination with other antihypertensives.

B. Adverse Effects

- Diarrhea – dose-related, occurs most frequently in females and older adult clients
- Risk for angioedema and rash caused by allergy to the medication
- Hyperkalemia

C. Diagnostic Tests

- The nurse should monitor serum electrolytes, paying close attention to potassium levels, because the client is at risk for hyperkalemia. This is especially important when the client takes ACE inhibitors concurrently, because these medications also raise potassium levels.

D. Client Teaching

- Advise clients not to take aliskiren with foods high in fat, which decreases absorption of the medication.
- Advise clients not to take potassium supplements or salt substitutes containing potassium.
- Female clients should be told that aliskiren should not be taken during pregnancy.
- Instruct the client that if rash or angioedema occur, aliskiren should be discontinued and the provider notified.
- The client should call 911 if severe manifestations of allergy are present.

Ⓝ NCLEX® Connection: Pharmacological Therapies, Expected Actions/Outcomes

chapter **20**

Overview

- Heart failure results from the inability of the heart muscle to pump enough blood to supply the whole body.

- The different determinants of cardiac output (CO), such as heart rate, stroke volume (SV), preload, and afterload, are affected in heart failure.

- Inability to pump sufficient blood results in:

  - Decreased tissue perfusion as evidenced by fatigue, weakness, and activity intolerance.

  - Left-sided heart failure (with pulmonary manifestations such as dyspnea, cough, and oliguria), or right-sided heart failure (systemic congestion with peripheral edema, jugular vein distention, weight gain).

- Diuretics, ACE inhibitors, angiotensin II receptor blockers (ARBs), and beta adrenergic blockers are the medications of choice for treatment of heart failure. Cardiac glycosides are indicated if these medications are unable to control effects of heart failure.

MEDICATION CLASSIFICATION: CARDIAC GLYCOSIDES

- Select Prototype Medication: digoxin (Lanoxin)

Purpose

- Expected Pharmacological Action

  - Positive inotropic effect – increased force of myocardial contraction

    - Increased force and efficiency of myocardial contraction improves the heart's effectiveness as a pump, improving stroke volume and cardiac output.

  - Negative chronotropic effect – decreased heart rate

    - At therapeutic levels, digoxin slows the rate of SA node depolarization and the rate of impulses through the conduction system of the heart.

    - A decreased heart rate gives the ventricles more time to fill with blood coming from the atria, which leads to increased SV and increased CO.

- Therapeutic Uses

  - Treatment of heart failure

  - Dysrhythmias (atrial fibrillation)

Complications

ADVERSE EFFECTS	NURSING INTERVENTIONS/CLIENT EDUCATION

› Dysrhythmias (caused by interfering with the electrical conduction in the myocardium)
 	
› Cardiotoxicity leading to bradycardia
	› Conditions that increase the risk of developing digoxin-induced dysrhythmias include hypokalemia, increased serum digoxin levels, and heart disease. Older adult clients are particularly at risk.
	
	› Monitor serum levels of K⁺ to maintain a level between 3.5 to 5.0 mEq/L.
	
	› Instruct clients to report indications of hypokalemia (nausea/vomiting, general weakness). Potassium supplements may be prescribed if clients are concurrently taking a diuretic.
	
	› Advise clients to consume high-potassium foods (green leafy vegetables, bananas, potatoes).
	
	› Monitor the client's digoxin level.
	  » Therapeutic serum levels can vary, but usually range from 0.5 to 2.0 ng/mL.
	  » Indications of toxicity can appear at levels less than 1.75 ng/mL.
	  » Clients who have heart failure respond best with serum medication levels between 0.5 to 0.8 ng/mL.
	  » Dosages should be based on serum levels and client response to medication.
	
	› Show clients how to monitor pulse rate, and recognize and report changes. The rate can be irregular with early or extra beats noted.

› GI effects include anorexia (usually the first indication), nausea, vomiting, and abdominal pain.	› Advise clients to monitor for these effects and report to the provider if they occur.
› CNS effects include fatigue, weakness, vision changes (diplopia, blurred vision, yellow-green or white halos around objects).	› Instruct clients to monitor for these effects and report to the provider if they occur.

Contraindications/Precautions

- Pregnancy Risk Category C.
- Contraindicated in clients who have disturbances in ventricular rhythm, including ventricular fibrillation, ventricular tachycardia, and second- and third-degree heart block.
- Use cautiously in clients who have hypokalemia, partial AV block, advanced heart failure, and renal insufficiency.

Interactions

MEDICATION/FOOD INTERACTIONS	NURSING INTERVENTIONS/CLIENT EDUCATION
› Thiazide diuretics, such as hydrochlorothiazide (HCTZ), and loop diuretics, such as furosemide (Lasix), can lead to hypokalemia, which increases the risk of developing dysrhythmias	› Monitor K⁺ level and maintain between 3.5 to 5.0 mEq/L. › Hypokalemia can be treated with potassium supplements or a potassium-sparing diuretic.
› ACE inhibitors and ARBs increase the risk of hyperkalemia, which can lead to decreased therapeutic effects of digoxin.	› Use cautiously if these medications are used with potassium supplements or a potassium-sparing diuretic. › Maintain K⁺ between 3.5 to 5.0 mEq/L.
› Sympathomimetic medications such as dopamine complement the inotropic action of digoxin and increase the rate and force of heart muscle contraction. › These medications can be beneficial, but also can increase the risk of tachydysrhythmias.	› Assist in monitoring ECG. Instruct clients to measure heart rate and report palpitations.
› Quinidine increases the risk of digoxin toxicity when used concurrently.	› Avoid concurrent use.
› Verapamil (Calan) increases plasma levels of digoxin.	› If used concurrently, digoxin dose should be decreased. Concurrent use usually is avoided because of verapamil cardiosuppression action counteracting the action of digoxin.
› Antacids decrease absorption of digoxin and can decrease its effectiveness.	› Advise clients to talk to the provider before taking any antacids.

Nursing Administration

- Advise clients to take the medication as prescribed. If a dose is missed, the next dose should not be doubled.

- Check the pulse rate and rhythm before administration of digoxin and record. Notify the provider of heart rate less than 60/min in an adult, less than 70/min in children, and less than 90/min in infants.

- Administer digoxin at the same time daily.

- Monitor digoxin levels periodically during treatment, and maintain therapeutic levels between 0.5 and 2.0 ng/mL to prevent digoxin toxicity.

- Avoid taking OTC medications to prevent adverse effects and medication interactions.

- Instruct clients to observe for manifestations of hypokalemia, such as muscle weakness, and to notify the provider if they occur.

- Instruct clients to observe for indications of digoxin toxicity (fatigue, weakness, vision changes, GI effects), and to notify the provider if they occur.

- Assist with management of digoxin toxicity.
  - Digoxin and potassium-wasting medication should be stopped immediately.
  - Monitor K$^+$ levels. For levels less than 3.5 mEq/L, monitor clients receiving potassium intravenously or by mouth. Do not give any further K$^+$ if the level is greater than 5.0 mEq/L.
  - Phenytoin (Dilantin) or lidocaine may be prescribed for dysrhythmias.
  - Atropine for may be prescribed bradycardia.
  - For excessive overdose, activated charcoal, cholestyramine, or Digibind can be used to bind digoxin and prevent absorption.

Nursing Evaluation of Medication Effectiveness

- Depending on therapeutic intent, effectiveness can be evidenced by:
  - Control of heart failure.
  - Absence of cardiac dysrhythmias.

MEDICATION CLASSIFICATION: ADRENERGIC AGONISTS

- Select Prototype Medication
  - Catecholamines
    - Epinephrine
    - Dopamine
    - Dobutamine
- Other Medications
  - Isoproterenol: catecholamine
  - Terbutaline: noncatecholamine

Purpose

RECEPTORS	SITE/RESPONSE
Alpha$_1$	› Activation of receptors in arterioles of skin, viscera and mucous membranes, and veins leads to vasoconstriction.
Beta$_1$	› Heart stimulation leads to increased heart rate, increased myocardial contractility, and increased rate of conduction through the AV node. › Activation of receptors in the kidney lead to the release of renin.
Beta$_2$	› Activation of receptors in the arterioles of the heart, lungs, and skeletal muscles leads to vasodilation. › Bronchial stimulation leads to bronchodilation. › Activation of receptors in uterine smooth muscle causes relaxation. › Activation of receptors in the liver cause glycogenolysis. › Skeletal muscle receptor activation leads to muscle contraction.
Dopamine	› Activation of receptors in the kidney cause the renal blood vessels to dilate.

RECEPTORS	PHARMACOLOGICAL ACTION	THERAPEUTIC USE
Epinephrine		
› Alpha$_1$	› Vasoconstriction	› Slows absorption of local anesthetics › Manages superficial bleeding › Decreased congestion of nasal mucosa › Increased blood pressure
› Beta$_1$	› Increased heart rate › Increased myocardial contractility › Increased rate of conduction through the AV node	› Treatment of AV block and cardiac arrest
› Beta$_2$	› Bronchodilation	› Asthma
Dopamine		
› Low dose » Dopamine	› Renal blood vessel dilation	› Shock › Heart failure

› Moderate dose
  » Dopamine
  » Beta$_1$
	› Renal blood vessel dilation
	› Increased heart rate
	› Increased myocardial contractility
	› Increased rate of conduction through the AV node	

› High dose
  » Dopamine
  » Beta$_1$
  » Alpha$_1$
	› Renal blood vessel constriction
	› Increased heart rate
	› Increased myocardial contractility
	› Increased rate of conduction through the AV node
	› Vasoconstriction, increased blood pressure	

Dobutamine		
› Beta$_1$	› Increased heart rate › Increased myocardial contractility › Increased rate of conduction through the AV node	› Heart failure

Complications

ADVERSE EFFECTS	NURSING INTERVENTIONS/CLIENT EDUCATION
Epinephrine	
› Vasoconstriction from activation of alpha$_1$ receptors in the heart can lead to hypertensive crisis.	› Assist with continuous cardiac monitoring. › Report changes in vital signs to the provider.
› Beta$_1$ receptor activation in the heart can cause dysrhythmias. Beta$_1$ receptor activation also increases the workload of the heart and increases oxygen demand, leading to the development of angina.	› Assist with continuous cardiac monitoring. › Notify the provider of changes in vital signs.
Dopamine	
› Beta$_1$ receptor activation in the heart can cause dysrhythmias. Beta$_1$ receptor activation also increases the workload of the heart and increases oxygen demand, leading to development of angina.	› Assist with continuous cardiac monitoring. › Notify the provider of increased HR and chest pain.
› Necrosis can occur from extravasation of high doses of dopamine.	› Monitor IV site carefully.
Dobutamine	
› Increased HR	› Assist with continuous cardiac monitoring. › Report changes in vital signs to the provider.

Contraindications/Precautions

- Epinephrine and dopamine are Pregnancy Risk Category C.
- Dobutamine is Pregnancy Risk Category B.
- Contraindicated in clients who have tachydysrhythmias and ventricular fibrillation.
- Use cautiously in clients who have hyperthyroidism, angina, history of myocardial infarction, hypertension, and diabetes.

Interactions

MEDICATION/FOOD INTERACTIONS	NURSING INTERVENTIONS/CLIENT EDUCATION
› MAOIs prevent inactivation of epinephrine and therefore prolong the effects of epinephrine. › MAOIs can increase cardiovascular effects of dopamine and dobutamine.	› Avoid use of MAOIs in clients receiving epinephrine. › Clients taking these medications concurrently many need a lowered dosage of dopamine and dobutamine.
› Tricyclic antidepressants block uptake of epinephrine, which will prolong and intensify effects of epinephrine. › Tricyclic antidepressants can increase cardiovascular effects of dopamine and dobutamine.	› Clients taking these medications concurrently may need a lowered dosage of epinephrine, dopamine, and dobutamine.
› General anesthetics can cause the heart to become hypersensitive to the effects of epinephrine, dopamine, and dobutamine, leading to dysrhythmias.	› Assist with continuous ECG monitoring.
› Alpha-adrenergic blocking agents, such as phentolamine, block action at alpha receptors.	› Phentolamine may be used to treat epinephrine toxicity.
› Beta-adrenergic blocking agents, such as propranolol, block action at beta receptors.	› Propranolol may be used to treat chest pain and dysrhythmias.
› Diuretics promote beneficial effects of dopamine.	› Monitor for therapeutic effects.

Nursing Administration

- Monitor clients receiving dopamine and dobutamine, which must be administered IV by continuous infusion.
- Monitor clients for chest pain. Notify the provider if chest pain occurs.
- Monitor urine output frequently for indications of decreased renal perfusion. Assist with monitoring ECG continuously for indications of tachycardia or dysrhythmias.

Nursing Evaluation of Medication Effectiveness

- Depending on therapeutic intent, effectiveness can be evidenced by improved perfusion as evidenced by urine output of greater than or equal to 30 mL/hr (with normal renal function), improved mental status, and systolic blood pressure maintained at greater than or equal to 90 mm Hg.

APPLICATION EXERCISES

1. A nurse in a provider's office is monitoring serum electrolytes for four older adult clients who take digoxin (Lanoxin) and furosemide (Lasix). Which of the following electrolyte values puts a client at risk for digoxin toxicity?

    A. Calcium 9.2 mg/dL

    B. Calcium 10.3 mg/dL

    C. Potassium 3.4 mEq/L

    D. Potassium 4.8 mEq/L

2. A nurse is caring for an older adult client who has a new prescription for digoxin and takes multiple other medications. Concurrent use of which of the following medications places the client at risk for digoxin toxicity?

    A. Phenytoin (Dilantin)

    B. Verapamil (Calan)

    C. Warfarin (Coumadin)

    D. Aluminum hydroxide (Amphojel)

3. A nurse is assisting with the monitoring of a client who is receiving a dopamine infusion at a moderate dose for the treatment of severe heart failure. Which of the following is an expected effect?

    A. Lowered heart rate

    B. Increased myocardial contractility

    C. Decreased conduction through the AV node

    D. Vasoconstriction of renal blood vessels

4. A nurse is reinforcing teaching to a client who has a new prescription for digoxin (Lanoxin). Which of the following can indicate digoxin toxicity and should be reported to the provider? (Select all that apply.)

    _____ A. Fatigue

    _____ B. Constipation

    _____ C. Anorexia

    _____ D. Rash

    _____ E. Diplopia

5. A nurse is monitoring the digoxin level for a client who has been taking a daily dose of digoxin for 1 month. The digoxin level is 0.25 ng/mL. The nurse should notify the provider and anticipate which of the following?

    A. An increase in the client's digoxin dose

    B. A decrease in the client's digoxin dose

    C. No change in the client's digoxin dose

    D. Discontinuation of the client's digoxin prescription

6. A nurse is caring for a client who has heart failure and has a new prescription for digoxin (Lanoxin) 0.125 mg PO daily. What should the nurse include when reinforcing teaching to the client about this medication? Use the ATI Active Learning Template: Medication to complete this item to include the following:

    A. Therapeutic Use

    B. Adverse Effects: Identify two.

    C. Diagnostic Tests: Describe two to monitor.

    D. Nursing Actions: Describe two.

APPLICATION EXERCISES KEY

1. A. INCORRECT: A calcium of 9.2 mg/dL is within the expected reference range and does not put a client at risk for digoxin toxicity.

    B. INCORRECT: A calcium of 10.3 mg/dL is within the expected reference range and does not put a client at risk for digoxin toxicity.

    C. **CORRECT:** A potassium of 3.4 mEq/L is below the normal range and puts a client at risk for digoxin toxicity. A low potassium can cause fatal dysrhythmias, especially in older clients who take digoxin. The nurse should notify the provider, who may prescribe a potassium supplement or a potassium-sparing diuretic for the client.

    D. INCORRECT: A potassium level of 4.8 mEq/L is within the expected reference range and does not put a client at risk for digoxin toxicity.

    Ⓝ NCLEX® Connection: Pharmacological Therapies, Adverse Effects/Contraindications/ Side Effects/Interactions

2. A. INCORRECT: Phenytoin, an antiseizure and antidysrhythmic medication, does not put a client at risk for digoxin toxicity. When given as an antidysrhythmic, phenytoin can treat dysrhythmias caused by digoxin toxicity.

    B. **CORRECT:** Verapamil, a calcium-channel blocker, can increase digoxin levels. If these medications are given concurrently, the digoxin dosage may need to be decreased and the nurse should monitor digoxin levels carefully.

    C. INCORRECT: Warfarin does not interact with digoxin to increase digoxin levels.

    D. INCORRECT: Antacids, such as aluminum hydroxide, decrease absorption of digoxin and can decrease digoxin levels and effectiveness.

    Ⓝ NCLEX® Connection: Pharmacological Therapies, Adverse Effects/Contraindications/ Side Effects/Interactions

3. A. INCORRECT: At a moderate dose, dopamine stimulates $beta_1$ receptors, which increase the heart rate. At high doses, dopamine stimulates $alpha_1$ receptors, which can decrease the heart rate.

    B. **CORRECT:** The nurse should expect dopamine to cause increased myocardial contractility, which also increases cardiac output. This occurs with the stimulation of $beta_1$ receptors and is a positive inotropic effect of dopamine when it is administered at a moderate dose.

    C. INCORRECT: At a moderate dose, dopamine stimulates $beta_1$ receptors, which increases conduction through the AV node.

    D. INCORRECT: At a moderate dose, dopamine stimulates $beta_1$ receptors, which dilates renal blood vessels. In high doses, dopamine stimulates $alpha_1$ receptors, which can constrict blood vessels.

    Ⓝ NCLEX® Connection: Pharmacological Therapies, Expected Actions/Outcomes

4. A. **CORRECT:** Fatigue and weakness are early CNS findings that can indicate digoxin toxicity.

    B. INCORRECT: Nausea, vomiting, and diarrhea, rather than constipation, are GI effects of digoxin toxicity.

    C. **CORRECT:** GI disturbances such as anorexia is an indication of digoxin toxicity.

    D. INCORRECT: Rash is not a manifestation of digoxin toxicity.

    E. **CORRECT:** Visual changes, such as diplopia and yellow-tinged vision, are manifestations of digoxin toxicity.

    Ⓝ NCLEX® Connection: Pharmacological Therapies, Adverse Effects/Contraindications/ Side Effects/Interactions

5. A. **CORRECT:** The client's digoxin level is below the therapeutic range. If the client's clinical findings correlate with the digoxin level, the nurse can expect an increase in the client's digoxin dose.

    B. INCORRECT: The nurse should not expect to receive a prescription to decrease the client's digoxin dose.

    C. INCORRECT: The nurse should not expect that the digoxin dose will remain unchanged.

    D. INCORRECT: The nurse should not expect that the digoxin prescription will be discontinued.

    Ⓝ NCLEX® Connection: Pharmacological Therapies, Adverse Effects/Contraindications/ Side Effects/Interactions

6. *Using the ATI Active Learning Template: Medication*

   A. Therapeutic Use

   - Digoxin improves the heart's pumping effectiveness, and increases cardiac output and stroke volume. It decreases heart rate by slowing depolarization through the SA node, thus allowing more time for the ventricles to fill with blood. Due to these effects, digoxin is used to treat heart failure, atrial fibrillation, and some other tachydysrhythmias.

   B. Adverse Effects

   - The client should monitor for indications of digoxin toxicity, which include GI effects (nausea/vomiting, diarrhea), CNS effects (fatigue and weakness), visual effects (yellow-tinged vision, halos around lights, and diplopia), pulse rate less than 60/min in adults, or skipped beats when checking the pulse.

   C. Diagnostic Tests

   - The nurse should monitor digoxin serum levels periodically during treatment. The expected reference range is 0.5 to 2.0 ng/mL. However, toxicity can occur around 1.75 ng/mL in some clients.

   - The nurse should monitor serum potassium levels because hypokalemia can cause cardiac dysrhythmias, especially in older adult clients. Assisting with monitoring ECG is also important to check for dysrhythmias.

   D. Nursing Actions

   - Advise the client to take oral digoxin at the same time each day. The client should not skip a dose or take more than the prescribed dose each day.

   - Instruct the client to monitor for indications of toxicity.

   - Advise the client to report any new medication and to report any OTC medications to the provider, because digoxin interacts with many other substances.

   Ⓝ NCLEX® Connection: Pharmacological Therapies, Expected Actions/Outcomes

chapter 21

Overview

- Anginal pain is a result of an imbalance between myocardial oxygen supply and demand. Pharmacological management is aimed at prevention of myocardial ischemia, pain, myocardial infarction, and death.

- Anginal pain is managed with organic nitrates, beta adrenergic blocking agents, calcium channel blockers, and ranolazine. Clients who have chronic stable angina should concurrently take an antiplatelet agent such as aspirin or clopidogrel (Plavix), a cholesterol-lowering agent, and an ACE inhibitor to prevent myocardial infarction and death.

- Antilipemic agents help lower low-density lipoprotein (LDL cholesterol) levels, raise high-density lipoprotein (HDL cholesterol) levels, and possibly decrease very low-density lipoprotein (VLDL) levels. These medications should be used along with lifestyle modifications such as regular activity, diet, and weight control.

- Prior to starting an antilipemic agent, obtain baseline levels of total cholesterol, LDL cholesterol level, HDL cholesterol, triglycerides (TGs), and liver and kidney function tests. These blood values should be monitored periodically throughout the course of therapy.

- Classifications of antilipemic agents include:

  - HMG-CoA reductase inhibitors (statins)

  - Cholesterol absorption inhibitors

  - Bile-acid sequestrants

  - Nicotinic acid, niacin

  - Fibrates

MEDICATION CLASSIFICATION: ORGANIC NITRATES

- Select Prototype Medication: nitroglycerin

  - Oral extended-release capsules: Nitro-Time

  - Sublingual tablet: Nitrostat

  - Translingual spray: Nitrolingual Pumpspray

  - Topical ointment

  - Transdermal patch: Nitro-Dur

  - Intravenous

- Other Medications

  - Sublingual: isosorbide dinitrate (Isordil)

  - Oral: isosorbide mononitrate (Monoket)

Purpose

- Expected Pharmacological Action

    - In chronic stable exertional angina, nitroglycerin (NTG) dilates veins and decreases venous return (preload), which decreases cardiac oxygen demand.

    - In variant (Prinzmetal's or vasospastic) angina, nitroglycerin prevents or reduces coronary artery spasm, thus increasing oxygen supply.

- Therapeutic Uses

    - Treatment of acute angina attack

    - Prophylaxis of chronic stable angina or variant angina

Complications

ADVERSE EFFECTS	NURSING INTERVENTIONS/CLIENT EDUCATION
› Headache	› Instruct clients to use aspirin or acetaminophen to relieve pain.
	› Clients should notify the provider if adverse effects do not resolve in a few weeks. Dosage might need to be reduced.
› Orthostatic hypotension	› Advise clients to sit or lie down if experiencing dizziness or faintness.
	› Clients should rise slowly and avoid sudden changes of position.
› Reflex tachycardia	› Monitor vital signs.
	› Administer a beta-blocker, such as metoprolol (Lopressor), if reflex tachycardia occurs.
› Tolerance	› Use lowest dose needed to achieve effect.
	› All long-acting forms of nitroglycerin should be taken with a medication-free period each day. This action reduces the risk of tolerance.

Contraindications/Precautions

- Pregnancy Risk Category C.

- This medication is contraindicated in clients who have hypersensitivity to nitrates.

- Nitroglycerin is contraindicated in clients who have traumatic head injury because the medication can increase intracranial pressure.

- Use cautiously in clients taking antihypertensive medications and clients who have kidney or liver dysfunction.

Interactions

MEDICATION/FOOD INTERACTIONS	NURSING INTERVENTIONS/CLIENT EDUCATION
› Use of alcohol can contribute to the hypotensive effect of nitroglycerin.	› Advise clients to avoid use of alcohol.
› Antihypertensive medications, such as beta-blockers, calcium channel blockers, and diuretics can contribute to hypotensive effect.	› Use nitroglycerin cautiously in clients receiving these medications.
› Use of PDE5 inhibitors (sildenafil [Viagra], tadalafil [Cialis], vardenafil [Levitra]) and nitroglycerin can result in life-threatening hypotension.	› Instruct clients not to take these medications if prescribed nitroglycerin.

Nursing Administration

SUBLINGUAL TABLET AND TRANSLINGUAL SPRAY	
Types	› Rapid onset › Short duration
Use	› Treat acute attack › Prophylaxis of acute attack

Nursing Interventions/ Client Education	› Use this rapid-acting nitrate at the first indication of chest pain. Do not wait until pain is severe.
	› Use prior to activity that is known to cause chest pain, such as climbing a flight of stairs.
	› For sublingual tablet
	   » Place the tablet under the tongue and allow it to dissolve.
	   » Tablets should be stored in original bottles, and in a cool, dark place.
	› Translingual spray should be sprayed against oral mucosa and not inhaled.

SUSTAINED-RELEASE ORAL CAPSULES	
Types	› Slow onset › Long duration
Use	› Long-term prophylaxis against anginal attacks
Nursing Interventions/ Client Education	› Swallow capsules without crushing or chewing. › Take capsules on an empty stomach with at least 8 oz of water.

TRANSDERMAL	
Types	› Slow onset › Long duration
Use	› Long-term prophylaxis against anginal attacks
Nursing Interventions/ Client Education	› To ensure appropriate dose, patches should not be cut. › Place the patch on a hairless area of skin (chest, back, or abdomen) and rotate sites to prevent skin irritation. › Remove old patch, wash skin with soap and water, and dry thoroughly before applying new patch. › Remove the patch at night to reduce the risk of developing tolerance to nitroglycerin. Be medication-free 10 to 12 hr/day.

TOPICAL OINTMENT	
Types	› Slow onset › Long duration
Use	› Long-term prophylaxis against anginal attacks
Nursing Interventions/ Client Education	› Remove the prior dose before a new dose is applied. Measure specific dose with applicator paper and spread over 2.5 to 3.5 inches of the paper. › Apply to a clean, hairless area of the body, and cover with clear plastic wrap. › Follow same guidelines for site selection as for transdermal patch. › Avoid touching ointment with the hands.

- Treatment of anginal attack using sublingual tablets or translingual spray

  ○ Stop activity. Sit or lie down.

  ○ Immediately put one sublingual tablet under the tongue and let it dissolve. Rest for 5 min.

  ○ If pain not relieved by first tablet, call 911, then take a second tablet.

  ○ After 5 more minutes, take a third tablet if pain is still not relieved. Do not take more than three sublingual tablets.

  ○ If using nitroglycerin translingual spray, one spray substitutes for one sublingual tablet when treating an anginal attack.

- Advise clients to follow the provider's instructions and not stop taking long-acting nitroglycerin abruptly.

- Advise clients who have angina to record pain frequency, intensity, duration, and location. The provider should be notified if attacks increase in frequency, intensity, and/or duration.

- Do not crush or chew oral nitroglycerin or isosorbide tablets.

Nursing Evaluation of Medication Effectiveness

- Depending on therapeutic intent, effectiveness can be evidenced by:

  ○ Prevention of acute anginal attacks.

  ○ Long-term management of stable angina.

  ○ Control of perioperative blood pressure.

  ○ Control of heart failure following acute MI.

MEDICATION CLASSIFICATION: ANTIANGINAL AGENT

- Select Prototype Medication: ranolazine (Ranexa)

Purpose

- Expected Pharmacological Action – lowers cardiac oxygen demand and thereby improves exercise tolerance and decreases pain
- Therapeutic Uses – chronic stable angina in combination with amlodipine (Norvasc), a beta adrenergic blocker or an organic nitrate

Complications

ADVERSE EFFECTS	NURSING INTERVENTIONS/CLIENT EDUCATION
› QT prolongation	› Monitor ECG.
› Elevated blood pressure	› Monitor blood pressure.

Contraindications/Precautions

- Pregnancy Risk Category C.
- Ranolazine is contraindicated in clients who have QT prolongation or in clients taking other medications that can result in QT prolongation.
- This medication is contraindicated in clients who have liver dysfunction.
- Use cautiously in older adult clients.

Interactions

MEDICATION/FOOD INTERACTIONS	NURSING INTERVENTIONS/CLIENT EDUCATION
› Inhibitors of CYP3A4 can increase levels of ranolazine and lead to torsades de pointes. Agents include grapefruit juice, HIV protease inhibitors, macrolide antibiotics, azole antifungals, and verapamil.	› Avoid concurrent use.
› Quinidine and sotalol (Betapace) can further prolong QT interval.	› Avoid concurrent use.
› Concurrent use of digoxin (Lanoxin) and simvastatin (Zocor) increases serum levels of digoxin and simvastatin.	› Monitor digoxin level. › Instruct client to report muscle weakness.

Nursing Administration

- Administer as an extended release oral tablet, twice daily with or without food. Do not crush or chew tablet.
- Obtain baseline and monitor ECG for QT prolongation.
- Obtain baseline and monitor digoxin level with concurrent use.
- Can be taken concurrently with other antianginal medications, such as nitroglycerin.

Nursing Evaluation of Medication Effectiveness

- Depending on therapeutic intent, effectiveness can be evidenced by:
  - Prevention of acute anginal attacks.
  - Long-term management of stable angina.

MEDICATION CLASSIFICATION: HMG-CoA REDUCTASE INHIBITORS (STATINS)

- Select Prototype Medication: atorvastatin (Lipitor)
- Other Medications
  - Simvastatin (Zocor)
  - Lovastatin (Altoprev)
  - Pravastatin (Pravachol)
  - Rosuvastatin (Crestor)
  - Fluvastatin (Lescol, Lescol XL)
- Combination Medications
  - Simvastatin and ezetimibe (Vytorin)
  - Simvastatin and niacin (Simcor)
  - Lovastatin and niacin (Advicor)

Purpose

- Expected Pharmacological Actions
  - Decrease manufacture of LDL cholesterol
  - Decrease manufacture of VLDL
  - Increase manufacture of HDL
  - Other beneficial effects include promotion of vasodilation, decrease in plaque site inflammation, and decreased risk of thromboembolism.
- Therapeutic Uses
  - Primary hypercholesterolemia
  - Prevention of coronary events (primary and secondary)
  - Protection against MI and stroke for clients who have diabetes
  - Increasing levels of HDL in clients who have primary hypercholesterolemia

Complications

ADVERSE EFFECTS	NURSING INTERVENTIONS/CLIENT EDUCATION
› Hepatotoxicity, as evidenced by increase in aspartate transaminase (AST)	› Obtain baseline liver function. › Monitor liver function tests after 12 weeks and then every 6 months. › Advise clients to observe for indications of liver dysfunction (anorexia, vomiting, nausea, jaundice), and notify the provider if manifestations occur. › Advise clients to avoid alcohol. › Medication may be discontinued if liver function tests are abnormal.
› Myopathy, as evidenced by muscle aches, pain, and tenderness › May progress to myositis or rhabdomyolysis.	› Obtain baseline CK level. › Monitor CK levels periodically. › Advise clients to report muscle aches, pain, and tenderness. › Medication may be discontinued if CK levels are elevated.
› Peripheral neuropathy, as evidenced by weakness, numbness, tingling, and pain in the hands and feet	› Advise clients to observe for adverse effects, and to notify the provider if manifestations occur.

Contraindications/Precautions

- Pregnancy Risk Category X.
- Contraindicated in clients who have hepatitis induced by viral infection or alcohol.
- Rosuvastatin should be avoided for clients of Asian descent or prescribed in a smaller dose than for other clients.

- Use cautiously in older adult clients, clients in debilitated condition, and those who have chronic kidney disease.

Interactions

MEDICATION/FOOD INTERACTIONS	NURSING INTERVENTIONS/CLIENT EDUCATION
› Fibrates (gemfibrozil, fenofibrate) and ezetimibe (Zetia) increase the risk of myopathy.	› Obtain baseline CK level. › Monitor CK levels periodically during treatment. › Advise client to report muscle aches and pain. › Medication may be discontinued if CK levels are elevated.
› Medications that suppress CYP3A4, such as erythromycin and ketoconazole, can increase levels of statins when taken concurrently.	› Avoid atorvastatin, lovastatin, and simvastatin. › Dosage of statin may need to be decreased. › Advise clients to inform the provider of all medications currently taken.
› Grapefruit juice suppresses CYP3A4 and can increase levels of statins.	› Advise clients to limit the amount of grapefruit juice consumed each day. Clients should not drink more than 1 qt/day.

Nursing Administration

- Administer statins by oral route.
- Administer lovastatin with evening meal. Other statins can be taken without food, but evening dosing is best because most cholesterol is synthesized during the night.
- Atorvastatin or fluvastatin should be used in clients who have renal insufficiency. For other statins, dosages will be reduced.
- Advise clients about the importance of obtaining baseline cholesterol, HDL, LDL, and triglyceride levels, as well as liver and kidney function tests, and monitoring periodically during treatment.

MEDICATION CLASSIFICATION: CHOLESTEROL ABSORPTION INHIBITOR

- Select Prototype Medication: ezetimibe (Zetia)

Purpose

- Expected Pharmacological Action – Ezetimibe inhibits absorption of cholesterol secreted in the bile and from food.
- Therapeutic Uses
  - ○ Clients who have modified diets can use this medication as an adjunct to help lower LDL cholesterol.
  - ○ Medication can be used alone or in combination with a statin medication.

Complications

ADVERSE EFFECTS	NURSING INTERVENTIONS/CLIENT EDUCATION
› Hepatitis	› Obtain baseline liver function.
	› Advise clients to observe for liver dysfunction (anorexia, vomiting, nausea, jaundice) and notify the provider if effects occur.
	› Advise clients to avoid alcohol.
	› Medication may be discontinued if liver function tests are abnormal.
› Myopathy	› Obtain baseline CK level.
	› Monitor CK levels while on treatment periodically.
	› Advise clients to notify the provider if manifestations such as muscle aches and pains occur.
	› Medication may be discontinued if CK levels are elevated.

Contraindications/Precautions

- Pregnancy Risk Category X.
- Contraindicated in clients who have active moderate-to-severe liver disorders, especially those taking a statin concurrently.
- Use cautiously in older adults and in clients who have mild liver disorders.

Interactions

MEDICATION/FOOD INTERACTIONS	NURSING INTERVENTIONS/CLIENT EDUCATION
› Bile acid sequestrants, such as cholestyramine, interfere with absorption.	› Advise clients to take ezetimibe 1 hr before or 4 hr after taking bile sequestrants.
› Statins, such as atorvastatin, can increase the risk of liver dysfunction and/or myopathy.	› Obtain baseline liver function tests and monitor periodically. Advise clients to observe for indications of liver damage (anorexia, vomiting, nausea). The provider should be notified, and the medication will most likely be discontinued. › Advise clients to notify the provider of manifestations such as muscle aches and pains. › Medication may be discontinued if CK levels are elevated.
› Concurrent use with fibrates, such as gemfibrozil, increases the risk of cholelithiasis and myopathy	› Ezetimibe is not recommended for use with fibrates.
› Levels of ezetimibe can be increased with concurrent use of cyclosporine	› Monitor for adverse effects (liver damage, myopathy).

Nursing Administration

- Advise client to report muscle aches and pain.
- Medication may be discontinued if CK levels are elevated.
- Advise clients about the importance of obtaining baseline cholesterol, HDL, LDL, and triglyceride levels, as well as liver and kidney function tests, and monitor periodically during treatment.
- Advise clients to follow a low-fat, low-cholesterol diet and to get involved in a regular exercise regimen.
- Clients can take this medication in a fixed-dose combination with simvastatin as Vytorin.

MEDICATION CLASSIFICATION: BILE-ACID SEQUESTRANTS

- Select Prototype Medication: colesevelam HCL (Welchol)
- Other Medication: colestipol (Colestid)

Purpose

- Expected Pharmacological Action – decrease in LDL cholesterol
- Therapeutic Use – Used as adjunct with a HMG-CoA reductase inhibitor, such as atorvastatin, and with dietary measures to lower cholesterol levels.

Complications

ADVERSE EFFECTS	NURSING INTERVENTIONS/CLIENT EDUCATION
› Constipation	› Advise clients to increase the intake of high-fiber food and oral fluids, if not restricted.

Contraindications/Precautions

- Colesevelam is Pregnancy Risk Category B. Colestipol is Pregnancy Risk Category C.
- Colesevelam is contraindicated in pancreatitis caused by high triglycerides and in bowel obstruction.
- Use cautiously in clients who have biliary disorders, diabetes mellitus, and in older adults.

Interactions

MEDICATION/FOOD INTERACTIONS	NURSING INTERVENTIONS/CLIENT EDUCATION
› Bile-acid sequestrants interfere with absorption of many medications, including levothyroxine (Synthroid); second-generation sulfonylureas, such as glipizide; phenytoin (Dilantin); fat-soluble vitamins (A, D, E, K); and oral contraceptives. They may interfere with absorption of other medications as well.	› Advise clients to take other medications 4 hr before taking bile sequestrants. › Advise clients to inform the provider of all medications currently taken.

Nursing Administration

- Colesevelam HCl is taken orally in tablet form. It should be taken with food and 8 oz of water, and not concurrently with other medications.
- Colestipol is supplied as oral tablet that should not be crushed or chewed. Give 30 min before a meal.
- Colestipol is also supplied in a powder formulation. Advise clients to use an adequate amount of fluid (4 to 8 oz) to dissolve the medication. This will prevent irritation or impaction of the esophagus.

OTHER MEDICATIONS: NICOTINIC ACID, NIACIN (NIACOR, NIASPAN)

Purpose

- Expected Pharmacological Action – decrease in LDL cholesterol and triglyceride levels
- Therapeutic Uses
    - For clients at risk for pancreatitis and elevated triglyceride levels
    - To lower elevated LDL cholesterol and triglycerides, and to raise HDL levels (Niaspan)

Complications

ADVERSE EFFECTS	NURSING INTERVENTIONS/CLIENT EDUCATION
› GI distress	› Usually self-limiting. Advise client to take with food.
› Facial flushing and feeling of warmth, tingling of hands and feet (temporary)	› Advise client to take aspirin 30 min before each dose.
› Hyperglycemia	› Monitor blood glucose levels.
› Hepatotoxicity	› Obtain baseline liver function tests and monitor periodically. › Advise clients to observe for indications of liver dysfunction (anorexia, vomiting, nausea, jaundice), and notify the provider if these occur. › Medication may be discontinued if liver function tests are abnormal.
› Hyperuricemia	› Monitor kidney function, BUN, and creatinine, I&O. › Encourage adequate fluid intake of 2 to 3 L of water each day from food and beverage sources unless contraindicated. › Administer allopurinol if uric acid level is elevated.

Contraindications/Precautions

- Pregnancy Risk Category C.
- Contraindicated in clients who have liver disease and gout.

Nursing Administration

- Administer by oral route, either in tablet or liquid form. Tablet may be standard form or time-released.
- Administer standard form three times a day with or after meals.
- Administer time-released formulations once in the evening.
- Advise clients that dosage is much larger than dosage when taken as vitamin supplement.

Nursing Evaluation of Medication Effectiveness

- Depending on therapeutic intent, effectiveness may be evidenced by:
  - Decreased LDL cholesterol level.
  - Decreased triglyceride (VLDL) levels.
  - Absence of cardiovascular events such as stroke, MI, or thrombosis.

MEDICATION CLASSIFICATION: FIBRATES

- Select Prototype Medication: gemfibrozil (Lopid)
- Other Medications: fenofibrate (Tricor)

Purpose

- Expected Pharmacological Action
  - Decrease in triglyceride levels (increase in VLDL excretion for clients unable to lower triglyceride levels with lifestyle modification or other antilipemic medications)
  - Increase in HDL levels by promoting production of precursors to HDLs
- Therapeutic Uses
  - Reduction of plasma triglycerides (VLDL)
  - Increased levels of HDL

Complications

ADVERSE EFFECTS	NURSING INTERVENTIONS/CLIENT EDUCATION
› GI distress	› Usually mild and self-limiting.
› Gallstones	› Advise clients to observe for indications of gallbladder disease (right upper quadrant pain, fat intolerance, bloating). › Advise clients to notify the provider if manifestations occur.
› Myopathy (muscle tenderness, pain)	› Obtain baseline CK level. › Monitor CK levels periodically during treatment. › Monitor for muscle aches, pain, and tenderness, and notify the provider if adverse effects occur. › Stop medication if CK levels are elevated.
› Hepatotoxicity	› Obtain baseline liver function tests, and monitor periodically. › Advise clients to observe for indications of liver dysfunction (anorexia, vomiting, nausea, jaundice), and notify the provider if manifestations occur. › Stop medication if liver function tests are abnormal.

Contraindications/Precautions

- Pregnancy Risk Category C.
- Contraindicated in clients who have liver disorders, severe renal dysfunction, and gallbladder disease.

Interactions

MEDICATION/FOOD INTERACTIONS	NURSING INTERVENTIONS/CLIENT EDUCATION
› With concurrent use, warfarin (Coumadin) increases the risk of bleeding	› Obtain baseline prothrombin time (PT) and INR, and perform periodic monitoring. › Advise clients to report indications of bleeding (bruising, bleeding gums), and notify the provider if these occur.
› Statins increase the risk of myopathy.	› Avoid using concurrently.

Nursing Administration

- Administer by oral route.
- Advise clients to take medication 30 min prior to breakfast and dinner.

APPLICATION EXERCISES

1. A nurse is reinforcing teaching for a client who has angina pectoris and is learning how to treat acute anginal attacks. The clients asks, "What is my next step if I take one tablet, wait 5 minutes, but still have anginal pain?" Which of the following replies by the nurse is appropriate?

    A. "Take two tablets at the same time and then call 911."

    B. "Call 911 and take a second sublingual tablet."

    C. "Take a sustained-release nitroglycerin capsule rather than a sublingual tablet and wait 5 more minutes before calling 911."

    D. "Wait another 5 minutes before taking a second sublingual tablet."

2. A nurse is reinforcing teaching for a client who is prescribed nitroglycerin (Nitro-Dur) transdermal patch for angina pectoris. Which of the following instructions should the nurse give the client?

    A. Remove the patch each evening and replace it with a new patch in the morning.

    B. Cut each patch in half if angina attacks are under control.

    C. Take off the nitroglycerin patch temporarily for 30 min if a headache occurs.

    D. Change the patch every 48 hr right after the first meal of the day.

3. A nurse is collecting medication history data from a client who has angina and is to begin taking ranolazine (Ranexa). The nurse should report which of the following medications in the client's history that can interact with ranolazine? (Select all that apply.)

    _____ A. Digoxin (Lanoxin)

    _____ B. Simvastatin (Zocor)

    _____ C. Verapamil (Calan)

    _____ D. Amlodipine (Norvasc)

    _____ E. Nitroglycerin transderm patch (Nitro-Dur)

4. A nurse is reinforcing teaching with a client who is taking digoxin (Lanoxin) and has a new prescription for colesevelam (Welchol). Which of the following instructions should the nurse include in the teaching?

    A. Take digoxin with your morning dose of colesevelam.

    B. Your sodium and potassium levels will be monitored periodically while taking colesevelam.

    C. Watch for bleeding or bruising while taking colesevelam.

    D. Take colesevelam with food and at least one glass of water.

5. A nurse is caring for a client who is starting niacin (Niaspan) to reduce cholesterol. The nurse should monitor the client for which of the following adverse effects? (Select all that apply.)

   _____ A. Muscle aches

   _____ B. Hyperglycemia

   _____ C. Hearing loss

   _____ D. Flushing of the skin

   _____ E. Jaundice

6. A nurse is providing care for a client who has elevated total cholesterol, LDL, and triglycerides, and has a new prescription for atorvastatin (Lipitor) once daily. The client has type 2 diabetes mellitus and hypertension. What should the nurse reinforce with the client about this atorvastatin? Use the ATI Active Learning Template: Medication to complete this item to include the following:

A. Therapeutic Use: Identify for atorvastatin.

B. Adverse Effects: Identify two.

C. Diagnostic Tests: Describe two to monitor.

D. Nursing Actions: Describe two.

APPLICATION EXERCISES KEY

1. A. INCORRECT: The client should not be instructed to take two sublingual doses at once.

    B. **CORRECT:** The next step is to call 911 and then take a second sublingual tablet. If the first tablet does not work, the client can be having a myocardial infarction, and should call for emergency care. The client may take a third tablet if the second one has not relieved the pain after waiting an additional 5 minutes.

    C. INCORRECT: Taking an oral sustained-release capsule is not appropriate when treating an anginal attack.

    D. INCORRECT: Waiting an additional 5 minutes before taking a second tablet is not appropriate. The client should call 911 because he can be having a myocardial infarction.

    Ⓝ NCLEX® Connection: Pharmacological Therapies, Medication Administration

2. A. **CORRECT:** In order to prevent tolerance to the nitroglycerin, the client should remove the patch for 10 to 12 hr during each 24-hr period.

    B. INCORRECT: Transdermal patches are used to prevent anginal attacks, so cutting the dose in half could bring on an attack. The client should always apply a whole patch. The patches are available in many dosages, and the client should use the prescribed dose.

    C. INCORRECT: The nurse should not instruct the client to remove patches for a 30-min period if a headache occurs. The client should notify the provider if headaches do not resolve because the dose of nitroglycerin can need to be decreased.

    D. INCORRECT: The nurse should not instruct the client to change the patch every 48 hr after breakfast.

    Ⓝ NCLEX® Connection: Pharmacological Therapies, Medication Administration

3. A. **CORRECT:** Concurrent use with ranolazine increases serum levels of digoxin, so digoxin toxicity may result.

   B. **CORRECT:** Concurrent use with ranolazine increases serum levels of simvastatin, so liver toxicity may result.

   C. **CORRECT:** Verapamil is an inhibitor of CYP3A4, which can increase levels of ranolazine and lead to the dysrhythmia, torsades de pointes.

   D. INCORRECT: Amlodipine, a calcium channel blocker used for hypertension and stable angina, may be prescribed along with ranolazine to treat angina.

   E. INCORRECT: Nitroglycerin transderm patches may be prescribed along with ranolazine to treat angina.

   Ⓝ NCLEX® Connection: Pharmacological and Parenteral Therapies, Medication Administration

4. A. INCORRECT: Many medications, including digoxin, should be taken 4 hr before colesevelam to prevent decreased absorption of the other medications.

   B. INCORRECT: Serum electrolytes are not checked periodically while taking colesevelam. However, total cholesterol, LDL, HDL, and triglycerides are checked, as well as blood glucose and HbA1C levels for clients who have diabetes mellitus.

   C. INCORRECT: Bleeding and bruising are not expect effects caused by colesevelam.

   D. **CORRECT:** Colesevelam should be taken with food and at least 8 oz of water.

   Ⓝ NCLEX® Connection: Pharmacological Therapies, Medication Administration

5. A. INCORRECT: Myopathy (muscles aches) may occur with statins and other antilipemic medications, but this is not an adverse effect of niacin.

    B. **CORRECT:** Hyperglycemia may occur as an adverse effect of niacin. The nurse should plan to monitor blood glucose periodically.

    C. INCORRECT: Hearing loss is not an adverse effect of taking niacin.

    D. **CORRECT:** Flushing of the skin, along with tingling of the extremities, occurs soon after taking niacin. The effect should decrease in a few weeks, and can be minimized by taking an aspirin tablet 30 min before the niacin.

    E. **CORRECT:** Niacin may cause liver disorders, so the nurse should monitor for jaundice, abdominal pain, and anorexia.

    (N) NCLEX® Connection: Pharmacological Therapies, Adverse Effects/Contraindications/Side Effects/ Interactions

6. *Using the ATI Active Learning Template: Medication*

    A. Therapeutic Use
    - Atorvastatin decreases LDL and triglycerides and elevates HDL. It reduces risk for cardiovascular events, such as myocardial infarction, and also provides secondary prevention in clients who have already had a cardiovascular event. In clients who have diabetes mellitus and hypertension, atorvastatin can reduce mortality by controlling cholesterol levels.

    B. Adverse Effects
    - Muscle pain/tenderness (myopathy)
    - Liver toxicity with findings such as jaundice, upper abdominal pain, anorexia, nausea

    C. Diagnostic Tests
    - Baseline and periodic cholesterol levels (including LDL, HDL, and triglycerides), creatine kinase (CK) levels for myopathy, and liver function tests for liver toxicity

    D. Nursing Actions
    - Instruct the client in additional ways to help decrease cholesterol and improve health, such as exercise, low-fat diet, weight control, and smoking cessation.
    - Instruct the client to take atorvastatin in the evening without regard to meals. (Antilipemic agents are given in the evening because cholesterol is mostly synthesized during the night.)

    (N) NCLEX® Connection: Pharmacological Therapies, Medication Administration

UNIT 5   Medications Affecting the Hematologic System

CHAPTERS
› Medications Affecting Coagulation
› Growth Factors

chapter 22

Overview

- Pharmaceutical agents that modify coagulation are used to prevent clot formation or break apart an already-formed clot. These medications work in the blood to alter the clotting cascade, prevent platelet aggregation, or dissolve a clot.
- The goal of medications that alter coagulation is to increase circulation and perfusion, decrease pain, and prevent further tissue damage.
- The groups of medications used include oral and parenteral anticoagulants, direct thrombin inhibitors, direct inhibitors of factor Xa, antiplatelet medications, and thrombolytic agents.

MEDICATION CLASSIFICATION: ANTICOAGULANTS – PARENTERAL

- Select Prototype Medication: heparin
- Low molecular weight heparins (LMWH)
  - Select Prototype Medication: enoxaparin (Lovenox)
  - Other Medications: dalteparin (Fragmin)
- Activated factor X (Xa) inhibitor
  - Select Prototype Medication: fondaparinux (Arixtra)

Purpose

- Expected Pharmacological Action: These parenteral anticoagulants prevent clotting by activating antithrombin, thus indirectly inactivating both thrombin and factor Xa. This inhibits fibrin formation.
- Therapeutic Uses
  - Heparin
    - In conditions necessitating prompt anticoagulant activity (evolving stroke, pulmonary embolism, massive deep-vein thrombosis)
    - As an adjunct for clients having open heart surgery or dialysis
    - As low-dose therapy for prophylaxis against postoperative venous thrombosis (i.e., hip/knee or abdominal surgery)
  - Low molecular weight heparins
    - Prevent deep-vein thrombosis (DVT) in postoperative clients
    - Treat DVT and pulmonary embolism
    - Prevent complications in certain types of myocardial infarction
  - Activated Factor X (Xa) inhibitor (fondaparinux)
    - Prevent DVT and pulmonary embolism in postoperative clients
    - Treat acute DVT or pulmonary embolism in conjunction with warfarin

Administration

- These medications cannot be absorbed by the intestinal tract and must be given by subcutaneous injection or IV infusion.

Complications

HEPARIN	
Adverse Effects	Nursing Interventions/Client Education
› Hemorrhage secondary to heparin overdose	› Monitor vital signs. › Advise clients to observe for bleeding (increased heart rate, decreased blood pressure, bruising, petechiae, hematomas, black tarry stools). › In the case of overdose, stop heparin, administer protamine, and avoid aspirin. › Monitor activated partial thromboplastin time (aPTT). Therapeutic value is 1.5 to 2 times the baseline.
› Heparin-induced thrombocytopenia, as evidenced by low platelet count and increased development of thrombi – mediated by antibody development (white clot syndrome)	› Monitor platelet count periodically throughout treatment, especially in the first month. › Stop heparin if platelet count is less than 100,000/mm³. Nonheparin anticoagulants, such as argatroban (Acova), can be used as a substitute if anticoagulation is still needed.
› Hypersensitivity reactions (chills, fever, urticaria)	› The client should receive a small test dose prior to the administration of heparin.
› Toxicity/overdose	› Assist in the administration of protamine, which binds with heparin and forms a heparin-protamine complex that has no anticoagulant properties.

ENOXAPARIN	
Adverse Effects	Nursing Interventions/Client Education
› Hemorrhage	› Monitor vital signs. › Advise clients to observe for bleeding (increased heart rate, decreased blood pressure, bruising, petechiae, hematomas, black tarry stools). › Monitor platelet count. Instruct client to avoid aspirin.
› Neurologic damage from hematoma formed during spinal or epidural anesthesia	› In clients who have spinal or epidural anesthesia: Monitor insertion site for indications of hematoma formation, such as redness or swelling. Monitor sensation and movement of lower extremities. Notify provider of abnormal findings.
› Thrombocytopenia, as evidenced by low platelet count	› Monitor platelets. Discontinue medication for platelet count less than 100,000/mm³.
› Toxicity/overdose	› Assist with the administration of protamine (heparin antagonist).

FONDAPARINUX	
Adverse Effects	Nursing Interventions/Client Education
› Hemorrhage	› Monitor vital signs. › Advise clients to observe for bleeding (increased heart rate, decreased blood pressure, bruising, petechiae, hematomas, black tarry stools). › Monitor platelet count. Instruct client to avoid aspirin.
› Neurologic damage from hematoma formed during spinal or epidural anesthesia	› In clients who have spinal or epidural anesthesia: Monitor insertion site for indications of hematoma formation such as redness or swelling. Monitor sensation and movement of lower extremities. Notify provider of abnormal findings.
› Thrombocytopenia, as evidenced by low platelet count	› Monitor platelets. Discontinue medication for platelet count less than 100,000/mm^3.

Contraindications/Precautions

- Parenteral anticoagulants are contraindicated in clients who have low platelet counts (thrombocytopenia) or uncontrollable bleeding.
- These medications should not be used during or following surgeries of the eye(s), brain, or spinal cord; lumbar puncture; or regional anesthesia.
- Use cautiously in clients who have hemophilia, increased capillary permeability, dissecting aneurysm, peptic ulcer disease, severe hypertension, hepatic or kidney disease, or threatened abortion.

Interactions

MEDICATION/FOOD INTERACTIONS	NURSING INTERVENTIONS/CLIENT EDUCATION
› Anti-platelet agents such as aspirin, NSAIDs, and other anticoagulants can increase risk for bleeding.	› Avoid concurrent use when possible. › Monitor carefully for evidence of bleeding. › Take precautionary measures to avoid injury (limit venipunctures and injections).

Nursing Administration

- Heparin
  - Obtain baseline vital signs.
  - Obtain baseline and monitor complete blood count (CBC), platelet count, and hematocrit levels.
  - Read label carefully. Heparin is dispensed in units and in different concentrations.
  - Check dosages with another nurse before administration.
  - Assist in monitoring the rate of IV infusion every 30 to 60 min.
  - Monitor aPTT every 4 to 6 hr until appropriate dose is determined, then monitor daily.

- ○ For subcutaneous injections, use a 20- to 22-gauge needle to withdraw medication from the vial. Then, change the needle to a smaller needle (25- or 26-gauge, ½ to 5/8 inches long).

- ○ Administer deep subcutaneous injections in the abdomen, ensuring a distance of 2 inches from the umbilicus. Do not aspirate.

- ○ Apply gentle pressure for 1 to 2 min after the injection. Rotate and record injection sites.

- ○ Instruct clients to monitor for indications of bleeding (bruising, gums bleeding, abdominal pain, nose bleeds, coffee-ground emesis, and tarry stools).

- ○ Instruct clients to avoid the use of over-the-counter NSAIDs, aspirin, or medications containing salicylates.

- ○ Advise clients to use an electric razor for shaving and to brush with a soft toothbrush.

- Enoxaparin/fondaparinux

  - ○ Monitoring is not required. These medications are acceptable for home use.

  - ○ Provide instruction regarding correct self-administration. Medications can be available in pre-filled syringes.

  - ○ For subcutaneous injections, use a 20- to 22-gauge needle to withdraw medication from the vial. Then, change to a small needle (25- or 26-gauge, ½ to 5/8 inches long).

  - ○ Do not expel the air bubble from the prefilled syringe. The air bubble should follow the medication to ensure the client receives the full dose of medication in the syringe.

  - ○ Administer subcutaneous enoxaparin in the anterolateral or posterolateral abdominal wall while the client is in a supine position. Do not aspirate.

  - ○ Administer subcutaneous fondaparinux in the abdomen, ensuring a distance of 2 inches from the umbilicus. Do not aspirate.

  - ○ Do not massage the site after the injection. Rotate and record injection sites.

  - ○ Instruct clients to monitor for indications of bleeding such as bruising, gums bleeding, abdominal pain, nose bleeds, coffee-ground emesis, and tarry stools.

  - ○ Instruct clients to avoid the use of over-the-counter NSAIDs, aspirin, or medications containing salicylates.

  - ○ Advise client to use an electric razor for shaving and to brush teeth with a soft toothbrush.

Nursing Evaluation of Medication Effectiveness

- Depending on therapeutic intent, effectiveness can be evidenced by the following:

  - ○ Heparin – Client aPTT levels of 60 to 80 seconds.

  - ○ Heparin, enoxaparin, and fondaparinux sodium – No development or no further development of venous thrombi or emboli.

MEDICATION CLASSIFICATION: ANTICOAGULANT – ORAL

- Select Prototype Medication: warfarin (Coumadin)

Purpose

- Expected Pharmacological Action: Oral anticoagulants antagonize vitamin K, thereby preventing the synthesis of four coagulation factors: factor VII, IX, X, and prothrombin.
- Therapeutic Uses
  - Treatment of venous thrombosis
  - Treatment of thrombus formation in clients who have atrial fibrillation or prosthetic heart valves
  - Prevention of recurrent myocardial infarction, transient ischemic attacks, pulmonary embolus, and DVT

Complications

ADVERSE EFFECTS	NURSING INTERVENTIONS/CLIENT EDUCATION
› Hemorrhage	› Monitor vital signs.
	› Advise clients to observe for bleeding (increased heart rate, decreased blood pressure, bruising, petechiae, hematomas, black tarry stools).
	› Obtain baseline prothrombin time (PT), and monitor levels of PT and international normalized ratio (INR) periodically.
	› In the case of a warfarin overdose, discontinue administration of warfarin, and administer vitamin K_1 (phytonadione [Mephyton]).
› Hepatitis	› Check liver enzymes. Monitor for jaundice.
› Toxicity/overdose	› Administer vitamin K_1 to promote synthesis of coagulation factors VII, IX, and X, and prothrombin.
	› Administer small doses of vitamin K_1 (2.5 mg PO) to prevent development of resistance to warfarin.
	› If vitamin K_1 cannot control bleeding, monitor clients receiving fresh frozen plasma or whole blood.

Contraindications/Precautions

- Classified as Pregnancy Risk Category X due to high risk of fetal hemorrhage, fetal death, and CNS defects. Advise clients to notify the provider if they become pregnant during warfarin therapy. If anticoagulation is needed during pregnancy, heparin can be used safely.
- Contraindicated in clients who have low platelet counts (thrombocytopenia) or uncontrollable bleeding.
- Contraindicated during or following surgeries of the eye(s), brain, or spinal cord; lumbar puncture; or regional anesthesia.
- Contraindicated in clients who have vitamin K deficiencies, liver disorders, and alcohol use disorder due to the additive risk of bleeding.
- Use cautiously in clients who have hemophilia, dissecting aneurysm, peptic ulcer disease, severe hypertension, or threatened abortion.

Interactions

MEDICATION/FOOD INTERACTIONS	NURSING INTERVENTIONS/CLIENT EDUCATION
› Concurrent use of heparin, aspirin, acetaminophen, glucocorticoids, sulfonamides, and parenteral cephalosporins increases effects of warfarin, which increases the risk for bleeding.	› Avoid concurrent use if possible. › Instruct clients to observe for inclusion of aspirin in over-the-counter medications. › If used concurrently, monitor carefully for indications of bleeding and increased prothrombin time (PT), INR, and aPTT levels. › Medication dosage should be adjusted accordingly.
› Concurrent use of phenobarbital, carbamazepine (Tegretol), phenytoin (Dilantin), oral contraceptives, and vitamin K decreases anticoagulant effects.	› Avoid concurrent use if possible. › If used concurrently, monitor carefully for reduced PT and INR levels. › Medication dosage should be adjusted accordingly.
› Foods high in vitamin K, such as dark green leafy vegetables (lettuce, cooked spinach), cabbage, broccoli, Brussels sprouts, mayonnaise, canola, and soybean oil, can decrease anticoagulant effects with excessive intake.	› Provide clients with a list of foods high in vitamin K. › Instruct clients to maintain a consistent intake of vitamin K to avoid sudden fluctuations that could affect the action of warfarin.
› Multiple other medications interact with warfarin.	› Take a complete medication history for clients prescribed warfarin and advise clients to inform provider if any new medication is started.

Nursing Administration

- Administration is usually oral, once daily, and at the same time each day.
- Obtain baseline vital signs.
- Monitor PT levels (therapeutic level 18 to 24 seconds) and INR levels (therapeutic levels 2 to 3). INR levels are the most accurate. Hold dose and notify the provider if levels exceed therapeutic ranges.
- Obtain baseline and monitor CBC, platelet count, and Hct levels.
- Instruct clients that anticoagulant effects can take 8 to 12 hr, and full therapeutic effect is not achieved for 3 to 5 days. For clients in the hospital setting, explain the need for continued heparin infusion when starting oral warfarin.
- Advise clients that anticoagulation effects can persist for up to 5 days following discontinuation of medication because of long half-life.
- Advise clients to avoid alcohol and over-the-counter medications to prevent adverse effects and medication interactions, such as risk of bleeding.
- Advise clients to employ nonmedication measures to avoid development of thrombi, including avoiding sitting for prolonged periods of time, not wearing constricting clothing, and elevating and moving legs when sitting.
- Advise clients to wear a medical alert bracelet indicating warfarin use.
- Have vitamin K_1 available in case of warfarin overdose.

- Reinforce teaching for clients to self-monitor PT and INR at home as appropriate.

- Advise clients to record dosage, route, and time of warfarin administration on a daily basis.

- Plan for frequent PT monitoring for clients who are prescribed medications that interact with warfarin. The client is at greatest risk for harm when the interacting medication is being deleted or added. Frequent PT monitoring will allow for dosage adjustments as necessary.

- Advise clients to notify the provider regarding warfarin use.

- Advise clients to use a soft-bristle toothbrush to prevent gum bleeding and an electric razor for shaving.

Nursing Evaluation of Medication Effectiveness

- Depending on therapeutic intent, effectiveness can be evidenced by:
  - PT 1.3 to 1.5 times control.
    - 1.5 to 2 times control for mechanical heart valves or for the treatment of recurrent systemic embolism
  - INR of 2 to 3 for treatment of acute myocardial infarction, atrial fibrillation, pulmonary embolism, venous thrombosis, and/or tissue heart valves.
  - INR of 3 to 4.5 for mechanical heart valve or recurrent systemic embolism.
  - No development or no further development of venous thrombi.

MEDICATION CLASSIFICATION: DIRECT THROMBIN INHIBITORS

- Select Prototype Medication: dabigatran (Pradaxa)
- Other Medications
  - Hirudin analogs: bivalirudin (Angiomax)
  - Argatroban (Acova)

Purpose

- Expected Pharmacological Action: These medications work by directly inhibiting thrombin, thus preventing a thrombus from developing.

- Therapeutic Uses
  - Dabigatran prevents stroke or embolism in clients who have atrial fibrillation not caused by valvular heart disease.
  - Bivalirudin is given concurrently with aspirin for clients who undergo coronary angioplasty.
  - Argatroban is used to prevent or treat thrombosis in clients who cannot take heparin due to heparin-induced thrombocytopenia.

Complications

ADVERSE EFFECTS	NURSING INTERVENTIONS/CLIENT EDUCATION
› Bleeding (GI, GU, cranial and other sites)	› Instruct clients to report manifestations of bleeding to provider. › For severe bleeding, no antidote to dabigatran is available. Dialysis or injections of recombinant factor VIIa may be used. › Clients who are about to undergo elective surgery should stop taking dabigatran before surgery.
› GI discomfort, nausea, vomiting, esophageal reflux, ulcer formation	› Take dabigatran with food. › Client can need a proton pump inhibitor, such as omeprazole (Prilosec) or an H_2 receptor antagonist, such as ranitidine (Zantac) for these manifestations.
› Bivalirudin also can cause hypotension and headache	› Check vital signs and monitor for headache when taking this medication.

Contraindications/Precautions

- Dabigatran and argatroban are Pregnancy Risk Category C. Bivalirudin is Pregnancy Risk Category B.
- Contraindicated in clients who have active bleeding or allergy to the medication.
- Use cautiously in clients who have liver impairment or who are at risk for bleeding.
- Use dabigatran and bivalirudin cautiously in clients who have impaired kidney function.

Interactions

MEDICATION/FOOD INTERACTIONS	NURSING INTERVENTIONS/CLIENT EDUCATION
› Rifampin (Rifadin) decreases levels of dabigatran.	› Use cautiously together and watch for therapeutic effect.
› Other thrombolytics and anticoagulants can increase risk for bleeding.	› Monitor coagulation studies carefully with concurrent use.

Nursing Administration

- Dabigatran is available in oral capsules that should be swallowed whole and can be taken with or without food. The container should be used within 30 days of opening. Discontinue other anticoagulants when starting dabigatran.
- Bivalirudin and argatroban are administered IV by direct bolus or continuous infusion.

MEDICATION CLASSIFICATION: DIRECT INHIBITOR OF FACTOR XA

- Select Prototype Medication: rivaroxaban (Xarelto)

Purpose

- Expected Pharmacological Action: Provides anticoagulation selectively and directly by inhibiting factor Xa.
- Therapeutic Uses: Prevents DVT and pulmonary embolism in clients who are undergoing total hip or knee arthroplasty surgery.

Complications

ADVERSE EFFECTS	NURSING INTERVENTIONS/CLIENT EDUCATION
› Bleeding (GI, GU, cranial, retinal)	› Instruct client to report bleeding, bruising, headache, or eye pain.
	› Monitor hemoglobin and hematocrit.
	› No antidote is available for severe bleeding; not removed by dialysis.
› Elevated liver enzymes (ALT, AST, GGT) and bilirubin	› Monitor baseline and periodic liver function.
	› Report elevated values to provider.

Contraindications/Precautions

- Pregnancy Risk Category C.
- Contraindicated with previous allergy to rivaroxaban, or in clients who have active bleeding, severe kidney impairment, or moderate to severe liver impairment.
- Use cautiously in clients taking anticoagulants, antiplatelet medications, or fibrinolytics, and in mild liver impairment or moderate kidney impairment.

Interactions

MEDICATION/FOOD INTERACTIONS	NURSING INTERVENTIONS/CLIENT EDUCATION
› Bleeding risk is increased when taking erythromycin, diltiazem, verapamil, quinidine, or amiodarone.	› Monitor carefully for bleeding if these medications are taken concurrently.
› Rifampin, carbamazepine, phenytoin, and St. John's wort can decrease rivaroxaban levels.	› Monitor for therapeutic effect in clients who take medications concurrently.

Nursing Administration

- Administer tablets orally, once daily, with or without food, and at the same time of day.
- Monitor hemoglobin, hematocrit, and liver and kidney function periodically during treatment.

MEDICATION CLASSIFICATION: ANTIPLATELETS

- Antiplatelet/salicylic
  - Select Prototype Medication: aspirin
- Antiplatelet/glycoprotein inhibitors
  - Select Prototype Medication: abciximab (ReoPro)
  - Other Medications: eptifibatide (Integrilin), tirofiban (Aggrastat)
- Antiplatelet/ADP inhibitors
  - Select Prototype Medications: clopidogrel (Plavix)
  - Other Medications: ticlopidine
- Antiplatelet/arterial vasodilator
  - Select Prototype Medication: pentoxifylline (Trental)
  - Other Medications: dipyridamole (Persantine), cilostazol (Pletal)

Purpose

- Expected Pharmacological Actions
  - Antiplatelets prevent platelets from clumping together by inhibiting enzymes and factors that normally lead to arterial clotting.
  - Antiplatelet medications inhibit platelet aggregation at the onset of the clotting process. These medications alter bleeding time.
- Therapeutic Uses
  - Primary prevention of acute myocardial infarction
  - Prevention of reinfarction in clients following an acute myocardial infarction
  - Prevention of ischemic stroke
  - Acute coronary syndromes (abciximab, tirofiban, eptifibatide, clopidogrel)
  - Intermittent claudication (cilostazol, pentoxifylline, dipyridamole)
- Route of administration
  - Aspirin: oral
  - Abciximab: IV
  - Clopidogrel: oral
  - Pentoxifylline: oral

Complications

ASPIRIN	
Adverse Effects	Nursing Interventions/Client Education
› GI effects (nausea, vomiting, dyspepsia)	› Advise clients to use enteric-coated tablets and to take aspirin with food. › Concurrent use of a proton pump inhibitor, such as omeprazole (Prilosec), can be appropriate.
› Hemorrhagic stroke	› Advise clients to observe for weakness, dizziness, and headache, and to notify the provider if effects occur.
› Prolonged bleeding time, gastric bleed, thrombocytopenia	› Monitor bleeding time. Monitor for gastric bleed, such as coffee-ground emesis or bloody, tarry stools. Monitor for bruising, petechiae, and bleeding gums.
› Tinnitus, hearing loss	› Monitor for hearing loss. › If manifestations occur, withhold dose and notify the provider.

ABCIXIMAB	
Adverse Effects	Nursing Interventions/Client Education
› Prolonged bleeding time, gastric bleed, thrombocytopenia	› Monitor bleeding time. › Monitor for gastric bleed (coffee-ground emesis or bloody, tarry stools). › Monitor for bruising, petechiae, and bleeding gums.

CLOPIDOGREL	
Adverse Effects	Nursing Interventions/Client Education
› Prolonged bleeding time, gastric bleed, thrombocytopenia	› Monitor bleeding time. › Monitor for gastric bleed (coffee-ground emesis or bloody, tarry stools). › Monitor for bruising, petechiae, and bleeding gums.
› GI effects – diarrhea, dyspepsia, pain	› Advise client to monitor for effects and notify provider.

PENTOXIFYLLINE	
Adverse Effects	Nursing Interventions/Client Education
› Dyspepsia, nausea, vomiting	› Take with food. › Do not crush or chew medication. › Monitor hydration if GI upset occurs.

Contraindications/Precautions

- Aspirin
  - ○ Pregnancy Risk Category D in the third trimester.
  - ○ Contraindicated in clients who have bleeding disorders and thrombocytopenia.
  - ○ Use cautiously in clients who have peptic ulcer disease and severe kidney and/or hepatic disorders. Do not give to children or adolescents who have a fever or recent chickenpox.

  - ○ Use with caution in older adults.
- Abciximab
  - ○ Pregnancy Risk Category C.
  - ○ Contraindications include clients who have bleeding disorders, thrombocytopenia, recent stroke, AV malformation, aneurysm, uncontrolled hypertension, and recent major surgery.
  - ○ Use cautiously in clients who have peptic ulcer disease and severe kidney and/or hepatic disorders.
- Clopidogrel
  - ○ Pregnancy Risk Category B.
  - ○ Contraindications include clients who have bleeding disorders, thrombocytopenia, peptic ulcer disease, and intracranial bleed.
  - ○ Use cautiously in clients who have peptic ulcer disease and severe kidney and/or hepatic disorders. Clients who are breastfeeding should not take this medication.
- Pentoxifylline
  - ○ Pregnancy Risk Category C.
  - ○ Contraindicated for clients who have bleeding disorders or retinal or cerebral bleeds.

Interactions

MEDICATION/FOOD INTERACTIONS	NURSING INTERVENTIONS/CLIENT EDUCATION
Aspirin	
› Concurrent use of other medications that enhance bleeding (NSAIDs, heparin, warfarin, thrombolytics, antiplatelets) increases risk for bleeding.	› Advise clients to avoid concurrent use. › If used concurrently, monitor carefully for indications of bleeding.
› Urine acidifiers (ammonium chloride) can increase aspirin levels.	› Monitor for aspirin toxicity (hearing loss, tinnitus).
› Concurrent use of aspirin can reduce hypertensive action of beta blockers.	› Monitor blood pressure.
› Corticosteroids can increase aspirin excretion and decrease aspirin effects. These medications can increase risk for GI bleed.	› Monitor for decreased aspirin effectiveness. › Monitor for gastric bleed (coffee-ground emesis and tarry or bloody stools).
› Caffeine can increase aspirin absorption.	› Monitor for toxicity.

MEDICATION/FOOD INTERACTIONS	NURSING INTERVENTIONS/CLIENT EDUCATION
Abciximab	
› Concurrent use of other medications that enhance bleeding (NSAIDs, heparin, warfarin, thrombolytics, antiplatelets) increases risk for bleeding.	› Advise clients to avoid concurrent use. › If used concurrently, monitor carefully for indications of bleeding.
Clopidogrel	
› Concurrent use of other medications that enhance bleeding (NSAIDs, heparin, warfarin, thrombolytics, antiplatelets) increases risk for bleeding.	› Advise clients to avoid concurrent use. › If used concurrently, monitor carefully for indications of bleeding.
› Proton pump inhibitors decrease effectiveness	› If needed for GI effects, pantoprazole (Protonix) interferes the least with platelet inhibition.
Pentoxifylline	
› Concurrent use of anticoagulants increases risk for bleeding.	› Monitor PT and INR. Clients can require reduced dosage.
› Pentoxifylline can increase levels of theophylline.	› Monitor theophylline level. Clients can require reduced dosage.

Nursing Administration

- Advise clients that prevention of strokes, myocardial infarctions, and reinfarction can be accomplished with low-dose aspirin (81 mg).

- Aspirin 325 mg should be taken during initial acute episode of myocardial infarction.

- Advise clients to notify the provider regarding aspirin use.

- Clopidogrel is sometimes prescribed concurrently with aspirin, which increases the risk for bleeding. Clopidogrel should be discontinued 7 days before an elective surgery.

Nursing Evaluation of Medication Effectiveness

- Depending on therapeutic intent, effectiveness can be evidenced by absence of arterial thrombosis, adequate tissue perfusion, and blood flow without occurrence of abnormal bleeding.

MEDICATION CLASSIFICATION: THROMBOLYTIC MEDICATIONS

- Select Prototype Medication: alteplase (Activase, Cathflo Activase) – often called tPA (tissue Plasminogen Activator)
- Other Medications
  - Tenecteplase (TNKase)
  - Reteplase (Retavase)

Purpose

- Expected Pharmacological Action: Thrombolytic medications dissolve clots that have already formed. Clots are dissolved by conversion of plasminogen to plasmin, which destroys fibrinogen and other clotting factors.
- Therapeutic Uses
  - Treat acute myocardial infarction (all three medications)
  - Treat massive pulmonary emboli (alteplase only)
  - Treat acute ischemic stroke (alteplase only)
  - Restore patency to central IV catheters (Cathflo Activase only)

Routes of Administration

- IV only

Complications

ALTEPLASE	
Adverse Effects	Nursing Interventions/Client Education
› Serious risk of bleeding from different sites – internal bleeding (GI or GU tracts and cerebral bleeding), as well as superficial bleeding (wounds, IV catheter sites)	› Limit venipunctures and injections. › Apply pressure dressings to recent wounds. › Assist in monitoring for changes in vital signs, alterations in level of consciousness, weakness, and indications of intracranial bleeding. › Notify the provider if indications of bleeding occur. › Monitor aPTT and PT, Hgb, and Hct.

Contraindications/Precautions

- Pregnancy Risk Category C.
- Because of the additive risk for serious bleeding, use is contraindicated in clients who have:
  - Any prior intracranial hemorrhage (hemorrhagic stroke).
  - Known structural cerebral vascular lesion (arteriovenous malformation).
  - Active internal bleeding.
  - History of significant closed head or spinal trauma within past 2 months.
  - Acute pericarditis or bacterial endocarditis.
  - Brain tumors.
  - Severe hepatic or kidney disorders.

- Use cautiously in clients who have severe hypertension, cerebral vascular disorders, recent GU or GI bleeding, major surgery within past 10 days, or in older adult clients.

Interactions

MEDICATION/FOOD INTERACTIONS	NURSING INTERVENTIONS/CLIENT EDUCATION
› Concurrent use of other medications that enhance bleeding (NSAIDs, heparin, warfarin, thrombolytics, antiplatelets) increases risk for bleeding.	› If used concurrently, monitor the client carefully for indications of bleeding.

Nursing Administration

- Use of thrombolytic agents should take place as soon as possible after onset of manifestations; within 2 hr is best.
- Clients receiving a thrombolytic agent should be monitored in a setting that provides for close supervision and continuous monitoring of vital signs, laboratory values, and hemodynamic status during and after administration of the medication.
- Minimize bruising or bleeding by limiting venipunctures and subcutaneous/intramuscular injections. Hold direct pressure to injection site or ABG site for up to 30 min until any oozing stops.

Nursing Evaluation of Medication Effectiveness

- Depending on therapeutic intent, effectiveness can be evidenced by evidence of thrombus lysis and restoration of circulation.

APPLICATION EXERCISES

1. A nurse is planning to administer subcutaneous enoxaparin (Lovenox) to an adult client following hip arthroplasty. Which of the following actions should the nurse plan to take?

    A. Choose a 22-gauge needle to administer the injection.

    B. Use a 5/8-inch needle to administer the injection.

    C. Administer the injection in the client's thigh.

    D. Aspirate carefully after inserting the needle into the client's skin.

2. A nurse is assisting with the care of a hospitalized client who is receiving IV heparin for a deep-vein thrombosis. The client begins vomiting blood. After the heparin has been stopped, which of the following medications should the client receive?

    A. Vitamin K_1 (phytonadione)

    B. Atropine

    C. Protamine

    D. Calcium gluconate

3. A nurse is caring for a client who has been taking a daily dose of warfarin as prescribed for the past 2 weeks following an acute myocardial infarction. The client's most recent INR is 1 to 2. The nurse should instruct the client to expect which of the following prescriptions from the provider?

    A. Continue the warfarin at the same dosage.

    B. Discontinue the warfarin.

    C. Increase the dosage of warfarin.

    D. Decrease the dosage of warfarin.

4. A nurse is monitoring a client who takes aspirin 81 mg PO daily. Which of the following clinical manifestations are adverse effects of daily aspirin therapy? (Select all that apply.)

    _____ A. Hypertension

    _____ B. Coffee-ground emesis

    _____ C. Tinnitus

    _____ D. Paresthesias of the extremities

    _____ E. Nausea

5. A nurse is caring for a client who has atrial fibrillation and has a new prescription for dabigatran (Pradaxa) to prevent development of thrombosis. Which of the following medications is prescribed concurrently to treat an adverse effect of dabigatran?

    A. Vitamin K_1 (phytonadione)

    B. Protamine

    C. Omeprazole (Prilosec)

    D. Probenecid (Benemid)

6. A nurse is reinforcing teaching for a client who has a new prescription for clopidogrel (Plavix) following a myocardial infarction. What should the nurse include in the teaching about this medication? Use the ATI Active Learning Template: Medications to complete this item to include the following:

    A. Therapeutic Use: Identify for clopidogrel in this client.

    B. Adverse Effects: Identify two for this medication.

    C. Diagnostic Tests: Describe one the nurse should monitor periodically.

    D. Nursing Actions: Describe two.

APPLICATION EXERCISES KEY

1.   A. INCORRECT: The nurse should use a 25- or 26-gauge needle to administer the injections. If drawing medication from a vial, the nurse might use a 20- or 22-gauge needle to draw up the medication, then change to a smaller clean needle for performing the injection.

   B. **CORRECT:** The nurse should plan to use a ½- to 5/8-inch needle to perform the injection.

   C. INCORRECT: A deep subcutaneous injection should be administered into the subcutaneous tissue of the anterolateral or posterolateral abdominal wall.

   D. INCORRECT: The nurse should not aspirate when administering enoxaparin or other heparin products subcutaneously.

   Ⓝ NCLEX® Connection: Pharmacological Therapies, Medication Administration

2.   A. INCORRECT: Vitamin K$_1$ is used to reverse the effects of warfarin (Coumadin).

   B. INCORRECT: Atropine is used to reverse bradycardia caused by beta adrenergic blockers.

   C. **CORRECT:** Protamine reverses the anticoagulant effect of heparin.

   D. INCORRECT: Calcium gluconate is used to treat magnesium sulfate toxicity.

   Ⓝ NCLEX® Connection: Pharmacological Therapies, Adverse Effects/Contraindications/
   Side Effects/Interactions

3.   A. INCORRECT: An INR of 1 to 2 is not therapeutic for a client following an acute myocardial infarction. It is not appropriate to continue the warfarin at the same dosage.

   B. INCORRECT: An INR of 1 to 2 is not therapeutic for a client following an acute myocardial infarction. It is not appropriate to discontinue the warfarin.

   C. **CORRECT:** The INR for a client who has had an acute myocardial infarction should be 2 to 3. The nurse should expect the provider to increase the dosage.

   D. INCORRECT: An INR of 1 to 2 is not therapeutic for a client following an acute myocardial infarction. It is not appropriate to decrease the dosage of warfarin.

   Ⓝ NCLEX® Connection: Pharmacological Therapies, Medication Administration

4.   A.   INCORRECT: Hypotension and shock can result if severe aspirin allergy occurs, but hypertension is not an adverse effect of aspirin therapy.

   B.   **CORRECT:** GI bleeding with dark stools or coffee-ground emesis can be an adverse effect of aspirin therapy.

   C.   **CORRECT:** Tinnitus and hearing loss can occur as an adverse effect of aspirin therapy

   D.   INCORRECT: Paresthesias of the extremities are not adverse effects of aspirin therapy.

   E.   **CORRECT:** Nausea, vomiting, and abdominal pain can occur as a result of aspirin therapy.

   Ⓝ NCLEX® Connection: Pharmacological Therapies, Adverse Effects/Contraindications/ Side Effects/Interactions

5.   A.   INCORRECT: Vitamin K_1 is used to treat hemorrhage or overdose of warfarin (Coumadin), but this medication is not an antidote for dabigatran.

   B.   INCORRECT: Protamine is used to treat severe hemorrhage or overdose of heparin, but is not an antidote for dabigatran.

   C.   **CORRECT:** Omeprazole or another proton pump inhibitor is prescribed for a client who is taking dabigatran and has abdominal pain and other GI findings that can occur as adverse effects of dabigatran. The nurse also should advise the client who has GI effects to take dabigatran with food.

   D.   INCORRECT: Probenecid is used to treat gout and gouty arthritis, and is not indicated to treat an adverse effect of dabigatran.

   Ⓝ NCLEX® Connection: Pharmacological Therapies, Adverse Effects/Contraindications/ Side Effects/Interactions

6. *Using the ATI Active Learning Template: Medications*

   A. Therapeutic Use

   - Clopidogrel inhibits platelet aggregation and prolongs bleeding time. It is used to prevent myocardial infarction (MI) or stroke in clients who have already had an MI or stroke.

   B. Adverse Effects

   - Like other platelet inhibitors, clopidogrel can cause bleeding due to thrombocytopenia. It also can cause GI effects, such as abdominal pain, nausea, and diarrhea.

   C. Diagnostic Tests

   - The nurse should plan to monitor the platelet count periodically while the client takes clopidogrel.

   D. Nursing Actions

   - Advise the client to monitor for bleeding. The client should watch for black stools, coffee-ground emesis, blood in the urine, nose bleeds, unusual bruising, or petechiae. The client should inform the provider if these occur and should also inform the provider about GI effects.

   - The nurse should be aware of all medications the client is taking, because risk for bleeding increases if the medication is taken with anticoagulants or antiplatelet medications. Clopidogrel is sometimes administered concurrently with aspirin, and that increases the risk for bleeding. The medication should be discontinued 7 days before any elective surgery.

   Ⓝ NCLEX® Connection: Pharmacological Therapies, Expected Actions/Outcomes

chapter 23

Overview

- Blood cells and platelets are produced in the body by the biological process hematopoiesis. In the body, this process is naturally controlled by hormones, also known as hematopoietic growth factors.
- Genetically engineered products are available for therapeutic purposes.
  - Replacement of neutrophils and platelets after chemotherapy
  - Hastening of bone marrow function after a bone marrow transplant
  - Increase in red blood cell production for clients who have chronic kidney failure
- There are three groups of hematopoietic growth factors.
  - Erythropoietic growth factors
    - Biological name – erythropoietin
  - Leukopoietic growth factors
    - Biological names
      - Granulocyte colony stimulating factor (G-CSF)
      - Granulocyte-macrophage colony-stimulating factor (GM-CSF)
  - Thrombopoietic growth factor
    - Interleukin-11

MEDICATION CLASSIFICATION: ERYTHROPOIETIC GROWTH FACTORS

- Select Prototype Medication: epoetin alfa (Epogen, Procrit)
- Other Medications
  - Darbepoetin alfa (Aranesp) – long-acting erythropoietin
  - Methoxy polyethylene glycol (MGEG)-epoetin beta (Mircera) – very long-acting erythropoietin

Purpose

- Expected Pharmacological Action – Hematopoietic growth factors act on the bone marrow to increase production of red blood cells.
- Therapeutic Uses – Anemia related to chronic kidney failure and use of zidovudine (Retrovir) in clients who have HIV infection, chemotherapy, and elective surgery.

Complications

ADVERSE EFFECTS	NURSING INTERVENTIONS/CLIENT EDUCATION
› Hypertension secondary to elevations in hematocrit level	› Monitor Hgb levels and blood pressure. If elevated, administer antihypertensive medications.
› Risk for a thrombotic event, such as myocardial infarction or stroke if the client has a Hgb of 11 g/dL or higher, or an increase of more than 1 g in 2 weeks. Seizures also can occur with a too-rapid rise in the blood counts.	› Decrease dosage when these limits are reached. Therapy may be resumed when Hgb drops to acceptable level, but dosage should be reduced.
› Increased risk for deep-vein thrombosis in preoperative clients	› Prophylactic use of an anticoagulant can be needed for preoperative clients.
› Headache and body aches	› Report headaches that are frequent or severe to provider. Hypertension can be the cause.

Contraindications/Precautions

- Pregnancy Risk Category C.

- Contraindicated in clients who have uncontrolled hypertension.

- Contraindicated in clients who have certain cancers because of possible increase in tumor growth.

Nursing Administration

- Obtain baseline blood pressure. In clients who have chronic kidney injury, control hypertension before the start of treatment.

- Monitor blood pressure frequently, because adjustments in antihypertensive medication can also be required as treatment progresses.

- Administer by subcutaneous injection. Monitor clients receiving IV bolus medication. Dosage is based on clients' weight.

- Do not agitate the vial of medication. Use each vial for one dose, and do not put the needle back into the vial when withdrawing the medication.

- Do not mix medication with any other medication in syringe.

- Dosing is usually three times/week, but may be once per week with some types of chemotherapy.

- Monitor iron levels, and implement measures to ensure a normal iron level. RBC growth is dependent upon adequate quantities of iron, folic acid, and vitamin B_{12}. Without adequate levels of these, erythropoietin is significantly less effective.

- Monitor Hgb and Hct twice per week until target range is reached.

- The longer-acting forms are administered less frequently (weekly or monthly), but can be prescribed for clients who have chronic kidney failure only.

Nursing Evaluation of Medication Effectiveness

- Depending on therapeutic intent, effectiveness can be evidenced by Hgb level of 10 to 11 g/dL and maximum Hct of 33%.

MEDICATION CLASSIFICATION: LEUKOPOIETIC GROWTH FACTORS

- Select Prototype Medication: filgrastim (Neupogen)
- Other Medication: pegfilgrastim (Neulasta)

Purpose

- Expected Pharmacological Action – Leukopoietic growth factors stimulate the bone marrow to increase production of neutrophils.
- Therapeutic Uses
  - Decreases the risk of infection in clients who have neutropenia from cancer and other conditions
  - To build up numbers of hematopoietic stem cells prior to harvesting for autologous transplant

Complications

ADVERSE EFFECTS	NURSING INTERVENTIONS/CLIENT EDUCATION
› Bone pain	› Monitor for bone pain and notify the provider. › Administer acetaminophen or opioid analgesic if acetaminophen is not effective.
› Leukocytosis	› Monitor CBC two times per week during treatment. › Decrease dose or interrupt treatment if WBC is greater than 100,000/mm³ or absolute neutrophil count exceeds 10,000/mm³.
› Splenomegaly and risk of splenic rupture with long-term use	› Evaluate reports of left upper quadrant abdominal pain or shoulder tip pain carefully and report to provider.

Contraindications/Precautions

- Contraindicated in clients who are sensitive to *Escherichia coli* protein.
- Use cautiously in clients who have cancer of the bone marrow.

Nursing Administration

- Administer filgrastim by subcutaneous infusion or subcutaneous injection. Monitor clients receiving medication by intermittent IV bolus or continuous IV.
- Do not agitate the vial of medication. Use each vial for one dose, and do not combine with other medications. Do not put the needle back into the vial when withdrawing the medication.
- Monitor CBC two times per week.
- If client will be administering subcutaneous filgrastim at home, reinforce teaching on self-administration procedures.

Nursing Evaluation of Medication Effectiveness

- Depending on therapeutic intent, effectiveness can be evidenced by:
  - Absence of infection.
  - WBC count and differential within expected reference ranges.

MEDICATION CLASSIFICATION:
GRANULOCYTE MACROPHAGE COLONY-STIMULATING FACTOR

- Select Prototype Medication: sargramostim (Leukine)

Purpose

- Expected Pharmacological Action – This medication acts on the bone marrow to increase production of white blood cells (neutrophils, monocytes, macrophages, eosinophils).
- Therapeutic Uses
  - Hastens bone marrow function after bone marrow transplant
  - Used in the treatment of failed bone marrow transplant

Complications

ADVERSE EFFECTS	NURSING INTERVENTIONS/CLIENT EDUCATION
› Diarrhea, weakness, rash, malaise, bone pain	› Monitor for adverse effects and notify the provider if they occur. › Administer acetaminophen.
› Leukocytosis, thrombocytosis	› Monitor CBC two times per week during treatment. › Reduce dose or interrupt treatment for absolute neutrophil count 20,000/mm³ or greater, WBC 50,000/mm³ or greater, or platelets 500,000/mm³ or greater.
› First IV dose effect: tachycardia, hypotension, chills, fever, diaphoresis, dyspnea	› Monitor carefully for these effects and notify provider if they occur.

Contraindications/Precautions

- Contraindicated in clients who are allergic to yeast products.
- Use cautiously in clients who have heart disease, hypoxia, peripheral edema, or pleural or pericardial effusion.
- Use cautiously in clients who have cancer of the bone marrow.

Nursing Administration

- Obtain baseline CBC, differential, and platelet count. Monitor periodically during treatment.
- When administered subcutaneously, reconstitute with sterile water. Mix contents gently, but do not shake vial.
- Monitor clients receiving IV infusion. Slow or discontinue infusion if client who has pre-existing heart failure or respiratory disorders experiences increase in dyspnea.

Nursing Evaluation of Medication Effectiveness

- Depending on therapeutic intent, effectiveness can be evidenced by:
  - Absence of infection.
  - WBC and differential within expected reference ranges.

MEDICATION CLASSIFICATION: THROMBOPOIETIC GROWTH FACTORS

- Select Prototype Medication: oprelvekin (Interleukin-11, Neumega)

Purpose

- Expected Pharmacological Action – Increases the production of platelets.

- Therapeutic Uses – Decreases thrombocytopenia and the need for platelet transfusions in clients receiving chemotherapy.

Complications

ADVERSE EFFECTS	NURSING INTERVENTIONS/CLIENT EDUCATION
› Fluid retention (peripheral edema, dyspnea on exertion)	› Monitor I&O. › If adverse effects occur, stop the medication and notify the provider.
› Cardiac dysrhythmias (tachycardia, atrial fibrillation, atrial flutter)	› Use cautiously in clients who have a history of cardiac dysrhythmias. › Monitor vital signs, heart rate, and rhythm. › If adverse effects occur, stop the medication and notify the provider.
› Conjunctival injection, transient blurring of vision, papilledema (inflammation of the eye and eyelid)	› Advise the client to observe for adverse effects. The medication should be withheld until notification of the provider.
› Allergic reactions, possible anaphylaxis	› Observe carefully for allergic reactions. Stop the medication and notify the provider if adverse effects occur.

Contraindications/Precautions

- Generally contraindicated in clients who have cancer of the bone marrow, because they can stimulate tumor growth.

- Use cautiously in clients who have heart failure and pleural effusion.

Nursing Administration

- Obtain baseline CBC, platelet count, and electrolytes.

- Oprelvekin should not be agitated and or combined with other medications.

- Administer oprelvekin once daily by subcutaneous injection until platelet count reaches prescribed level.

Nursing Evaluation of Medication Effectiveness

- Depending on therapeutic intent, effectiveness can be evidenced by platelet count greater than 50,000/mm^3.

APPLICATION EXERCISES

1. A nurse is caring for a client who is receiving daily doses of oprelvekin (Interleukin-11). Which of the following laboratory values should the nurse monitor to determine effectiveness of this medication?

    A. Hemoglobin

    B. Absolute neutrophil count

    C. Platelet count

    D. Total white blood count

2. A nurse is preparing to administer filgrastim (Neupogen) for the first time to a client who has just undergone a bone marrow transplant. Which of the following interventions is appropriate?

    A. Administer intramuscularly in a large muscle mass to prevent injury.

    B. Ensure that the medication is refrigerated until just prior to administration.

    C. Shake vial gently to mix well before withdrawing dose.

    D. Discard vial after removing one dose of the medication.

3. A nurse is monitoring a client who is receiving epoetin alfa (Epogen) for adverse effects. Which of the following is an adverse effect of this medication?

    A. Leukocytosis

    B. Hypertension

    C. Edema

    D. Blurred vision

4. A nurse is checking a client who has chronic neutropenia and who has been receiving filgrastim (Neupogen). Which of the following actions should the nurse take?

    A. Check for bone pain.

    B. Check for right lower quadrant pain.

    C. Auscultate for crackles in the bases of the lungs.

    D. Auscultate the chest to listen for a heart murmur.

5. A nurse is reinforcing teaching with a client who has chronic kidney injury and who is starting subcutaneous epoetin alfa (Epogen) three times weekly. What should the nurse instruct the client about this medication? Use the ATI Active Learning Template: Medication to complete this item to include the following:

A. Therapeutic Use: Identify for epoetin alfa in this client.

B. Adverse Effects: Identify two the client should watch for.

C. Diagnostic Tests: Describe two the nurse should monitor periodically.

D. Nursing Actions: Describe two.

APPLICATION EXERCISES KEY

1. A. INCORRECT: Hemoglobin levels should be monitored for a client receiving epoetin alfa (Epogen).

    B. INCORRECT: Absolute neutrophil count should be monitored for a client receiving filgrastim (Neupogen).

    C. **CORRECT:** The expected outcome for oprelvekin is a platelet count greater than 50,000/mm^3.

    D. INCORRECT: A total WBC should be monitored for a client receiving sargramostim (Leukine).

    (N) NCLEX® Connection: Pharmacological Therapies, Expected Actions/Outcomes

2. A. INCORRECT: Filgrastim is not administered by the IM route.

    B. INCORRECT: The nurse can allow the medication to reach room temperature prior to administration.

    C. INCORRECT: Before withdrawing a dose of filgrastim, the nurse should take care not to shake the medication vial.

    D. **CORRECT:** Only one dose of filgrastim should be withdrawn from the vial. The vial should then be discarded.

    (N) NCLEX® Connection: Pharmacological Therapies, Medication Administration

3. A. INCORRECT: Leukocytosis is an adverse effect of filgrastim (Neupogen), rather than for epoetin alfa (Epogen).

    B. **CORRECT:** Hypertension is an adverse effect of epoetin alfa that the nurse should monitor for throughout treatment.

    C. INCORRECT: Edema is an adverse effect of oprelvekin (Interleukin-11) caused by fluid retention, rather than of epoetin alfa.

    D. INCORRECT: Blurred vision is an adverse effect of oprelvekin, rather than of epoetin alfa.

    (N) NCLEX® Connection: Pharmacological Therapies, Adverse Effects/Contraindications/ Side Effects/Interactions

4. A. **CORRECT:** Bone pain is a dose-related adverse effect of filgrastim. It can be treated with acetaminophen and, if necessary, an opioid analgesic.

    B. INCORRECT: Palpating gently for right lower quadrant pain can be a necessary part of the nurse's examination, but will not determine an adverse effect of filgrastim.

    C. INCORRECT: Auscultating for crackles in the bases of the lungs can be a necessary part of the nurse's examination, but will not determine an adverse effect of filgrastim.

    D. INCORRECT: Auscultating the chest to listen for a heart murmur can be a necessary part of the nurse's examination, but will not check for an adverse effect of filgrastim.

    Ⓝ NCLEX® Connection: Pharmacological Therapies, Adverse Effects/Contraindications/ Side Effects/Interactions

5. *Using the ATI Active Learning Template: Medication*

    A. Therapeutic Use
    - Erythropoietin, a substance that stimulates bone marrow to produce red blood cells, is produced by the kidney. In clients who have kidney failure, erythropoietin is no longer present and anemia results. Epoetin alfa stimulates production of red blood cells in these clients.

    B. Adverse Effects
    - Headaches and myalgia (body aches)
    - Thrombotic events, such as myocardial infarction and cerebral vascular accident
    - Hypertension (common, sometimes serious)
    - A too-rapid increase (Hgb greater than 1 g/dL over 2 weeks, or Hgb greater than 10 to 11 g/dL) can worsen hypertension, increase risk of thrombosis, and cause seizures.

    C. Diagnostic Tests
    - Baseline iron levels, CBC with differential, and platelet count
    - Hgb and Hct twice weekly until blood counts stabilize

    D. Nursing Actions
    - Calculate dosages carefully. Both subcutaneous and IV epoetin alfa have dosages based on the client's weight. Do not shake the epoetin alfa vial, and discard vial after one dose is removed.
    - Monitor blood pressure carefully and report increases to the provider. Question client about frequency and severity of headaches, which could be an indication of increasing BP or a simple adverse effect.

    Ⓝ NCLEX® Connection: Pharmacological Therapies, Expected Actions/Outcomes

UNIT 6   Medications Affecting the Gastrointestinal System and Nutrition

CHAPTERS

› Peptic Ulcer Disease
› Gastrointestinal Disorders
› Vitamins, Minerals, and Supplements

NCLEX® CONNECTIONS

When reviewing the chapters in this unit, keep in mind the relevant sections of the NCLEX® outline, in particular:

Client Needs: Pharmacological Therapies

› Relevant topics/tasks include:

» Adverse Effects/Contraindications/Side Effects/Interactions

› Monitor and document the side effects of medications.

» Expected Actions/Outcomes

› Evaluate the client's response to medications (adverse reactions, interactions, therapeutic effects).

» Medication Administration

› Administer medication by gastrointestinal tube (g-tube, nasogastric tube, g-button or j-tube).

UNIT 6   MEDICATIONS AFFECTING THE GASTROINTESTINAL SYSTEM AND NUTRITION

CHAPTER 24   Peptic Ulcer Disease

Overview

- Pharmacological management of peptic ulcer disease addresses the imbalance between gastric mucosal defenses and antagonistic factors such as *H. pylori* infection, NSAIDs, and secretions including gastric acid and pepsin.
- Therapeutic management outcomes
    - Lessening of manifestations
    - Encouragement of healing
    - Decreased risk of complications
    - Stopping reoccurrence
- Groups of medications used in the management of peptic ulcer disease
    - Antibiotics
    - Antisecretory agents (H_2 receptor antagonists and proton pump inhibitors)
    - Mucosal protectants
    - Antacids
- The disease process is only altered by the use of antibiotics. All other medications make an environment that is conducive to healing.

MEDICATION CLASSIFICATION: ANTIBIOTICS

- Select Prototype Medications
    - Amoxicillin (Amoxil)
    - Bismuth (Pepto-Bismol)
    - Clarithromycin (Biaxin)
    - Metronidazole (Flagyl)
    - Tetracycline

Purpose

- Expected Pharmacological Action – eradication of *H. pylori* bacteria
- Therapy should include combination of two or three antibiotics for 14 days to increase effectiveness and to minimize the development of medication resistance.
- Nursing Administration Considerations
    - Advise clients that adverse effects of nausea and diarrhea are common.
    - Remind clients to take the full course of prescribed medications.
        - Refer to the chapter on antibiotics for more information regarding adverse effects, contraindications, and interactions.

MEDICATION CLASSIFICATION: HISTAMINE$_2$-RECEPTOR ANTAGONISTS

- Select Prototype Medication: ranitidine (Zantac)
- Other Medications
    - Cimetidine (Tagamet)
    - Famotidine (Pepcid)
    - Nizatidine (Axid) – PO use only

Purpose

- Expected Pharmacological Action
    - Histamine$_2$-receptor antagonists suppress the secretion of gastric acid by selectively blocking H$_2$ receptors in parietal cells lining the stomach.
- Therapeutic Uses
    - Histamine$_2$-receptor antagonists are prescribed for gastric and peptic ulcers, GERD, and hypersecretory conditions, such as Zollinger-Ellison syndrome.
    - Histamine$_2$-receptor antagonists are used in conjunction with antibiotics to treat ulcers caused by *H. pylori*.

Complications

ADVERSE EFFECTS	NURSING INTERVENTIONS/CLIENT EDUCATION
› Cimetidine can block androgen receptors, resulting in decreased libido and impotence.	› Inform clients of these possible effects.
› Cimetidine can cause CNS effects (lethargy, depression, confusion)	› These effects are seen more often in older adults who have kidney or liver dysfunction.
	› The use of cimetidine should be avoided in older adults.

- Ranitidine and famotidine have few adverse effects and interactions.

Contraindications/Precautions

- These medications are Pregnancy Risk Category B.
- The risk of CNS effects (confusion) is greater in older adult clients.
- H$_2$-receptor antagonists decrease gastric acidity, which promotes bacterial colonization of the stomach and secondarily of the respiratory tract. Use cautiously in clients who are at a high risk for pneumonia, such as clients who have chronic obstructive pulmonary disease (COPD).

Interactions

MEDICATION/FOOD INTERACTIONS	NURSING INTERVENTIONS/CLIENT EDUCATION
› Cimetidine can inhibit medication-metabolizing enzymes and thus increase the levels of warfarin (Coumadin), phenytoin (Dilantin), theophylline, and lidocaine.	› In clients taking warfarin, monitor for indications of bleeding. › Monitor international normalized ratio (INR) and prothrombin time (PT) levels, and adjust warfarin dosages accordingly. › In clients taking phenytoin, theophylline, and lidocaine, monitor serum levels and adjust dosages accordingly.
› Concurrent use of antacids can decrease absorption of histamine₂-receptor antagonists.	› Advise clients not to take an antacid 1 hr before or after taking a histamine₂-receptor antagonist.

Nursing Administration

- Advise clients to practice good nutrition.
- Instruct clients to avoid foods that promote gastric secretion, to eat meals on a regular schedule in a relaxed setting, and to not overeat.
- Inform clients that adequate rest and reduction of stress can promote healing.
- Clients should avoid smoking, because smoking can delay healing.
- Encourage clients to avoid aspirin and other NSAIDs unless taking low-dose aspirin therapy for prevention of cardiovascular disease.
- If alcohol exacerbates peptic ulcer disease, advise clients to avoid drinking alcohol.
- Availability of these medications OTC can discourage clients from seeking appropriate health care. Encourage clients to see the provider if problems persist.
- The medication regimen can be complex, often requiring clients to take two to three different medications for an extended period of time. Encourage clients to adhere to the medication regimen, and provide support.
- Ranitidine can be taken with or without food.
- Treatment of peptic ulcer disease is usually started as an oral dose twice a day until the ulcer is healed, followed by a maintenance dose, which usually is taken once a day at bedtime.
- Instruct clients to notify the provider for any indication of obvious or occult GI bleeding, such as coffee-ground emesis.

MEDICATION CLASSIFICATION: PROTON PUMP INHIBITORS

- Select Prototype Medication: omeprazole (Prilosec)
- Other Medications
  - Pantoprazole (Protonix)
  - Lansoprazole (Prevacid) and dexlansoprazole (Dexilant)
  - Rabeprazole sodium (AcipHex)
  - Esomeprazole (Nexium)

Purpose

- Expected Pharmacological Action
  - Proton pump inhibitors reduce gastric acid secretion by irreversibly inhibiting the enzyme that produces gastric acid.
  - Proton pump inhibitors reduce basal and stimulated acid production.
- Therapeutic Use
  - Proton pump inhibitors are prescribed for gastric and duodenal ulcers, erosive esophagitis, GERD, and hypersecretory conditions such as Zollinger-Ellison syndrome.

Complications

- Insignificant adverse effects with short-term treatment
- Low incidence of headache, diarrhea, nausea, and vomiting

Contraindications/Precautions

- These medications are Pregnancy Risk Category B, except for omeprazole, which is Category C.
- Contraindicated for clients hypersensitive to medication and during lactation.
- Use cautiously in children and with clients who have dysphagia or liver disease.
- These medications increase the risk for pneumonia. Use cautiously in clients at high risk for pneumonia, such as clients who have COPD.
- Long-term use of proton pump inhibitors increases the risk of osteoporosis.

Interactions

MEDICATION/FOOD INTERACTIONS	NURSING INTERVENTIONS/CLIENT EDUCATION
› Diazepam (Valium), phenytoin (Dilantin), and warfarin (Coumadin) levels can be increased when used concurrently with omeprazole.	› Monitor phenytoin levels carefully if prescribed concurrently.
› Absorption of ketoconazole, itraconazole (Sporanox), and atazanavir (Reyataz) is extremely decreased when taken concurrently with proton pump inhibitors.	› Concurrent use should be avoided. If necessary to administer concurrently, separate medication administration by 2 to 12 hr.

Nursing Administration

- Do not crush, chew, or break sustained-release capsules.
- Clients may sprinkle the contents of the capsule over food to facilitate swallowing.
- Clients should take omeprazole once a day prior to eating in the morning.
- Encourage clients to avoid alcohol and irritating medications such as NSAIDs.
- Active ulcers should be treated for 4 to 6 weeks.
- Pantoprazole (Protonix) can be prescribed intravenously. There can be irritation at the injection site leading to thrombophlebitis. Monitor the IV site for inflammation (redness, swelling, local pain).
- Instruct clients to notify the provider for any indication of obvious or occult GI bleeding, such as coffee-ground emesis.

MEDICATION CLASSIFICATION: MUCOSAL PROTECTANT

- Select Prototype Medication: sucralfate (Carafate)

Purpose

- Expected Pharmacological Action
  - The acidic environment of the stomach and duodenum changes sucralfate into a thick substance that adheres to an ulcer. This protects the ulcer from further injury that can be caused by acid and pepsin.
  - This viscous substance can stick to the ulcer for up to 6 hr.
- Therapeutic Uses
  - Sucralfate is used for clients who have acute duodenal ulcers and those requiring maintenance therapy.
  - Investigational use of sucralfate includes gastric ulcers and GERD.

Complications

- To prevent constipation, encourage clients to increase dietary fiber and drink at least 1,500 mL/day if fluids are not restricted.
- Sucralfate has no systemic effects.

Contraindications/Precautions

- Pregnancy Risk Category B.
- Contraindicated in clients who are hypersensitive to the medication.
- Use cautiously in clients who have chronic kidney disease.

Interactions

MEDICATION/FOOD INTERACTIONS	NURSING INTERVENTIONS/CLIENT EDUCATION
› Sucralfate can interfere with the absorption of phenytoin, digoxin, warfarin, and ciprofloxacin.	› Maintain a 2-hr interval between these medications and sucralfate to minimize this interaction.
› Antacids interfere with the absorption of sucralfate.	› Antacids should not be administered within 30 min of sucralfate.

Nursing Administration

- Assist clients with the medication regimen.
- Instruct clients that sucralfate should be taken four times a day, 1 hr before meals, and again at bedtime.
- Clients can break or dissolve the medication in water, but should not crush or chew the tablet.
- Encourage clients to complete the course of treatment.

MEDICATION CLASSIFICATION: ANTACIDS

- Select Prototype Medication: aluminum hydroxide (Amphojel)
- Other Medications
  - Aluminum carbonate (Basaljel)
  - Magnesium hydroxide (Milk of Magnesia)
  - Sodium bicarbonate
  - Calcium carbonate (Tums)

Purpose

- Expected Pharmacological Action
  - Antacids neutralize gastric acid and inactivate pepsin.
  - Mucosal protection can occur by the antacid's ability to stimulate the production of prostaglandins.
- Therapeutic Uses
  - Antacids are used to treat peptic ulcer disease (PUD) by promoting healing and relieving pain.
  - Antacids provide clients with relief from the manifestations of GERD.

Complications

ADVERSE EFFECTS	NURSING INTERVENTIONS/CLIENT EDUCATION
› Aluminum and calcium compounds cause constipation. Magnesium compounds cause diarrhea.	› Advise clients that use of these compounds can be alternated to offset intestinal effects and normalize bowel function. › If a client has difficulty managing bowel function, recommend a combination product that contains aluminum hydroxide, magnesium hydroxide, and simethicone.
› Antacids containing sodium can result in fluid retention. › Sodium bicarbonate can cause systemic alkalosis in clients who have impaired kidney function.	› Advise clients who have hypertension, heart failure, or impaired kidney function to avoid antacids that contain sodium.
› Aluminum hydroxide can lead to hypophosphatemia and hypomagnesemia.	› Monitor electrolyte levels.
› Magnesium compounds can lead to toxicity in clients who have impaired kidney function.	› Advise clients who have impaired kidney function to avoid antacids that contain magnesium.

Contraindications/Precautions

- Aluminum hydroxide and sodium bicarbonate are Pregnancy Risk Category C medications.
- Antacids should be not administered to clients who have GI perforation or obstruction.
- Use cautiously in clients who have abdominal pain.

Interactions

MEDICATION/FOOD INTERACTIONS	NURSING INTERVENTIONS/CLIENT EDUCATION
› Aluminum compounds bind to warfarin and tetracycline and interfere with absorption.	› Instruct clients to take these medications 1 hr apart.

Nursing Administration

- Clients taking tablets should be instructed to chew the tablets thoroughly and then drink at least 8 oz water or milk.
- Instruct clients to shake liquid formulations to ensure even dispersion of the medication.
- Compliance is difficult for clients because of the frequency of administration. Medication can be administered seven times a day: 1 hr before and 3 hr after meals, and again at bedtime. Encourage compliance by reinforcing the intended effect of the antacid (i.e., relief of pain, healing of ulcer).
- Advise clients to take other medications at least 1 hr before or after taking an antacid.

MEDICATION CLASSIFICATION: PROSTAGLANDIN E ANALOG

- Select Prototype Medication: misoprostol (Cytotec)

Purpose

- Expected Pharmacological Action
  - Prostaglandin E analog acts as an endogenous prostaglandin in the GI tract to decrease acid secretion, increase the secretion of bicarbonate and protective mucus, and promote vasodilation to maintain submucosal blood flow. These actions all serve to prevent gastric ulcers.
- Therapeutic Uses
  - Prostaglandin E analog is used in clients taking long-term NSAIDs to prevent gastric ulcers.
  - Prostaglandin E analog is used in clients who are pregnant to induce labor by causing cervical ripening.

Complications

ADVERSE EFFECTS	NURSING INTERVENTIONS/CLIENT EDUCATION
› Concurrent use of magnesium antacids can increase diarrhea.	› Instruct clients to notify the provider of diarrhea or abdominal pain. › Dosage might need to be reduced.
› Women can experience dysmenorrhea and spotting.	› Instruct clients to notify the provider if dysmenorrhea and spotting occur. › The provider can discontinue the medication. › Advise women of childbearing age to avoid pregnancy while taking misoprostol.

Contraindications/Precautions

- Pregnancy Risk Category X

Nursing Administration

- Advise clients to take misoprostol with meals and at bedtime.

Nursing Evaluation of Medication Effectiveness

- Depending on therapeutic intent, effectiveness can be evidenced by
  - Reduced frequency or absence of GERD manifestations (heartburn, bloating, belching)
  - Absence of GI bleeding
  - Healing of gastric and duodenal ulcers
  - No reoccurrence of ulcer

APPLICATION EXERCISES

1. A nurse is reinforcing teaching for a client who has a prescription for metronidazole (Flagyl) to treat peptic ulcer. The client asks the nurse why this medication has been prescribed. Which of the following responses by the nurse is correct?

    A. "The purpose of this medication is to get rid of the infection from giardiasis."

    B. "The purpose of this medication is to get rid of the infection from *H. pylori.*"

    C. "The purpose of this medication is to increase the pH of gastric juices in the stomach."

    D. "The purpose of this medication is to decrease the pH of gastric juices in the stomach."

2. A nurse is caring for a client who is starting omeprazole (Prilosec) PO for management of GERD. The nurse should recognize that this medication works by

    A. improving gastric motility.

    B. decreasing the production of gastric acid.

    C. neutralizing gastric acid.

    D. antagonizing serotonin receptors.

3. A client taking sucralfate (Carafate) PO for PUD has been started on phenytoin (Dilantin) to control seizures. Which of the following should be included when reinforcing teaching for the client?

    A. Take both of these medications at the same time.

    B. Take sucralfate with a glass of milk.

    C. Allow a 2-hr interval between these medications.

    D. Chew the sucralfate thoroughly before swallowing.

4. For which of the following clients who have PUD is misoprostol (Cytotec) contraindicated?

    A. 27-year-old client who is pregnant

    B. 75-year-old client who has osteoarthritis

    C. 37-year-old client who has a kidney stone

    D. 46-year-old client who has a urinary tract infection

5. A nurse is reinforcing teaching for a client who has peptic ulcer disease about managing his condition. Which of the following instructions should the nurse include? (Select all that apply.)

_____ A. "Eat six small meals a day."

_____ B. "Drink milk to aid in healing your ulcer."

_____ C. "Low-dose aspirin therapy should be avoided."

_____ D. "Seek measures to reduce stress."

_____ E. "Avoid smoking."

6. A nurse is caring for a female client who has a prescription for aluminum hydroxide (Amphojel) suspension to treat peptic ulcer disease (PUD). Use the ATI Active Learning Template: Medication to complete this item to include the following sections:

A. Therapeutic Uses: Identify the therapeutic use of aluminum hydroxide.

B. Client Education: Identify three instructions the nurse should reinforce regarding taking this medication.

APPLICATION EXERCISES KEY

1. A. INCORRECT: Although metronidazole is used to treat giardiasis, this is not the reason this medication has been prescribed for this client.

    B. **CORRECT:** *H. pylori* is a gram-negative organism that can reside in the client's stomach and duodenum. Metronidazole and other antibiotics are used to eradicate *H. pylori*, which greatly reduces the recurrence of peptic ulcer disease.

    C. INCORRECT: Metronidazole does not increase the pH of the gastric juices in the stomach.

    D. INCORRECT: Metronidazole does not decrease the pH of the gastric juices in the stomach.

    (N) NCLEX® Connection: Pharmacological Therapies, Expected Actions/Outcomes

2. A. INCORRECT: Gastric motility is improved by metoclopramide (Reglan), a prokinetic agent.

    B. **CORRECT:** Omeprazole reduces gastric acid secretion by inhibiting the enzyme that produces gastric acid.

    C. INCORRECT: Gastric acid is neutralized by aluminum hydroxide, an antacid.

    D. INCORRECT: Ondansetron (Zofran), an antiemetic, antagonizes serotonin receptors, decreasing nausea and vomiting.

    (N) NCLEX® Connection: Pharmacological Therapies, Expected Actions/Outcomes

3. A. INCORRECT: Sucralfate can interfere with the absorption of phenytoin, so the client should allow a 2-hr interval between the sucralfate and phenytoin.

    B. INCORRECT: Sucralfate should be taken on an empty stomach.

    C. **CORRECT:** Sucralfate can interfere with the absorption of phenytoin, so the client should allow a 2-hr interval between the sucralfate and phenytoin.

    D. INCORRECT: Sucralfate should be swallowed whole.

    (N) NCLEX® Connection: Pharmacological Therapies, Medication Administration

4. A. **CORRECT:** Misoprostol can induce labor, and therefore is contraindicated in pregnancy.

    B. INCORRECT: There are no contraindications for use in clients who have osteoarthritis.

    C. INCORRECT: There are no contraindications for use in clients who have kidney stones.

    D. INCORRECT: There are no contraindications for use in clients who have urinary tract infections.

    Ⓝ NCLEX® Connection: Pharmacological Therapies, Adverse Effects/Contraindications/
    Side Effects/Interactions

5. A. INCORRECT: Eating six small meals a day can stimulate production of gastric acid and delay
    healing of the ulcer.

    B. INCORRECT: The client should avoid excessive intake of milk and cream, which can stimulate
    production of gastric acid and delay healing of the ulcer.

    C. INCORRECT: Although frequent use of NSAIDs can decrease prostaglandin production resulting in
    injury to gastric tissue, low-dose aspirin therapy is permitted.

    D. **CORRECT:** Reducing stress is beneficial for healing of the ulcer and prevention of complications.

    E. **CORRECT:** Smoking inhibits healing of the ulcer.

    Ⓝ NCLEX® Connection: Pharmacological Therapies, Expected Actions/Outcomes

6. *Using the ATI Active Learning Template: Medication*

    A. Therapeutic Uses
    - Aluminum hydroxide raises the pH of gastric contents, which reduces irritation of stomach
      mucosa, resulting in relief of pain.

    B. Client Education
    - Aluminum hydroxide is a Pregnancy Risk Category C medication. Discontinue use and notify
      your provider if you become pregnant.
    - Shake the medication prior to taking each dose in order to disperse the medication.
    - Take other medications at least 1 hr before or 3 hr after taking aluminum hydroxide.
    - Aluminum hydroxide can cause constipation. Notify your provider if it persists. You might need
      to alternate this antacid with one that has diarrhea as an adverse effect.
    - Continue to take the medication even after you no longer have manifestations so that the ulcer
      will continue to heal.
    - The medication is prescribed at frequent dosing intervals to promote healing of the ulcer. Seven
      times a day, 1 hr before, 3 hr after meals, and at bedtime is a common dosing schedule.

    Ⓝ NCLEX® Connection: Pharmacological Therapies, Expected Actions/Outcomes

chapter 25

Overview

- The medications in this section affect some aspect of the gastrointestinal tract to treat or prevent nausea, vomiting, motion sickness, diarrhea, constipation, or to treat GERD by increasing gastric motility.

- Medications include antiemetics, laxatives, antidiarrheals, prokinetic agents, and medications for irritable bowel syndrome (IBS).

- Many medications used to treat cancer often cause chemotherapy-induced nausea and vomiting (CIVN). To prevent CIVN, antiemetics are administered before chemotherapy. A single medication or a combination of medications may be used according to need.

MEDICATION CLASSIFICATION: ANTIEMETICS

- Select Prototype Medications
  - Glucocorticoids: dexamethasone
  - Substance P/neurokinin$_1$ antagonists: aprepitant (Emend)
  - Serotonin antagonists: ondansetron (Zofran), granisetron (Kytril)
  - Dopamine antagonists: prochlorperazine, metoclopramide (Reglan)
  - Cannabinoids: dronabinol (Marinol)
  - Anticholinergics: scopolamine (Transderm Scop)
  - Antihistamines: dimenhydrinate, hydroxyzine (Vistaril)
  - Benzodiazepines: lorazepam (Ativan)

Purpose

EXPECTED PHARMACOLOGICAL ACTION	THERAPEUTIC USES
Glucocorticoids: dexamethasone, methylprednisolone (Solu-Medrol)	
› The antiemetic mechanism of dexamethasone is unknown.	› Dexamethasone and methylprednisolone usually are used in combination with other antiemetics to treat chemotherapy-induced nausea and vomiting (CINV). › Administer IV.
Substance P/neurokinin₁ antagonists: aprepitant, fosaprepitant	
› Aprepitant inhibits substance P/neurokinin₁ in the brain.	› For best results, it should be used in combination with a glucocorticoid or serotonin antagonist to prevent postoperative nausea, vomiting, and CINV. › Extended duration of action makes it effective for acute use and delayed response with CINV. › Administer PO or IV.
Serotonin antagonist: ondansetron	
› Ondansetron prevents emesis by blocking the serotonin receptors in the chemoreceptor trigger zone (CTZ), and antagonizing the serotonin receptors on the afferent vagal neurons that travel from the upper GI tract to the CTZ.	› Ondansetron prevents emesis related to chemotherapy, radiation therapy, and postoperative recovery. › Administer PO or IV.
Dopamine antagonists: prochlorperazine (a subset of phenothiazine)	
› Antiemetic effects of prochlorperazine result from blockade of dopamine receptors in the CTZ.	› Prochlorperazine prevents emesis related to chemotherapy, opioids, and postoperative recovery. › Administer PO or IV.
Cannabinoids: dronabinol	
› Antiemetic mechanism of dronabinol is unknown.	› Dronabinol is used to control CINV and to increase appetite in clients who have AIDS. › Administer PO.
Anticholinergic: scopolamine	
› Scopolamine interferes with the transmission of nerve impulses traveling from the vestibular apparatus of the inner ear to the vomiting center (VC) in the brain.	› Scopolamine treats motion sickness. › Administer topical, PO, or subcutaneously.
Antihistamines: dimenhydrinate	
› Muscarinic and histaminergic receptors in nerve pathways that connect the inner ear and VC are blocked by dimenhydrinate.	› Dimenhydrinate treats motion sickness. › Administer PO, IM, or IV.
Benzodiazepines: lorazepam	
› Lorazepam depresses nerve function at multiple CNS sites.	› It is used in combination with other medications to suppress CINV.

Complications

ADVERSE EFFECTS	NURSING INTERVENTIONS/CLIENT EDUCATION
Substance P/neurokinin1 antagonist: aprepitant	
› Fatigue, diarrhea, dizziness, possible liver damage	› Treat headache with nonopioid analgesics. › Monitor stool pattern.
Serotonin antagonist: ondansetron	
› Headache, diarrhea, dizziness	› Treat headache with nonopioid analgesics. › Monitor stool pattern.
Dopamine antagonists: prochlorperazine	
› Extrapyramidal symptoms (EPS)	› Inform clients of possible adverse effects (restlessness, anxiety, spasms of face and neck). › Advise clients to stop the medication and inform the provider if EPSs occur. › Administer an anticholinergic medication, such as diphenhydramine or benztropine (Cogentin), to treat manifestations.
› Hypotension	› Monitor clients receiving antihypertensive medications for low blood pressure.
› Sedation	› Inform clients of the potential for sedation. › Advise clients to avoid activities that require alertness, such as driving.
› Anticholinergic effects (dry mouth, urinary retention, constipation)	› Instruct clients to increase fluid intake. › Instruct clients to increase physical activity by engaging in regular exercise. › Tell clients to suck on hard candy or chew gum to help relieve dry mouth. › Administer a stimulant laxative such as senna (Senokot) to counteract a decrease in bowel motility, or stool softeners such as docusate sodium (Colace) to prevent constipation. › Advise clients to void every 4 hr. Monitor I&O and palpate the lower abdomen area every 4 to 6 hr to assess the bladder.
Cannabinoids: dronabinol	
› Potential for dissociation, dysphoria › Abuse potential: mimic subjective effects of marijuana	› Avoid using in clients who have mental health disorders.
› Hypotension, tachycardia	› Use cautiously in clients who have cardiovascular disorders.
› Drowsiness	› Do not combine with alcohol, sedatives, or CNS depressants.
Anticholinergics: scopolamine and antihistamines: dimenhydrinate	
› Sedation	› Inform clients of the potential for sedation. › Advise clients to avoid activities that require alertness, such as driving.
› Anticholinergic effects (dry mouth, urinary retention, constipation)	› Instruct clients to increase fluid intake. › Instruct clients to increase physical activity by engaging in regular exercise. › Tell clients to suck on hard candy or chew gum to help relieve dry mouth. › Administer a stimulant laxative such as senna to counteract a decrease in bowel motility, or stool softeners such as docusate sodium to prevent constipation. › Advise clients to void every 4 hr. Monitor I&O, and palpate the lower abdomen area every 4 to 6 hr to assess the bladder.

Contraindications/Precautions

- Ondansetron should not be given to clients who have long QT syndrome.

- Use dopamine antagonists cautiously, if at all, with children and older adults due to the increased risk of EPSs.

- Dopamine antagonists, antihistamines, and anticholinergic antiemetics should be used cautiously in clients who have urinary retention or obstruction, asthma, and narrow angle glaucoma.

- Aprepitant should be used cautiously in children, and clients who have severe liver and kidney disease.

- Promethazine is contraindicated in children under 2 years old and should be used with extreme caution in older children.

Interactions

MEDICATION/FOOD INTERACTIONS	NURSING INTERVENTIONS/CLIENT EDUCATION
› CNS depressants, such as opioids and alcohol, can intensify CNS depression of antiemetics.	› Advise clients that CNS depression is more likely and to avoid activities that require mental alertness.
› Concurrent use of antihypertensives can intensify hypotensive effects of antiemetics.	› Advise clients to sit or lie down if lightheadedness or dizziness occur. Clients should avoid sudden changes in position by moving slowly from a lying to a sitting or standing position. › Provide assistance with ambulation as needed.
› Concurrent use of anticholinergic medications (antihistamines) can intensify anticholinergic effects of antiemetics.	› Provide teaching to reduce anticholinergic effects (sipping on fluids, use of laxatives, voiding on a regular basis).

Nursing Administration

- Antiemetics prevent or treat nausea and vomiting from various causes. Nursing assessment can identify the underlying related factors and verify that the appropriate medication is used.

- When a client is receiving a chemotherapy agent that causes severe nausea, combining three antiemetics and administering them prior to chemotherapy is more effective than treating nausea that is already occurring.

Nursing Evaluation of Medication Effectiveness

- Depending on therapeutic intent, effectiveness can be evidenced by absence of nausea and vomiting.

MEDICATION CLASSIFICATION: LAXATIVES

- Select Prototype Medications
  - Psyllium (Metamucil)
  - Docusate sodium (Colace)
  - Bisacodyl (Dulcolax)
  - Magnesium hydroxide (Milk of Magnesia)
- Other Medications: senna (Senokot), lactulose (Cephulac)

Purpose

EXPECTED PHARMACOLOGICAL ACTION	THERAPEUTIC USES
Bulk-forming laxatives: psyllium	
› Bulk-forming laxatives soften fecal mass and increase bulk, which is identical to the action of dietary fiber.	› Decrease diarrhea in clients who have diverticulosis and IBS › Control stool for clients who have an ileostomy or colostomy › Promote defecation in older adults with decrease in peristalsis due to age-related changes in the GI tract
Surfactant laxatives: docusate sodium	
› Surfactant laxatives lower surface tension of the stool to allow penetration of water. › Can act on intestinal wall to inhibit fluid absorption out of intestine and stimulate secretion of water and electrolytes into intestine.	› Relieve constipation related to pregnancy or opioid use › Prevent painful elimination in clients who have conditions such as hemorrhoids or following a procedure such as episiotomy › Prevent straining in clients who have conditions such as cerebral aneurysm or post-MI › Decrease the risk of fecal impaction in immobile clients and promote defecation in older adults with decreased peristalsis due to age-related changes in the GI tract
Stimulant laxatives: bisacodyl	
› Stimulant laxatives have two effects on the bowel: stimulation of intestinal peristalsis and increase the amount of water and electrolytes within the intestinal lumen.	› Prepare client prior to surgery or diagnostic tests such as a colonoscopy › Short-term treatment of constipation caused by high-dose opioid use
Osmotic laxatives: magnesium hydroxide	
› Osmotic laxatives draw water into the intestine to increase the mass of stool, stretching musculature, which results in peristalsis.	› Low dose – Prevent painful elimination (clients who have episiotomy or hemorrhoids) › High dose – Client preparation prior to surgery or diagnostic tests such as a colonoscopy › Rapid evacuation of the bowel after ingestion of poisons or following anthelmintic therapy to rid the body of dead parasites

Complications

ADVERSE EFFECTS	NURSING INTERVENTIONS/CLIENT EDUCATION
› GI irritation	› Instruct clients not to crush or chew enteric-coated tablets.
› Rectal burning sensation, leading to proctitis	› Discourage clients from using bisacodyl suppositories on a regular basis.
› Laxatives with magnesium salts, such as magnesium hydroxide, can lead to accumulation of toxic levels of magnesium.	› Advise clients who have renal dysfunction to read labels carefully and to avoid laxatives that contain magnesium.
› Laxatives with sodium salts, such as sodium phosphate, place clients at risk for sodium absorption and fluid retention.	› Advise clients who have heart disease to read labels carefully and to avoid laxatives that contain sodium.
› Osmotic diuretics may cause dehydration.	› Monitor I&O. › Monitor for manifestations of dehydration, such as poor skin turgor. › Encourage clients to increase water intake to at least 8 to 10 glasses/day.
› Chronic use of laxatives can diminish defecatory reflexes, leading to further reliance on laxatives with possible severe pathologic changes in the bowel.	› Clients should be advised that if a laxative must be used, it should be used briefly and in the smallest effective dose.

Contraindications/Precautions

- Laxatives are contraindicated in clients who have fecal impaction, bowel obstruction, and acute surgical abdomen to prevent perforation.
- Laxatives are contraindicated in clients who have nausea, cramping, and abdominal pain.
- Laxatives, with the exception of bulk-forming laxatives, are contraindicated in clients who have ulcerative colitis and diverticulitis.
- Use cautiously during pregnancy and lactation. Bisacodyl and docusate are Pregnancy Risk Category C.

Interactions

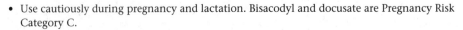

MEDICATION/FOOD INTERACTIONS	NURSING INTERVENTIONS/CLIENT EDUCATION
› Milk and antacids can destroy enteric coating of bisacodyl.	› Instruct clients to take bisacodyl at least 1 hr apart from these medications.

Nursing Administration

- Obtain a complete history of laxative use, and provide teaching as appropriate.
- Teach clients that chronic laxative use can lead to fluid and electrolyte imbalances.
- To promote defecation and resumption of normal bowel function, instruct clients to increase high-fiber foods, such as bran, fresh fruits and vegetables, in the diet and to increase amounts of fluids. Recommend at least 2 to 3 L/day from beverages and food sources.
- Encourage clients to maintain a regular exercise regimen to improve bowel function.
- Instruct clients to take bulk-forming and surfactant laxatives with a glass of water.

Nursing Evaluation of Medication Effectiveness

- Depending on therapeutic intent, effectiveness can be evidenced by:
  - Return to regular bowel function.
  - Evacuation of bowel in preparation for surgery or diagnostic tests.

MEDICATION CLASSIFICATION: ANTIDIARRHEALS

- Select Prototype Medication: diphenoxylate plus atropine (Lomotil)
- Other Medications: loperamide (Imodium), paregoric (Camphorated Tincture of Opium)

Purpose

- Expected Pharmacological Action
  - Antidiarrheals activate opioid receptors in the GI tract to decrease intestinal motility and to increase the absorption of fluid and sodium in the intestine.
- Therapeutic Uses
  - Specific antidiarrheal agents may be used to treat the underlying cause of diarrhea. For example, antibiotics may be used to treat diarrhea caused by a bacterial infection.
  - Nonspecific antidiarrheal agents provide symptomatic treatment of diarrhea (decrease in frequency and fluid content of stool).

Complications

- At recommended doses for diarrhea, diphenoxylate does not affect the CNS system.
- At high doses, clients can experience typical opioid effects, such as euphoria or CNS depression. However, the addition of atropine, which has unpleasant adverse effects (blurred vision, dry mouth, urinary retention, constipation, tachycardia) in diphenoxylate discourages ingestion of doses higher than those prescribed.

Contraindications/Precautions

- There is an increased risk of megacolon in clients who have inflammatory bowel disorders. This could lead to a serious complication, such as perforation of the bowel.

- Diphenoxylate is contraindicated in severe electrolyte imbalance or dehydration. It is a Controlled Substance Category V medication.

- Paregoric is contraindicated in clients who have COPD.

- Antidiarrheals are Pregnancy Risk Category C medications.

Interactions

- Alcohol or other CNS depressants can enhance CNS depression.

Nursing Administration

- Administer initial dose of diphenoxylate 4 mg. Follow each loose stool with additional dose of 2 mg, but do not exceed 16 mg/day.

- Loperamide is an analog of the opioid meperidine. This medication is not a controlled substance, and at high doses does not mimic morphine-like symptoms.

- Advise clients who have diarrhea to drink small amounts of clear liquids or a commercial oral electrolyte solution to maintain electrolyte balance for the first 24 hr.

- Advise clients to avoid drinking plain water because it does not contain necessary electrolytes that have been lost in the stool.

- Advise clients to avoid caffeine. Caffeine exacerbates diarrhea by increasing GI motility.

- Clients who have severe cases of diarrhea may be hospitalized for management of dehydration.

- Management of dehydration should include monitoring of weight, I&O, and vital signs. A hypotonic solution, such as 0.45% sodium chloride, may be prescribed.

Nursing Evaluation of Medication Effectiveness

- Depending on therapeutic intent, effectiveness can be evidenced by return of normal bowel pattern as evidenced by decrease in frequency and fluid volume of stool.

MEDICATION CLASSIFICATION: PROKINETIC AGENTS

- Select Prototype Medication: metoclopramide (Reglan)

Purpose

- Expected Pharmacological Action
  - ○ Metoclopramide controls nausea and vomiting by blocking dopamine and serotonin receptors in the CTZ.
  - ○ Metoclopramide augments action of acetylcholine, which causes an increase in upper GI motility.
- Therapeutic Uses
  - ○ Control of postoperative and chemotherapy-induced nausea and vomiting as well as facilitation of intubation and examination of the GI tract.
  - ○ Oral form is used for diabetic gastroparesis and management of GERD.

Complications

ADVERSE EFFECTS	NURSING INTERVENTIONS/CLIENT EDUCATION
› Extrapyramidal symptoms (EPS)	› Inform clients of the possible adverse effects, such as restlessness, anxiety, and spasms of face and neck.
	› Administer an antihistamine, such as diphenhydramine, to minimize EPSs.
› Sedation	› Inform clients of the potential for sedation.
	› Advise clients to avoid activities that require alertness, such as driving.
› Diarrhea	› Monitor bowel function and for manifestations of dehydration.

Contraindications/Precautions

- Contraindicated in clients who have GI perforation, GI bleeding, bowel obstruction, and hemorrhage.
- Contraindicated in clients who have a seizure disorder due to increased risk of seizures.

- Use cautiously in children and older adults due to the increase risk for EPSs.

Interactions

MEDICATION/FOOD INTERACTIONS	NURSING INTERVENTIONS/CLIENT EDUCATION
› Concurrent use of alcohol and other CNS depressants increases the risk of seizures and sedation.	› Advise clients to avoid the use of alcohol.
	› Use cautiously with other CNS depressants.
› Opioids and anticholinergics decrease the effects of metoclopramide.	› Advise clients to avoid using opioids and medications with anticholinergic effects.

Nursing Administration

- Monitor clients for CNS depression and EPSs.

- The medication can be given orally or intravenously. If IV dose 10 mg or less, it may be administered IVP undiluted over 2 min. If the dose is greater than 10 mg, it should be diluted and infused over 15 min. Dilute medication in at least 50 mL of dextrose 5% in water or lactated Ringer's.

Nursing Evaluation of Medication Effectiveness

- Depending on therapeutic intent, effectiveness can be evidenced by absence of nausea and vomiting.

MEDICATION CLASSIFICATION: MEDICATIONS FOR IRRITABLE BOWEL SYNDROME WITH DIARRHEA (IBS-D)

- Select Prototype Medication: alosetron (Lotronex)

Purpose

- Expected Pharmacological Action

  ○ Selective blockade of 5-HT3 receptors, which innervate the viscera and result in increased firmness in stool and decrease in urgency and frequency of defecation.

- Therapeutic Uses

  ○ Approved only for female clients who have severe IBS-D that has lasted more than 6 months and has been resistant to conventional management.

Complications

ADVERSE EFFECTS	NURSING INTERVENTIONS/CLIENT EDUCATION
› Constipation, which can result in GI toxicity such as ischemic colitis, bowel obstruction, impaction, or perforation	› Only clients who meet specific criteria and are willing to sign a treatment agreement may be prescribed medication. › Instruct clients to watch for rectal bleeding, bloody diarrhea, or abdominal pain and report to the provider. Medication should be discontinued.

Contraindications/Precautions

- Contraindicated for clients who have chronic constipation, history of bowel obstruction, Crohn's disease, ulcerative colitis, impaired intestinal circulation, thrombophlebitis, diverticulitis, toxic megacolon, and GI adhesions.

Interactions

MEDICATION/FOOD INTERACTIONS	NURSING INTERVENTIONS/CLIENT EDUCATION
› Medications that induce cytochrome P450 enzymes, such as phenobarbital, can decrease levels of alosetron.	› Monitor effectiveness of the medication.

Nursing Administration

- Instruct clients that symptoms should decline within 1 to 4 weeks but will return 1 week after medication is discontinued.
- Dosage will start as once a day and may be increased to twice daily.

Nursing Evaluation of Medication Effectiveness

- Depending on therapeutic intent, effectiveness can be evidenced by relief of diarrhea, and decrease in urgency and frequency of defecation.

MEDICATION CLASSIFICATION: MEDICATIONS FOR IRRITABLE BOWEL SYNDROME WITH CONSTIPATION (IBS-C)

- Select Prototype Medication: lubiprostone (Amitiza)

Purpose

- Expected Pharmacological Action
  - Increases fluid secretion in the intestine to promote intestinal motility
- Therapeutic Uses
  - Irritable bowel syndrome with constipation in women age 18 and older
  - Chronic constipation

Complications

ADVERSE EFFECTS	NURSING INTERVENTIONS/CLIENT EDUCATION
› Diarrhea	› Monitor frequency of stools. Notify the provider if severe diarrhea occurs.
› Nausea	› Instruct clients to take the medication with food.

Contraindications/Precautions

- Pregnancy Risk Category C
- Contraindicated for clients who have a history of bowel obstruction, Crohn's disease, ulcerative colitis, or diverticulitis

Interactions

- No significant interactions

Nursing Administration

- Instruct clients to take the medication with food to decrease nausea.
- Oral dosage should be taken twice a day.

Nursing Evaluation of Medication Effectiveness

- Depending on therapeutic intent, effectiveness can be evidenced by relief of constipation.

MEDICATION CLASSIFICATION: 5-AMINOSALICYLATES

- Select Prototype Medication: sulfasalazine (Azulfidine)
- Other Medications for IBS
    - 5-aminosalicylates: mesalamine (Asacol, Rowasa), olsalazine (Dipentum)
    - Glucocorticoids: hydrocortisone
    - Immunosuppressants: azathioprine (Imuran)
    - Immunomodulators: infliximab (Remicade)
    - Antibiotics: metronidazole (Flagyl)

Purpose

- Expected Pharmacological Action
    - Decrease inflammation by inhibiting prostaglandin synthesis
- Therapeutic Uses
    - IBS, Crohn's disease, ulcerative colitis.
    - IBS is controlled, rather than cured, by these medications, which often are used in combination therapy.

Complications

ADVERSE EFFECTS	NURSING INTERVENTIONS/CLIENT EDUCATION
› Blood disorders including agranulocytosis, and hemolytic and macrocytic anemia	› Monitor complete blood count.
› Nausea, cramps, rash, arthralgia	› Notify provider if manifestations persist.

Contraindications/Precautions

- Women who are pregnant, plan to become pregnant, or who are breastfeeding should consult their provider about continued use of sulfasalazine.

- 5-aminosalicylates are contraindicated in clients who have sensitivity to sulfonamides, salicylates, or thiazide diuretics.

 • Use cautiously in older adults and in clients who have liver or kidney disease or blood dyscrasias.

Interactions

- Iron and antibiotics can alter the absorption of sulfasalazine.

- Mesalamine can decrease the absorption of digoxin.

Nursing Administration

- Ensure that controlled-release and enteric-coated forms of the medications are not crushed or chewed.

Nursing Evaluation of Medication Effectiveness

- Depending on therapeutic intent, effectiveness can be evidenced by:
  - Decreased bowel inflammation and relief of GI distress.
  - Return to normal bowel function.

MEDICATION CLASSIFICATION: PROBIOTICS – DIETARY SUPPLEMENTS

Purpose

- Expected Pharmacological Action
  - Various preparations of bacteria and yeast, which are normal flora of the gut, help to metabolize foods, promote nutrient absorption, and reduce colonization by pathogenic bacteria. They also can increase nonspecific cellular and humoral immunity.

- Therapeutic Use
  - Probiotics are used to treat the symptoms of IBS, ulcerative colitis, and *Clostridium difficile*-associated diarrhea (CDAD), and can help treat rotavirus diarrhea in children.

Complications

- Adverse Effects – flatulence and bloating

Interactions

- If antibiotics or antifungals are used concurrently, they should be administered at least 2 hr apart from the probiotics.

APPLICATION EXERCISES

1. A nurse is caring for a client who was administered prochlorperazine 4 hr ago. The client reports spasms of his face. The nurse should anticipate a prescription for which of the following medications?

    A. Fomepizole (Antizol)

    B. Naloxone

    C. Phytonadione (vitamin K_1)

    D. Diphenhydramine

2. A nurse is providing instruction to a client who has a new prescription for ondansetron (Zofran). The nurse should advise the client that which of the following is an adverse effect of the medication?

    A. Headache

    B. Urinary retention

    C. Tachycardia

    D. Black stools

3. A nurse is providing instructions about the use of laxatives to a client who has heart failure. The nurse should tell the client he should avoid which of the following laxatives?

    A. Sodium phosphate (Fleet Phospho-Soda)

    B. Psyllium (Metamucil)

    C. Bisacodyl (Dulcolax)

    D. Polyethylene glycol (MiraLAX)

4. A nurse is taking a history for a female client who has irritable bowel syndrome with constipation. Which of the following in the client's history is a contraindication to lubiprostone (Amitiza)?

    A. Myocardial infarction

    B. Crohn's disease

    C. Diabetes mellitus

    D. Rheumatoid arthritis

5. A nurse is providing information about probiotic supplements to a male client. Which of the following information should the nurse include? (Select all that apply.)

_____ A. "Probiotics are micro-organisms that are normally found in the GI tract."

_____ B. "Probiotics are used to treat *Clostridium difficile.*"

_____ C. "Probiotics are used to treat benign prostatic hyperplasia."

_____ D. "You may experience bloating while taking probiotic supplements."

_____ E. "If you are prescribed an antibiotic, you should take it at the same time you take your probiotic supplement."

6. A nurse is caring for a client who has a prescription for sulfasalazine (Azulfidine). Use the ATI Active Learning Template: Medication to complete this item to include the following sections:

A. Therapeutic Uses: Identify two therapeutic uses for sulfasalazine.

B. Adverse Effects: Identify two blood disorders that occur as a complication with the use of sulfasalazine.

C. Nursing Administration: Identify how frequently the client should take the medication.

APPLICATION EXERCISES KEY

1.   A.   INCORRECT: Fomepizole is an antidote used to treat ethylene glycol poisoning.

     B.   INCORRECT: Naloxone is used to treat opioid overdose.

     C.   INCORRECT: Vitamin K$_1$ is used to treat warfarin overdose.

     D.   **CORRECT:** An adverse effect of prochlorperazine is acute dystonia, which is evidenced by spasms of the muscles in the face, neck, and tongue. Diphenhydramine is used to suppress extrapyramidal effects of prochlorperazine.

     Ⓝ   NCLEX® Connection: Pharmacological Therapies, Adverse Effects/Contraindications/ Side Effects/Interactions

2.   A.   **CORRECT:** Headache is a common adverse effect of ondansetron. The client can require a nonopioid analgesic to treat the headache.

     B.   INCORRECT: Urinary retention is a common adverse effect of anticholinergics, such as scopolamine.

     C.   INCORRECT: Tachycardia is a common adverse effect of cannabinoids, such as dronabinol.

     D.   INCORRECT: Black stools occur when a client takes bismuth (Pepto-Bismol).

     Ⓝ   NCLEX® Connection: Pharmacological Therapies, Adverse Effects/Contraindications/ Side Effects/Interactions

3.   A.   **CORRECT:** Typically, clients who have heart failure are on a sodium-restricted diet. Absorption of sodium from sodium phosphate causes fluid retention and is contraindicated for clients who have heart failure.

     B.   INCORRECT: Psyllium is not absorbed by the intestine and is not contraindicated for clients who have heart failure.

     C.   INCORRECT: Bisacodyl does not appear to have systemic effects and is not contraindicated for clients who have heart failure.

     D.   INCORRECT: Polyethylene glycol is contraindicated in a number of GI conditions, but it is not contraindicated for clients who have heart failure.

     Ⓝ   NCLEX® Connection: Pharmacological Therapies, Adverse Effects/Contraindications/ Side Effects/Interactions

4.   A. INCORRECT: Lubiprostone is not contraindicated for a client who has a history of myocardial infarction.

   B. **CORRECT:** Lubiprostone enhances intestinal motility and is therefore contraindicated in clients who have Crohn's disease.

   C. INCORRECT: Lubiprostone is not contraindicated for a client who has diabetes mellitus.

   D. INCORRECT: Lubiprostone is not contraindicated for a client who has rheumatoid arthritis.

   Ⓝ NCLEX® Connection: Pharmacological Therapies, Adverse Effects/Contraindications/ Side Effects/Interactions

5.   A. **CORRECT:** Probiotics consist of lactobacilli, bifidobacteria, and *Saccharomyces boulardii*, which normally are found in the digestive tract.

   B. **CORRECT:** Probiotics are used to treat a number of GI conditions, including irritable bowel syndrome, diarrhea associated with *Clostridium difficile*, and ulcerative colitis.

   C. INCORRECT: Saw palmetto is used to treat benign prostatic hyperplasia.

   D. **CORRECT:** Flatulence and bloating are adverse effects of probiotic supplements.

   E. INCORRECT: The client should take the probiotic supplement at least 2 hr after taking an antibiotic or antifungal medication. Antibiotics and antifungal medications destroy bacteria and yeast found in probiotic supplements.

   Ⓝ NCLEX® Connection: Pharmacological Therapies, Expected Actions/Outcomes

6.   *Using the ATI Active Learning Template: Medication*

   A. Therapeutic Uses
      • Crohn's disease and ulcerative colitis.

   B. Adverse Effects
      • Complications that occur with the use of sulfasalazine include agranulocytosis, and hemolytic and macrocytic anemia.

   C. Nursing Administration
      • The client should take sulfasalazine four times per day in divided doses.

   Ⓝ NCLEX® Connection: Pharmacological Therapies, Expected Actions/Outcomes

chapter 26

Overview

- The vitamins and minerals described in this section affect production of red blood cells (RBCs) and help prevent various types of anemia.
- Potassium and magnesium help regulate nerve transmission and muscle contractility. Supplements of these substances prevent multiple serious conditions.
- Categories of medications in this section
  - Vitamins, including vitamin B_{12} and folic acid
  - Iron supplements
  - Potassium and magnesium supplements
  - Various herbal supplements

MEDICATION CLASSIFICATION: IRON PREPARATIONS

- Select Prototype Medications
  - Oral: ferrous sulfate (Feosol, Slow FE)
  - Parenteral: iron dextran (INFeD, DexFerrum)
- Other Medications
  - Oral: ferrous gluconate (Fergon), ferrous fumarate (Feostat, Femiron)
  - Parenteral: ferumoxytol (Feraheme), iron sucrose (Venofer), sodium-ferric gluconate complex (SFGC) (Ferrlecit)

Purpose

- Expected Pharmacological Action
  - Iron preparations provide iron needed for RBC development and oxygen transport to cells. During times of increased growth (in growing children or during pregnancy) or when RBCs are in high demand (after blood loss), the need for iron can be greatly increased. Iron is poorly absorbed by the body, so relatively large amounts must be ingested orally to increase Hgb and Hct levels.
- Therapeutic Uses
  - Iron preparations are used to treat iron-deficiency anemia.
    - Ferumoxytol is limited to clients who have chronic kidney disease, regardless of whether on dialysis or administered erythropoietin.
    - Iron sucrose and SFGC are used solely for clients who are undergoing long-term hemodialysis and are deficient in iron.
  - Iron preparations are used to prevent iron deficiency anemia for clients who are at an increased risk, such as pregnant women, infants, and children.
  - Parenteral forms should be used only in clients who are unable to take oral medications, in which case the IV route is preferred.

Complications

ADVERSE EFFECTS	NURSING INTERVENTIONS/CLIENT EDUCATION
› GI distress (nausea, constipation, heartburn)	› If intolerable, administer medication with food, but this greatly reduces absorption. › May need to reduce dosage. › Monitor bowel pattern and intervene as appropriate. This adverse effect usually resolves with continued use.
› Teeth staining (liquid form)	› Advise clients to dilute liquid iron with water or juice, drink with a straw, and rinse mouth after swallowing.
› Staining of skin and other tissues with IM injections	› Give IM doses deep IM using Z-track technique. › Avoid this route if possible.
› Anaphylaxis risk with parenteral administration of iron dextran. › Anaphylaxis is triggered by the dextran in iron dextran, not by the iron. › Anaphylaxis is minimal with SFGC, iron sucrose, and ferumoxytol.	› IV route is safer than IM. › If IM iron dextran is prescribed, administer a test dose and observe the client closely. › Be prepared with life-support equipment.
› Hypotension, which can progress to circulatory collapse with parenteral administration	› Monitor vital signs when administering parenteral iron.
› Fatal iron toxicity in children can occur when an overdose of iron (2 to 10 g) is ingested.	› Indications of toxicity include severe GI distress, shock, acidosis, and liver and heart failure. The chelating agent deferoxamine (Desferal), given parenterally, is used to treat toxicity. › Avoid combining oral iron when administering parenteral iron.

Contraindications/Precautions

- Contraindicated for clients who have
  - Previous hypersensitivity to iron
  - Hemolytic anemia, peptic ulcer disease, and severe liver disease

Interactions

MEDICATION/FOOD INTERACTIONS	NURSING INTERVENTIONS/CLIENT EDUCATION
› Coadministration of antacids or tetracyclines reduces absorption of iron.	› Separate use by at least 2 hr.
› Vitamin C increases absorption, but also increases incidence of GI complications.	› Avoid vitamin C intake when taking medication if GI upset occurs.

Patient-Centered Care

- Instruct clients to take iron on an empty stomach, such as 1 hr before meals, to maximize absorption. Stomach acid increases absorption.

- Instruct clients to take iron with food if GI adverse effects occur. This can increase adherence to therapy even though absorption is also decreased.

- Instruct clients to space doses at approximately equal intervals throughout day to most efficiently increase RBC production. Inform clients to anticipate a harmless dark-green or black color of stool.

- Advise clients to dilute liquid iron with water or juice, drink with a straw, and rinse the mouth after swallowing.

- Instruct clients to increase water and fiber intake (unless contraindicated) and to maintain an exercise program to counter the constipation effects.

- Advise clients that therapy can last 1 to 2 months. Usually, dietary intake will be sufficient after Hgb has returned to an appropriate level.

- Encourage concurrent intake of appropriate quantities of foods high in iron (liver, egg yolks, muscle meats, yeast, grains, green leafy vegetables).

Nursing Evaluation of Medication Effectiveness

- Depending on therapeutic intent, effectiveness can be evidenced by
  - Increased reticulocyte count is expected at least 1 week after beginning iron therapy.
  - Increase in hemoglobin of 2 g/dL is expected 1 month after beginning therapy.
  - Fatigue and pallor (skin, mucous membranes) subside, and the client reports increased energy level.

MEDICATION CLASSIFICATION: VITAMIN B$_{12}$ – CYANOCOBALAMIN

- Select Prototype Medication: vitamin B$_{12}$
- Other Medications: intranasal cyanocobalamin (Nascobal)

Purpose

- Expected Pharmacological Action
  - Vitamin B$_{12}$ is necessary to convert folic acid from its inactive form to its active form. All cells rely on folic acid for DNA production.
  - Vitamin B$_{12}$ can be administered to prevent or correct deficiency, which results in megaloblastic anemia (macrocytic) and can cause fatal heart failure if not corrected.
  - Damage to rapidly multiplying cells can affect the skin and mucous membranes, causing GI disturbances. Neurologic damage, which includes numbness and tingling of extremities and CNS damage caused by demyelination of neurons, can result from deficiency of this vitamin.

○ In addition, a deficiency affects all blood cells produced in the bone marrow.

   ▪ Loss of erythrocytes leads to heart failure, cerebral vascular insufficiency, and hypoxia.

   ▪ Loss of leukocytes leads to infections.

   ▪ Loss of thrombocytes leads to bleeding and hemorrhage.

○ Loss of intrinsic factor within the cells of the stomach causes inability to absorb vitamin B_{12}, making it necessary to administer parenteral or intranasal vitamin B_{12} or high doses of oral B_{12} for the rest of the client's life.

- Therapeutic uses

  ○ Treatment of vitamin B_{12} deficiency

  ○ Megaloblastic (macrocytic) anemia related to vitamin B_{12} deficiency

Complications

ADVERSE EFFECTS	NURSING INTERVENTIONS/CLIENT EDUCATION
› Hypokalemia secondary to the increased RBC production effects of vitamin B_{12}	› Monitor potassium levels during the start of treatment. › Observe for findings of potassium deficiency (muscle weakness, abnormal cardiac rhythm). › Clients can require potassium supplements.

Contraindications/Precautions

- Vitamin B_{12} deficiency should never be treated only with folic acid, which can result in neurological damage. If folic acid is used for a client who has a vitamin B_{12} deficiency, ensure that dosage is adequate.

- Oral and intranasal cyanocobalamin are Pregnancy Risk Category A medications.

- Parenteral formulation is a Pregnancy Risk Category C medication.

Interactions

MEDICATION/FOOD INTERACTIONS	NURSING INTERVENTIONS
› Masking of indications of vitamin B_{12} deficiency with concurrent administration of folic acid	› Make sure that clients receive adequate doses of vitamin B_{12} when using folic acid.

Patient-Centered Care

- Obtain baseline vitamin B_{12}, Hgb, Hct, RBC, reticulocyte counts, and folate levels. Monitor periodically.

- Monitor for indications of vitamin B_{12} deficiency, such as beefy red tongue, pallor, or neuropathy.

- Cyanocobalamin can be administered intranasally, orally, or by IM or SC injection. Injections are painful and are usually reserved for clients who have significant reduced ability to absorb vitamin B_{12}, such as lack of intrinsic factor (pernicious anemia), enteritis, and partial removal of the stomach.

- Clients who have malabsorption syndrome can use intranasal or parenteral preparations.

- Intranasal cyanocobalamin should be administered 1 hr before or after eating hot foods, which can cause the medication to be removed from nasal passages without being absorbed because of increased nasal secretions.

- Clients who have irreversible malabsorption syndrome (parietal cell atrophy or total gastrectomy) will need lifelong treatment, usually parenterally. If oral therapy is used, doses must be very high.

  - Encourage concurrent intake of appropriate quantities of foods high in vitamin B_{12}, such as dairy products.

  - Perform Schilling test to determine vitamin B_{12} absorption in the gastrointestinal tract. Measurement of plasma B_{12} levels helps to determine need for therapy.

  - Advise clients to adhere to prescribed laboratory tests. Blood counts and vitamin B_{12} levels should be monitored every 3 to 6 months.

Nursing Evaluation of Medication Effectiveness

- Depending on therapeutic intent, effectiveness is evidenced by

  - Improvement of megaloblastic anemia as evidenced by increased reticulocyte count, absence of megaloblast in bone marrow, macrocytes in blood, and normal or increased Hgb and Hct levels.

  - Improvement of neurologic effects, such as absence of tingling sensation of hands and feet and numbness of extremities. Improvement can take months, and some clients never attain full recovery.

MEDICATION CLASSIFICATION: FOLIC ACID

- Select Prototype Medication: folic acid

Purpose

- Expected Pharmacological Action
  - Folic acid is essential in the production of DNA and erythropoiesis (RBC, WBC, and platelets).
- Therapeutic Uses
  - Treatment of megaloblastic (macrocytic) anemia secondary to folic acid deficiency
  - Prevention of neural tube defects during pregnancy (thus needed for all women of child-bearing age who can become pregnant)
  - Treatment of malabsorption syndrome, such as sprue
  - Alcohol use disorder (supplementation required due to poor dietary intake of folic acid and injury to the liver)

Contraindications/Precautions

- Indiscriminate use of folic acid is inappropriate because of the risk of masking indications of vitamin B_{12} deficiency.

Interactions

MEDICATION/FOOD INTERACTIONS	NURSING INTERVENTIONS/CLIENT EDUCATION
› Folate can decrease phenytoin serum levels because of increased metabolism.	› Avoid concurrent with phenytoin (Dilantin).

Patient-Centered Care

- Monitor for manifestations of megaloblastic anemia (pallor, easy fatigability, palpitations, paresthesias of hands or feet).
- Obtain baseline folic acid levels, RBC and reticulocyte counts, and Hgb and Hct levels. Monitor periodically.
- Advise clients who have a folic acid deficiency to concurrently increase intake of food sources of folic acid, such as green leafy vegetables, citrus fruits, and dried peas and beans. Monitor for risk factors indicating that folic acid therapy is needed, such as heavy alcohol use and child-bearing age.

Nursing Evaluation of Medication Effectiveness

- Depending on therapeutic intent, effectiveness can be evidenced by
  - Folate level within normal reference range
  - Return of RBC, reticulocyte count, and Hgb and Hct to levels within expected reference range
  - Improvement of anemia findings such as absence of pallor, dyspnea, and easy fatigability
  - Absence of neural tube defects in newborns

MEDICATION CLASSIFICATION: POTASSIUM SUPPLEMENTS

- Select Prototype Medication: potassium chloride (K-Dur, Klor-Con)
- Other Medications
  - Potassium gluconate
  - Potassium phosphate
  - Potassium bicarbonate

Purpose

- Expected Pharmacological Action
  - Potassium is essential for conducting nerve impulses, maintaining electrical excitability of muscle, and regulation of acid/base balance.
- Therapeutic uses
  - Potassium supplements are used to treat hypokalemia (potassium less than 3.5 mEq/L).
  - Potassium supplements are used:
    - For clients receiving diuretics resulting in potassium loss, such as furosemide (Lasix).
    - For clients who have potassium loss due to excessive or prolonged vomiting, diarrhea, overuse of laxatives, intestinal drainage, and GI fistulas.

Complications

ADVERSE EFFECTS	NURSING INTERVENTIONS/CLIENT EDUCATION
› Local GI ulceration and GI distress, such as nausea, vomiting, diarrhea, abdominal discomfort, and esophagitis with oral administration	› Instruct clients to take the medication with meals or a full glass of water to minimize GI discomfort and prevent ulceration. › Advise clients not to dissolve the tablet in the mouth because oral ulceration will develop.
› Hyperkalemia (potassium greater than 5.0 mEq/L)	› Hyperkalemia rarely occurs with oral administration. › Monitor clients receiving IV potassium for manifestations of hyperkalemia, such as bradycardia, hypotension, and ECG changes.

Contraindications/Precautions

- Contraindicated for clients who have severe kidney disease, hypoaldosteronism.

Interactions

MEDICATION/FOOD INTERACTIONS	NURSING INTERVENTIONS/CLIENT EDUCATION
› Concurrent use of potassium-sparing diuretics, such as spironolactone (Aldactone) or ACE inhibitors (lisinopril [Prinivil]), increases the risk of hyperkalemia.	› Concurrent use should be avoided.

Nursing Administration

- Oral formulations

    - Mix powdered formulations in at least 4 oz of liquid.

    - Advise clients to take potassium chloride with a glass of water or with a meal to reduce the risk of adverse GI effects.

    - Instruct clients not to crush extended-release tablets.

    - Instruct clients to notify the provider if they have difficulty swallowing the pills. Medication can be supplied as a powder or a sustained-release tablet that is easier to tolerate.

- IV administration

    - Monitor the IV site for local irritation, phlebitis, and infiltration.

Nursing Evaluation of Medication Effectiveness

- Depending on therapeutic intent, effectiveness can be evidenced by serum potassium level within expected reference range (3.5 to 5.0 mEq/L).

MEDICATION CLASSIFICATION: MAGNESIUM SULFATE

- Select Prototype Medication

    - Parenteral: magnesium sulfate

    - Oral: magnesium hydroxide (Milk of Magnesia [MOM]) and magnesium oxide (Uro-Mag, Maox), magnesium citrate (Citrate of Magnesia, Citroma, Citro-Nesia)

        - Magnesium hydroxide and magnesium oxide act as antacids when administered in a low dose, and all three act as laxatives.

Purpose

- Expected Pharmacological Action

    - Magnesium activates many intracellular enzymes and plays a role in regulating skeletal muscle contractility and blood coagulation.

- Therapeutic Uses

    - Magnesium supplements are used for clients who have hypomagnesemia (magnesium level less than 1.3 mEq/L).

    - Oral preparations of magnesium sulfate are used to prevent or treat low magnesium levels and as laxatives.

    - Parenteral magnesium is used for clients who have severe hypomagnesemia.

    - IV magnesium sulfate is used to stop preterm labor and as an anticonvulsant during labor and delivery.

Complications

ADVERSE EFFECTS	NURSING INTERVENTIONS/CLIENT EDUCATION
› Muscle weakness, flaccid paralysis, painful muscle contractions, cardiac disorders, and respiratory depression	› Monitor the cardiac and neuromuscular status of clients receiving IV administration. › Monitor serum magnesium levels.
› Diarrhea	› Monitor serum magnesium levels for magnesium loss from diarrhea. › Monitor I&O and observe for manifestations of dehydration.

Contraindications/Precautions

- Magnesium is a Pregnancy Risk Category A medication.
- Use cautiously with clients who have AV block, rectal bleeding, nausea/vomiting, and abdominal pain.
- Use cautiously with clients who have renal or cardiac disease.

Interactions

- Magnesium sulfate can decrease the absorption of tetracyclines.
- Monitor the therapeutic effect to determine if absorption has been affected.

Patient-Centered Care

- Monitor serum magnesium, calcium, and phosphorus.
- Monitor blood pressure, heart rate, and respiratory rate for the client receiving IV administration.
- Monitor for depressed or absent deep-tendon reflexes as an indication of toxicity.
- Calcium gluconate is given for magnesium sulfate toxicity.
- Instruct clients about dietary sources of magnesium (whole grain cereals, nuts, legumes, green leafy vegetables, bananas).

Nursing Evaluation of Medication Effectiveness

- Depending on therapeutic intent, effectiveness can be evidenced by serum magnesium levels within expected reference range (1.3 to 2.1 mEq/L).

HERBAL SUPPLEMENTS

Overview

- Herbal supplements are widely used but frequently less tested and regulated than conventional medications. Dosages are less precise than for more regulated medications. Because formulations are not standardized, it can be difficult to know which preparations can provide therapeutic effects.

- New supplements must be approved by the FDA for safety, and the supplement must have documentation of reasonable evidence that it is safe and effective to consume.

ALOE, ALOE VERA (ALOE GEL, ALOE LATEX)	
Action	› Topical antimicrobial, anti-inflammatory, analgesic, and cathartic. › Soothes pain, heals burns (aloe gel). › Softens skin, laxative (aloe latex).
Adverse Effects and Precautions	› Skin preparations: possible hypersensitivity. › Laxative: possible fluid and electrolyte imbalances. › Increases menstrual flow when taken during menses. › Avoid taking if the client has kidney disorders.
Interactions	› Interacts with digoxin, diuretics, corticosteroids and antidysrhythmics.
Nursing Administration	› Reinforce teaching for clients about recognizing manifestations of fluid and electrolyte imbalance if using as a laxative.
BLACK COHOSH	
Action	› Estrogen substitute. › Mechanism of action is unknown. › Treats manifestations of menopause.
Adverse Effects and Precautions	› GI distress, lightheadedness, headache, rash, weight gain. › Avoid taking during the first two trimesters of pregnancy. › Limit use to 6 months due to lack of information regarding long-term effects.
Interactions	› Increases effects of antihypertensive medications. › Can increase effect of estrogen medications. › Increases hypoglycemia in clients taking insulin or other medications for diabetes mellitus. › Interacts with St. John's wort.
Nursing Administration	› Question clients who take antihypertensives, insulin, or hypoglycemic agents or who may be pregnant about possible use of black cohosh.

ECHINACEA

Action	› Stimulates the immune system › Decreases inflammation › Topically heals skin disorders, wounds, and burns › Possibly treats viruses (common cold, herpes simplex) › Increases T-lymphocyte, tumor necrosis factor, and interferon production
Adverse Effects and Precautions	› Bitter taste. › Mild GI upset or fever can occur. › Allergic reactions, especially in clients who are allergic to plants such as ragweed or others in the daisy family.
Interactions	› With chronic use (more than 6 months), echinacea can decrease positive effects of medications for tuberculosis, HIV, or cancer.
Nursing Administration	› Echinacea is available in many forms, including dried roots, plants, extracts, and teas. › Question clients who have tuberculosis, cancer, HIV, lupus erythematosus, and rheumatoid arthritis about concurrent use and advise them to talk to their provider.

FEVERFEW

Action	› Can block platelet aggregation › Can block a factor that causes migraines › Can decrease the number and severity of migraine headaches (does not treat an existing migraine)
Adverse Effects and Precautions	› Mild GI effects. › Post-feverfew syndrome can occur, causing agitation, tiredness, inability to sleep, headache, and joint discomfort. › Can cause allergic reactions in clients allergic to ragweed or echinacea.
Interactions	› Can cause increased risk of bleeding in clients taking NSAIDs, heparin, and warfarin. › Discontinue 2 weeks before elective surgery.
Nursing Administration	› Question clients about concurrent use of NSAIDs, heparin, and warfarin.

GARLIC

Action	› Forms the enzyme allicin when crushed › Blocks LDL cholesterol and raises HDL cholesterol; lowers triglycerides › Suppresses platelet aggregation and disrupts coagulation › Acts as a vasodilator (can lower BP)
Adverse Effects and Precautions	› GI effects
Interactions	› Due to antiplatelet qualities, can increase risk of bleeding in clients taking NSAIDs, warfarin, and heparin › Can increase hypoglycemic effects of diabetes medications › Decreases levels of saquinavir, a medication for HIV treatment
Nursing Administration	› Question clients about concurrent use of NSAIDs, heparin, and warfarin. › Have clients taking antiplatelet or anticoagulant medication or saquinavir to contact their provider.

GINGER ROOT

Action	› Relieves vertigo and nausea
	› Increases intestinal motility
	› Increases gastric mucous production
	› Decreases GI spasms
	› Produces an anti-inflammatory effect
	› Suppresses platelet aggregation
	› Used to treat morning sickness, motion sickness, nausea from surgery
	› Can decrease pain and stiffness of rheumatoid arthritis
Adverse Effects and Precautions	› Use cautiously in pregnancy because high doses can cause uterine spasms.
	› Adverse effects unknown, with potential CNS and cardiac problems with very large overdose.
Interactions	› Interacts with medications that interfere with coagulation (NSAIDS, warfarin, and heparin).
Nursing Administration	› Question clients about concurrent use with NSAIDs, heparin, and warfarin.
	› Monitor for hypoglycemia if taking insulin or other medication for diabetes mellitus.

GINKGO BILOBA

Action	› Promotes vasodilation – Decreases leg pain caused from occlusive arterial disorders
	› Decreases platelet aggregation – Can decrease risk of thrombosis
	› Decreases bronchospasm
	› Increases blood flow to the brain – Improves memory (dementia, Alzheimer's disease)
Adverse Effects and Precautions	› Mild GI upset, headache, lightheadedness, which can be decreased by reducing dose
	› Should be taken with caution in those at risk for seizure
Interactions	› Can interact with medications that lower the seizure threshold, such as antihistamines, antidepressants, and antipsychotics
	› Can interfere with coagulation
Nursing Administration	› Question clients regarding history of antidepressant use (imipramine hydrochloride [Tofranil]), which causes a decrease in seizure threshold.
	› Question clients about concurrent use with NSAIDs, heparin, and warfarin.

GLUCOSAMINE

Action	› Stimulates cells to make cartilage and synovial fluid
	› Suppresses inflammation of the joints and cartilage degradation
	» Treats osteoarthritis of the knee, hip, and wrist
Adverse Effects and Precautions	› Mild GI upset (nausea, heartburn)
	› Use with caution with shellfish allergy.
Interactions	› Use caution if taking antiplatelet or anticoagulant medication.
Nursing Administration	› Question clients about concurrent use with NSAIDs, heparin, and warfarin.

KAVA (KAVA KAVA)

Action	› SHOULD BE AVOIDED – causes liver injury
	› Possibly acts on GABA receptors in the CNS
	› Promotes sleep
	› Decreases anxiety
	› Promotes muscle relaxation without affecting concentration
Adverse Effects and Precautions	› Chronic use causes dry, flaky skin and jaundice.
	› Chronic use and large doses can cause liver damage, including severe liver failure.
Interactions	› Can cause sedation when taken concurrently with CNS depressants.
Nursing Administration	› Question clients taking any CNS depressant, including alcohol, about use of kava.
	› Ask clients who have any liver condition about concurrent use.

MA HUANG (EPHEDRA SINICA)

Action	› SHOULD BE AVOIDED – Because it contains ephedrine, ma huang can stimulate the cardiovascular system and, at high doses, can cause hypertension and dysrhythmias resulting in possible MI and death.
	› Stimulates the CNS
	» Suppresses the appetite
	» Used for weight loss
	› Constricts arterioles – Increases heart rate and BP
	› Bronchodilates – Treats colds, influenza, and allergies
Adverse Effects and Precautions	› Can cause death from hypertension and dysrhythmias.
	› Stimulation of CNS can cause euphoria and, in high doses, psychosis.
Interactions	› Interacts with CNS stimulants to potentiate their effect
	› Can cause severe hypertension when taken with MAOI antidepressants
	› Interacts with antihypertensive medications, decreasing effects
Nursing Administration	› Question clients carefully about other medications.
	› Products that include more than 10 mg/dose are banned from sale in the U.S.

ST. JOHN'S WORT

Action	› Affects serotonin, producing antidepressant effects – Used for mild depression
	› Used orally as an analgesic to relieve pain and inflammation
	› Applied topically for infection
Adverse Effects and Precautions	› Mild adverse effects, including dry mouth, lightheadedness, constipation, and GI upset
	› Skin rash when exposed to sunlight
Interactions	› Can cause serotonin syndrome when combined with other antidepressants, amphetamine, and cocaine
	› Decreases effectiveness of oral contraceptives, cyclosporine, warfarin, digoxin, calcium-channel blockers, steroids, HIV protease inhibitors, and some cancer chemotherapy medications
Nursing Administration	› Question clients taking any of the medications with which this substance interacts about concurrent use.
	› Encourage clients using St. John's wort to prevent prolonged sun exposure and use sunscreen.

SAW PALMETTO	
Action	› Can decrease prostate manifestations of hyperplasia
Adverse Effects and Precautions	› Few adverse effects; can cause mild GI effects › Precaution: Can decrease prostate-specific antigen (PSA), the marker used to detect prostate cancer
Interactions	› Possible additive effects with finasteride (Proscar) › Can interact with antiplatelet and anticoagulant medications › FDA Pregnancy Risk Category X
Nursing Administration	› Question male clients about use before they have PSA tests. › Question clients about concurrent use with aspirin (ASA), heparin, and warfarin.
VALERIAN	
Action	› Increases gamma-aminobutyric acid (GABA) to prevent insomnia (similar to benzodiazepines) » Reduces anxiety-related restlessness » Drowsiness effect increases over time
Adverse Effects and Precautions	› Can cause drowsiness, lightheadedness, depression. › Risk of physical dependence. › Precaution: Clients who have mental health disorders should use with caution. › Should be avoided by pregnant and lactating women.
Interactions	› Not known if valerian potentiates effects of CNS depressants
Nursing Administration	› Clients taking valerian should be warned about possibility of drowsiness when operating motor vehicles and other equipment.

APPLICATION EXERCISES

1. A nurse is reinforcing teaching for a client who has anemia and has a new prescription for an iron supplement. Which of the following should be included in the teaching? (Select all that apply.)

_____ A. Add foods that are high in fiber to the diet.

_____ B. Rinse the mouth after taking the liquid formulation.

_____ C. Expect stools to be green or black in color.

_____ D. Take the medication on a full stomach.

_____ E. Add additional red meat to the diet.

2. A nurse is evaluating a group of clients at a health fair in relation to the need for folic acid therapy. Which of the following clients can benefit from folic acid therapy? (Select all that apply.)

_____ A. A 12-year-old child who has iron deficiency anemia

_____ B. A 24-year-old female who has no health problems

_____ C. A 44-year-old male who has hypertension

_____ D. A 55–year-old female who has alcohol use disorder

_____ E. A 35-year-old male who has type 2 diabetes mellitus

3. A nurse is caring for a client who has increased liver enzymes and is taking herbal supplements. The use of which of the following herbal supplements should be reported to the provider?

A. Ma huang

B. Saw palmetto

C. Kava

D. St. John's wort

4. A client requests information from a nurse on the use of the herbal supplement feverfew. Which of the following is an appropriate response by the nurse?

A. It is used to treat topical microbial infections.

B. It decreases the frequency of migraine headaches.

C. It lessens the nasal congestion of the common cold.

D. It relieves nausea of morning sickness during pregnancy.

5. A nurse is collecting data about a client's current medications. The client states she also takes gingko biloba. Which of the following medications is contraindicated for a client taking gingko biloba?

    A. Acetaminophen (Tylenol)

    B. Warfarin (Coumadin)

    C. Digoxin (Lanoxin)

    D. Lisinopril (Zestril)

6. A nurse is reinforcing teaching for a client about a new prescription for cyanocobalamin. Which of the following should the nurse include in the teaching? Using the ATI Active Learning Template: Medication to complete this item to include the following:

    A. Expected Pharmacological Action: Define.

    B. Nursing Interventions/Client Education: Describe four educational points to reinforce in the teaching.

    C. Evaluation of Medication Effectiveness: Describe two nursing interventions.

APPLICATION EXERCISES KEY

1.   A. **CORRECT:** Foods high in fiber can prevent constipation, which can occur when taking iron supplements.

    B. **CORRECT:** Iron supplements can stain a client's teeth when taken in a liquid form. The client should rinse orally after taking the medication.

    C. **CORRECT:** Green- or black-colored stools can occur when taking iron supplements, and the client should anticipate this effect.

    D. INCORRECT: Iron supplements are maximally absorbed when taken on an empty stomach or 1 hr before meals.

    E. **CORRECT:** Red meats are high in iron and recommended in a client's diet to improve anemia when taken concurrently with iron supplements.

    Ⓝ NCLEX® Connection: Pharmacological Therapies, Medication Administration

2.   A. INCORRECT: The client who has iron deficiency anemia requires treatment with iron supplements, not folic acid therapy.

    B. **CORRECT:** The female client of childbearing age should take folic acid to prevent neural tube defects in the fetus.

    C. INCORRECT: The client who has hypertension requires treatment with diet, exercise, and antihypertensive medication, not folic acid therapy.

    D. **CORRECT:** The client who has alcohol use disorder can require folic acid therapy. Excess alcohol consumption leads to poor dietary intake of folic acid and injury to the liver.

    E. INCORRECT: The client who has type 2 diabetes mellitus requires treatment with diet, exercise, and hyperglycemic medication, not folic acid therapy.

    Ⓝ NCLEX® Connection: Pharmacological Therapies, Expected Actions/Outcomes

3.   A. INCORRECT: Ma huang stimulates the CNS, suppresses appetite, and causes bronchodilation, but it does not affect the liver.

    B. INCORRECT: Saw palmetto can cause mild GI effects, but it does not affect the liver.

    C. **CORRECT:** Chronic use or high doses of kava can cause liver damage, including severe liver failure.

    D. INCORRECT: St. John's wort can cause GI upset and constipation, but it does not affect the liver.

    Ⓝ NCLEX® Connection: Pharmacological Therapies, Adverse Effects/Contraindications/ Side Effects/Interactions

4. A. INCORRECT: Aloe is a topical antimicrobial, anti-inflammatory, and analgesic used to treat tissue injury.

    B. **CORRECT:** Feverfew can decrease the frequency of migraine headaches, but it has not been proven to relieve an existing migraine headache.

    C. INCORRECT: Ma huang relieves manifestations of the common cold and suppresses the appetite.

    D. INCORRECT: Ginger root relieves nausea caused from morning sickness during pregnancy.

    Ⓝ NCLEX® Connection: Pharmacological Therapies, Expected Actions/Outcomes

5. A. INCORRECT: Acetaminophen is not contraindicated for a client taking gingko biloba.

    B. **CORRECT:** Warfarin is contraindicated for a client taking gingko biloba due to the risk of bleeding or hemorrhage.

    C. INCORRECT: Digoxin is not contraindicated for a client taking gingko biloba.

    D. INCORRECT: Lisinopril is not contraindicated for a client taking gingko biloba.

    Ⓝ NCLEX® Connection: Pharmacological Therapies, Adverse Effects/Contraindications/Side Effects/ Interactions

6. *Using the ATI Active Learning Template: Medication*

    A. Expected Pharmacological Action
    - Cyanocobalamin converts folic acid from an inactive form to an active form.
    - Cyanocobalamin corrects megaloblastic anemia related to a deficiency of vitamin B_{12}.

    B. Nursing Interventions/Client Education
    - Review manifestations of hypokalemia.
    - Discuss the appropriate use of potassium supplements, if prescribed.
    - Discuss dietary sources of potassium.
    - Encourage foods high in vitamin B_{12}.
    - Administer intranasal cyanocobalamin 1 hr before or after eating hot foods when nasal secretions are decreased.
      - Periodic laboratory testing of Hgb, Hct, RBC, reticulocyte count, and folate levels is advised.

    C. Evaluation of Medication Effectiveness
    - Review laboratory values for increased reticulocyte count and macrocytes and normal Hgb and Hct levels.
      - Monitor for improvement of neurologic effects (numbness, tingling of hands and feet).

    Ⓝ NCLEX® Connection: Pharmacological Therapies, Expected Actions/Outcomes

UNIT 7   Medications Affecting the Reproductive System

CHAPTERS

› Medications Affecting the Reproductive Tract

NCLEX® CONNECTIONS

When reviewing the chapters in this unit, keep in mind the relevant sections of the NCLEX® outline, in particular:

Client Needs: Pharmacological Therapies

› Relevant topics/tasks include:

  » Adverse Effects/Contraindications/Side Effects/Interactions

    › Monitor the client for actual and potential adverse effects of medications (prescribed, over-the-counter and/or herbal supplements).

  » Medication Administration

    › Collect required data prior to medication administration.

chapter 27

Overview

- Medications that affect the reproductive system include hormones that stimulate puberty, such as estrogen and progesterone in females and testosterone in males. These hormones also are used to replace a hormonal deficiency (male or female) or prevent pregnancy in women (oral contraceptives).

- Medications that are used to treat benign prostatic hyperplasia (BPH) include 5-alpha reductase inhibitors and alpha$_1$-adrenergic antagonists. Medications used to treat erectile dysfunction include the phosphodiesterase type 5 (PDE5) inhibitors.

MEDICATION CLASSIFICATION: ESTROGENS

- Select Prototype Medications: conjugated equine estrogens (Premarin)
- Other Medications: estradiol (Estrace, Vagifem), estradiol hemihydrate (Estrasorb)

Purpose

- Expected Pharmacological Action
  - Estrogens are hormones needed for growth and maturation of the female reproductive tract and secondary sex characteristics. Estrogens block bone resorption and reduce low-density lipoprotein (LDL) levels. At high levels, estrogens suppress the release of a follicle-stimulating hormone (FSH) needed for conception.

- Therapeutic Uses
  - Estrogens uses
    - Contraception
    - Treatment of acne
    - Relief of moderate to severe postmenopausal symptoms, such as hot flashes and mood changes
    - Prevention of postmenopausal osteoporosis
    - Treatment of dysfunctional uterine bleeding
    - Treatment of prostate cancer
    - Treatment of moderate to severe symptoms of vulvar atrophy

- Route of administration: oral, transdermal, intravaginal, IM, and IV
  - Transdermal therapy reduces incidents of nausea and vomiting.
    - A smaller dose can be prescribed to reduce fluctuation of blood estrogen levels and risk of complications.
  - IV and IM use is rare. IV use is generally limited to acute, emergency control of heavy uterine bleeding.

Complications

ADVERSE EFFECTS	NURSING INTERVENTIONS/CLIENT EDUCATION
› Endometrial and ovarian cancers when prolonged estrogen is the only postmenopausal therapy	› Administer progestins along with estrogen. › Instruct clients to report persistent vaginal bleeding if they have an intact uterus. › Advise clients to have an endometrial biopsy every 2 years and pelvic exam yearly.
› Potential risk for estrogen-dependent breast cancer	› Rule out estrogen-dependent breast cancer prior to starting therapy. › Encourage clients to examine their breasts regularly. Also, obtain yearly breast exams by a provider, and receive periodic mammograms.
› Embolic events such as MI, pulmonary embolism, DVT, stroke) › Women over 60 have increased risk of myocardial infarction and coronary heart disease (CHD)	› Encourage clients to avoid all nicotine products. › Monitor for pain, swelling, warmth, or erythema of lower legs. › Teach clients how to reduce risk of cardiovascular disease.

Contraindications/Precautions

- Pregnancy Risk Category X medication.
- Contraindicated for clients who have:
  - ○ Client or family history of heart disease.
  - ○ Abnormal vaginal bleeding that is undiagnosed.
  - ○ Breast or estrogen-dependent cancer.
  - ○ History or risk of thromboembolic disease.
- Use cautiously during breastfeeding because estrogens decrease quantity and quality of milk and can be excreted in breast milk.
- Use cautiously in prepubescent girls. If administered, monitor bone growth and check periodically for early epiphyseal plate closure.

Interactions

MEDICATION/FOOD INTERACTIONS	NURSING INTERVENTIONS/CLIENT EDUCATION
› Estrogens can reduce the effectiveness of warfarin (Coumadin).	› If used concurrently, monitor international normalized ratio (INR) and prothrombin time (PT). › Warfarin doses may need to be adjusted.
› Concurrent use of phenytoin (Dilantin) can decrease the effectiveness of estrogens.	› Monitor for decreased estrogen effects.
› Corticosteroids can increase effects of estrogen.	› Monitor for increased estrogen effects.
› Smoking increases risk for thrombophlebitis.	› Advise clients not to smoke. Use alternative treatment if smoking persists.

Nursing Administration

- Instruct clients to take the medication at the same time each day (e.g., at bedtime).
- Apply estrogen patches to the skin of the trunk. Avoid the breasts and waistline.
- Instruct clients to report menstrual changes such as dysmenorrhea, amenorrhea, breakthrough bleeding, or breast changes.
- Encourage clients to perform monthly breast self-examinations and schedule annual gynecologic and breast examinations with the provider.
- Advise clients to notify the provider of any swelling or redness in legs, shortness of breath, or chest pain.
- Discontinue prior to knee or hip surgery or any surgical procedures that can cause extensive immobilization.

Nursing Evaluation of Medication Effectiveness

- Depending on therapeutic intent, effectiveness may be evidenced by:
  - No evidence of conception.
  - Relief of severe postmenopausal symptoms (hot flashes, mood changes).
  - Reduction in dysfunctional uterine bleeding.
  - Decrease in spread of prostate cancer.

MEDICATION CLASSIFICATION: PROGESTERONES

- Select Prototype Medication: medroxyprogesterone (Provera)
- Other Medications: norethindrone (Micronor), megestrol acetate (Megace)

Purpose

- Expected Pharmacological Action
  - Progesterones induce favorable conditions for fetal growth and development and maintain pregnancy. A drop in progesterone levels results in menstruation.
- Therapeutic Uses
  - Use progestins alone or with estrogens for contraception. (See next section.)
  - Progesterones counter adverse effects of estrogen in hormone therapy for treatment of:
    - Dysfunctional uterine bleeding due to hormonal imbalance.
    - Amenorrhea due to hormonal imbalance.
    - Endometriosis.
    - Advanced cancer of the endometrium, breast, and kidney.
  - Can use in women who are undergoing in vitro fertilization, in some clients to prevent preterm birth, and to support early pregnancy.
- Routes of administration: oral, IM, subcutaneous, transdermal, and intravaginal

Complications

ADVERSE EFFECTS	NURSING INTERVENTIONS/CLIENT EDUCATION
› Breast cancer	› Encourage clients to perform regular breast self-examinations and get mammograms.
› Thromboembolic events (MI, pulmonary embolism, thrombophlebitis, stroke)	› Discourage clients from smoking. › Monitor for pain, swelling, warmth, or erythema of lower legs. › Advise client to notify the provider of chest pain or shortness of breath.
› Breakthrough bleeding, amenorrhea, and breast tenderness	› Obtain baseline breast exam and Papanicolaou (Pap) test. › Instruct clients to report abnormal vaginal bleeding.
› Edema	› Monitor blood pressure, I&O, and weight gain.
› Jaundice	› Monitor for indications of jaundice, such as yellowing of the skin and sclera of the eyes. Monitor liver enzymes.
› Migraine headaches	› Notify the provider of severe headache.

Contraindications/Precautions

- Pregnancy Risk Category X medication.
- Contraindicated in clients who have:
  - Undiagnosed vaginal bleeding.
  - History of thromboembolic disease, cardiovascular, or cerebrovascular disease.
  - History of breast or genital cancers.
- Use cautiously in clients who have diabetes mellitus, seizures disorders, and migraine headaches.

Interactions

MEDICATION/FOOD INTERACTIONS	NURSING INTERVENTIONS/CLIENT EDUCATION
› Use of carbamazepine (Tegretol), phenobarbital, phenytoin (Dilantin), and rifampin may decrease contraceptive effectiveness.	› Additional contraceptive measures may be needed with concurrent use of these medications.
› Concurrent use with bromocriptine (Parlodel) may cause amenorrhea.	› Do not use concurrently.
› Smoking increases risk for thrombophlebitis.	› Advise clients not to smoke. Use alternative treatment if smoking persists.

Nursing Administration

- Instruct clients to anticipate withdrawal bleeding 3 to 7 days after stopping the medication.
- Instruct clients to stop taking the medication immediately if pregnancy is suspected. Conception should be delayed for 3 months following use.

Nursing Evaluation of Medication Effectiveness

- Depending on therapeutic intent, effectiveness can be evidenced by:
  - Restoration of hormonal balance with control of uterine bleeding.
  - Restoration of menses.
  - Decrease in endometrial hyperplasia in postmenopausal women receiving concurrent estrogen.
  - Control of the spread of endometrial cancer.

MEDICATION CLASSIFICATION: HORMONAL CONTRACEPTIVES

- Select Prototype Medications
  - Estrogen-progestin combinations contain estrogen and progesterone and are referred to as combination oral contraceptives (OCs). OCs that contain progestin only often are referred to as "minipills."
  - Combination oral contraceptives with estrogen plus a progestin
    - Ethinyl estradiol and norethindrone (Ovcon 35, Necon 1/35)
    - Ethinyl estradiol and drospirenone (Yasmin)
  - Progestin-only oral contraceptives
    - Norethindrone (Micronor)
- Combination oral contraceptives are classified as monophasic, biphasic, triphasic, or quadriphasic. With monophasic OCs, the dosage of estrogen to progestin remains the same throughout the cycle. With the other classifications, the estrogen/progestin changes to duplicate a typical menstrual cycle.
- Other Medications
  - Transdermal patch: ethinyl estradiol and norelgestromin (Ortho Evra)
  - Vaginal contraceptive ring: ethinyl estradiol and etonogestrel (NuvaRing)
  - Parenteral: depot medroxyprogesterone acetate (DMPA), available as Depo-Provera for IM use and Depo-SubQ for subcutaneous use

Purpose

- Expected Pharmacological Action: Oral contraceptives stop conception by preventing ovulation. They also thicken the cervical mucus and alter the endometrial lining to reduce the chance of fertilization.
- Therapeutic Uses: Hormonal contraceptives are used to prevent pregnancy.
- Route of administration: oral, transdermal, intravaginal, intrauterine, IM, subcutaneous, subdermal.
- Combination oral contraceptives (OC) are given in a cyclic pattern, usually in a 28-day regimen. They also can be given in newer extended-cycle schedules.

Complications

ADVERSE EFFECTS	NURSING INTERVENTIONS/CLIENT EDUCATION
› Thromboembolic events (MI, pulmonary embolism, thrombophlebitis, stroke) – unlikely with progestin-only OCs.	› Discourage clients from smoking. › Instruct clients to report warmth, edema, tenderness, or pain in the lower legs.
› Hypertension	› Monitor blood pressure, and take actions to maintain normal blood pressure.
› Breakthrough or abnormal uterine bleeding	› Instruct clients to record duration and frequency of breakthrough bleeding. › Evaluate for possible pregnancy if two or more menstrual periods are missed.
› Breast cancer	› Oral contraceptives can increase growth of a pre-existing breast cancer. Do not give to women who have breast cancer.

Contraindications/Precautions

- Pregnancy Risk Category X medication.
- Contraindicated for clients who:
  - Are smokers and over the age of 35.
  - Have a history of thrombophlebitis and cardiovascular events.
  - Have a family history or risk factors for breast cancer.
  - Are experiencing abnormal vaginal bleeding.
- Use cautiously in clients who have hypertension, diabetes mellitus, gall bladder disease, uterine leiomyoma, seizures, and migraine headaches.

Interactions

MEDICATION/FOOD INTERACTIONS	NURSING INTERVENTIONS/CLIENT EDUCATION
› Oral contraceptive effectiveness decreases with use of carbamazepine (Tegretol); phenobarbital; antibiotics, especially penicillins and cephalosporins; phenytoin (Dilantin); and rifampin.	› Additional contraceptive measures may be needed with concurrent use of these medications.
› Oral contraceptives decrease the effects of warfarin (Coumadin) and oral hypoglycemics.	› Monitor INR and PT levels, and adjust warfarin dosages accordingly.

Nursing Administration

- Check for pregnancy prior to start of therapy.
- Instruct clients to take pills at the same time each day.
- Instruct clients to take medication for 21 days followed by 7 days of no medication (or inert pill). For the traditional 28-day cycle OCs, begin the sequence on the fifth day after the onset of menses.
- Monitor for hypertension.
- For one missed dose, instruct clients to take two together at the next scheduled dose. For two missed doses, instruct the client to double up for 2 days. For three missed doses, because of an increased risk of ovulation and resulting pregnancy, instruct clients to use an additional form of birth control and to start a new cycle of medications after waiting 7 days.
- Extended cycle OCs are taken for longer periods than the typical 28-day cycle. Eighty-four days is common, but some preparations are taken continuously.
  - For example, Seasonale is taken for 84 days. The client has withdrawal bleeding four times a year. Lybrel is taken continuously, and the client does not have withdrawal bleeding.
- Encourage clients who smoke to quit.
- Advise clients to report swelling or redness in legs, shortness of breath, severe headache, sudden chest pain, or sudden visual disturbance.

Nursing Evaluation of Medication Effectiveness

- Depending on therapeutic intent, effectiveness can be evidenced by no evidence of conception.

MEDICATION CLASSIFICATION: ANDROGENS

- Select Prototype Medication: testosterone (Androderm-50, Testopel)
- Other Medications: methyltestosterone (Android, Testred)

Purpose

- Expected Pharmacological Action
  - The hormone-receptor complex acts on cellular DNA to promote synthesis of specific mRNA molecules and production of proteins, resulting in:
    - Development of sex traits in men and the production and maturation of sperm.
    - Increase in skeletal muscle and bone growth.
    - Increase in synthesis of erythropoietin.
- Therapeutic Uses
  - Used to treat:
    - Hypogonadism in males.
    - Delayed puberty in boys.
    - Androgen replacement in testicular failure and restoration of libido.
    - Anemia not responsive to traditional therapy.
    - Postmenopausal breast cancer.
    - Muscle wasting in male clients who have AIDS.
- Route of administration: IM, transdermal, implantable pellets, buccal tablets

Complications

ADVERSE EFFECTS	NURSING INTERVENTIONS/CLIENT EDUCATION
› Androgenic (virilization) effects » In women, these medications can cause irregularity or cessation of menses, hirsutism, weight gain, acne, lowering of voice, growth of clitoris, vaginitis, and baldness. » In boys or men, these medications can cause acne, increased facial and body hair, penile enlargement, increased frequency of erections, and priapism (persistent erection).	› Advise clients of possible medication effects. › Advise women to report occurrence of these effects. › Medication may be discontinued to prevent permanent changes.
› Epiphyseal closure – Premature closure of epiphysis in boys can reduce mature height.	› Monitor epiphysis with serial X-rays.
› Cholestatic hepatitis, jaundice	› Monitor for indications of jaundice, such as yellowing of the skin and sclera of the eyes. › Monitor liver enzymes.
› Hypercholesterolemia – These medications can decrease high-density lipoproteins (HDL) and increase low-density lipoproteins (LDL).	› Monitor cholesterol levels. › Advise clients to adjust diet to reduce cholesterol levels.
› Increase in growth of prostate cancer	› Do not give to clients who have prostate cancer. › Monitor for prostate cancer.
› Polycythemia	› Monitor hemoglobin and hematocrit.
› Edema from salt and water retention	› Instruct clients to monitor for weight gain and swelling of extremities and report to the provider. › Medication may be discontinued.
› High abuse potential (often abused to enhance athletic performance)	› Identify high-risk groups and educate regarding abuse potential and potential health risks.

Contraindications/Precautions

- Pregnancy Risk Category X.
- Contraindicated in men with prostate or breast cancer, clients who have hypercalcemia, and older adult clients.
- Use cautiously in clients who have heart failure; hypertension; and cardiac, kidney, or liver disease.

Interactions

MEDICATION/FOOD INTERACTIONS	NURSING INTERVENTIONS/CLIENT EDUCATION
› Androgens can alter effects of oral anticoagulants.	› Monitor PT and INR.
› Androgens can alter effects of insulins and antidiabetic agents.	› Monitor glucose level and adjust dosages.
› Concurrent use of androgens and hepatotoxic medications can increase risk for hepatotoxicity.	› Monitor liver enzymes. Monitor for jaundice.

Nursing Administration

- Instruct clients using gel formulations to wash their hands after every application because of the possibility of skin-to-skin transfer to others.
- Inject IM formulations into a large muscle and rotate injection sites.
- Monitor women for indications of masculinization (facial hair, baldness, deepened voice, acne).
- Advise clients to use a barrier method of birth control.
- Advise clients to reduce cholesterol in the diet.
- Advise clients at risk about abuse potential.

Nursing Evaluation of Medication Effectiveness

- Depending on therapeutic intent, effectiveness can be evidenced by the following.
  - Puberty will be induced in boys and testosterone will be increased in men.
  - There will be a decrease in the progression of breast cancer in women. Medication will produce expected results with minimal adverse effects.
  - Maintenance of adult male sexual characteristics.

MEDICATION CLASSIFICATION: 5-ALPHA REDUCTASE INHIBITORS

- Select Prototype Medications: finasteride (Proscar, Propecia)
- Other Medications: dutasteride (Avodart)

Purpose

- Expected Pharmacological Action – Decreases usable testosterone by inhibiting the converting enzyme, and causes a reduction of the prostate size (thereby decreasing mechanical obstruction of the urethra) and increases hair growth.
- Therapeutic Uses
  - Benign prostatic hyperplasia (BPH)
  - Male pattern baldness
- Route of administration: oral

Complications

ADVERSE EFFECTS	NURSING INTERVENTIONS/CLIENT EDUCATION
› Decreased libido, ejaculate volume	› Advise client to notify the provider if adverse effects occur.
› Gynecomastia	› Advise clients to notify the provider if adverse effects occur.
› Orthostatic hypotension	› Advise the client to change positions slowly.

Contraindications/Precautions

- Pregnancy Risk Category X medication.
- Contraindicated in clients who have medication hypersensitivity.
- Use with caution in clients who have liver disease.

Interactions

- None significant

Nursing Administration

- PSA levels should be determined prior to and 6 months after treatment.
- Advise clients that therapeutic effects can take 6 months or longer.
- Pregnant women should not handle crushed or broken medication.
- Advise clients not to donate blood unless medication has been discontinued for at least 1 month.

Nursing Evaluation of Medication Effectiveness

- Depending on therapeutic intent, effectiveness can be evidenced by the following.
  - Prostate size is decreased, and client is able to urinate effectively.
  - Prostate-specific antigen (PSA) levels have decreased from baseline.
  - Client has increased hair growth.

MEDICATION CLASSIFICATION: ALPHA$_1$-ADRENERGIC ANTAGONISTS

- Select Prototype Medication: selective alpha$_1$ receptor antagonist: tamsulosin (Flomax)
- Other Medications
  - Selective alpha$_1$ receptor antagonist: silodosin (Rapaflo)
  - Nonselective alpha$_1$ receptor antagonists
    - Alfuzosin (Uroxatral)
    - Terazosin
    - Doxazosin (Cardura)

Purpose

- Expected Pharmacological Action
  - These agents decrease mechanical obstruction of the urethra by relaxing smooth muscles of the bladder neck and prostate.
  - Nonselective agents also affect blood vessels, resulting in lowered blood pressure. These agents can be used for clients who have BPH and hypertension.
- Therapeutic Uses
  - Benign prostatic hyperplasia (BPH), thus increasing urinary flow
- Route of administration: oral

Complications

ADVERSE EFFECTS	NURSING INTERVENTIONS/CLIENT EDUCATION
› Hypotension, dizziness, nasal congestion, sleepiness, faintness (more likely with nonselective antagonists)	› Monitor blood pressure. › Advise clients to rise slowly from sitting or lying position. › Advise clients not to drive or operate machinery when starting therapy or with change in dose until response is known.
› Problems with ejaculation (failure, decreased volume)	› Advise clients of possible adverse effect.

Contraindications/Precautions

- Contraindicated in clients who have medication sensitivity.
- Contraindicated for women.
- Silodosin should be used cautiously in clients who have renal impairment.
- Exercise caution when combining with other medications that lower blood pressure.

Interactions

MEDICATION/FOOD INTERACTIONS	NURSING INTERVENTIONS/CLIENT EDUCATION
› Cimetidine can decrease clearance of tamsulosin.	› Use together with caution.
› Antihypertensives, PDE5 inhibitors, and nitroglycerin used concurrently with nonselective agents can cause severe hypotension.	› Use with caution. › Monitor blood pressure.
› Erythromycin and HIV protease inhibitors (Ritonavir) increase levels of alfuzosin and silodosin when used concurrently.	› Avoid concurrent use.

Nursing Administration

- Monitor blood pressure, especially at the start of therapy and with changes of dose.
- Advise clients to take medication daily as prescribed.
  - Tamsulosin – 30 min after a meal at the same time each day
  - Silodosin – with same meal each day
  - Alfuzosin – right after the same meal each day
  - Terazosin – at bedtime
  - Doxazosin – at same time each day

Nursing Evaluation of Medication Effectiveness

- Depending on therapeutic intent, effectiveness can be evidenced by improved urinary flow with minimal adverse effects.

MEDICATION CLASSIFICATION: PHOSPHODIESTERASE TYPE 5 (PDE5) INHIBITORS

- Select Prototype Medications: sildenafil (Viagra)
- Other Medications: tadalafil (Cialis), vardenafil (Levitra)

Purpose

- Expected Pharmacological Action – Augments the effects of nitric oxide released during sexual stimulation, resulting in enhanced blood flow to the corpus cavernosum and penile erection.
- Therapeutic Uses – erectile dysfunction

Complications

ADVERSE EFFECTS	NURSING INTERVENTIONS/CLIENT EDUCATION
› MI, hypotension, sudden death	› Monitor risk factors and history with regard to cardiovascular health.
› Priapism	› Instruct clients to notify the provider if erection lasts more than 4 hr.

Contraindications/Precautions

- Contraindicated in clients taking any medications in the nitrate family, such as nitroglycerin.
- Use cautiously in clients who have cardiovascular disease, including QT prolongation.
- Advise clients that grapefruit juice can increase plasma concentrations and possible adverse effects of medication.

Interactions

MEDICATION/FOOD INTERACTIONS	NURSING INTERVENTIONS/CLIENT EDUCATION
› Organic nitrates, such as nitroglycerin (Nitrostat) and isosorbide dinitrate (Isordil), can lead to fatal hypotension.	› Discourage concurrent use of organic nitrates or alpha blockers.
› Ketoconazole, erythromycin, cimetidine, ritonavir, and grapefruit juice inhibit metabolism of sildenafil, thereby increasing plasma levels of medication.	› Use these medications cautiously in clients taking PDE5 inhibitors.

Nursing Administration

- Administer by oral route.
- Instruct clients that tadalafil is approved to be taken daily or prior to sexual activity.

Nursing Evaluation of Medication Effectiveness

- Depending on therapeutic intent, effectiveness can be evidenced by sexual arousal and erection sufficient for sexual intercourse.

APPLICATION EXERCISES

1. A nurse is reviewing the health care record of a client who has a prescription for conjugated equine estrogens (Premarin). In which of the following conditions is the use of estrogens contraindicated?

    A. Atrophic vaginitis

    B. Dysfunctional uterine bleeding

    C. Osteoporosis

    D. Thrombophlebitis

2. A nurse is explaining the mechanism of action of combination oral contraceptives to a group of clients. The nurse should tell the clients that which of the following actions occur with the use of combination oral contraceptives? (Select all that apply.)

    _____ A. Thickening the cervical mucus

    _____ B. Inducing maturation of ovarian follicle

    _____ C. Increasing the development of the corpus luteum

    _____ D. Altering the endometrial lining

    _____ E. Inhibiting ovulation

3. A nurse is reinforcing teaching with a female client who is taking testosterone (Andronaq-50) to treat advanced breast cancer. The nurse should tell the client that which of the following are adverse effects of this medication? (Select all that apply.)

    _____ A. Deepening voice

    _____ B. Male pattern baldness

    _____ C. Sedation

    _____ D. Constipation

    _____ E. Facial hair

4. A nurse is reinforcing teaching with a client who is to start alfuzosin (Uroxatral) for treatment of benign prostatic hyperplasia. Which of the following is an adverse effect of this medication?

    A. Rash

    B. Edema

    C. Hypotension

    D. Jaundice

5. A nurse is caring for a client who has angina and asks about obtaining a prescription for sildenafil (Viagra) to treat erectile dysfunction. Which of the following medications should not be taken concurrently with sildenafil?

  A. Ranolazine (Ranexa)

  B. Isosorbide (Isordil)

  C. Clopidogrel (Plavix)

  D. Lisinopril (Zestril)

6. A nurse in a provider's office is instructing a client who has a new prescription for finasteride (Proscar) to treat benign prostatic hyperplasia. Use the ATI Active Learning Template: Medication to complete this item to include the following:

  A. Expected Pharmacology

  B. Adverse Effects: Identify two.

APPLICATION EXERCISES KEY

1. A. INCORRECT: Atrophic vaginitis occurs when there is estrogen deficiency. This medication is used to treat atrophic vaginitis.

    B. INCORRECT: Dysfunctional uterine bleeding can occur when there is estrogen deficiency. This medication is used to treated dysfunctional uterine bleeding.

    C. INCORRECT: Women are at risk for osteoporosis after the onset of menopause. Estrogen is used to slow the progression of osteoporosis.

    D. **CORRECT:** Estrogen increases the risk of thrombolytic events. Estrogen used is contraindicated for a client who has a history of thrombophlebitis.

    Ⓝ NCLEX® Connection: Pharmacological Therapies, Adverse Effects/Contraindications/ Side Effects/Interactions

2. A. **CORRECT:** Oral contraceptives cause thickening of the cervical mucus, which slows sperm passage.

    B. INCORRECT: Inducing maturation of the ovarian follicle is not an action of oral contraceptives.

    C. INCORRECT: Increasing the development of the corpus luteum is not an action of oral contraceptives.

    D. **CORRECT:** Oral contraceptives alter the lining of the endometrium, which inhibits implantation of the fertilized egg.

    E. **CORRECT:** Oral contraceptives prevent pregnancy by inhibiting ovulation.

    Ⓝ NCLEX® Connection: Pharmacological Therapies, Expected Actions/Outcomes

3. A. **CORRECT:** Virilization, the development of adult male characteristics in a female, is an adverse effect of testosterone. The nurse should tell the client that a deepening voice is an adverse effect of testosterone.

    B. **CORRECT:** Male pattern baldness is associated with virilization. The nurse should tell the client that male pattern baldness is an adverse effect of this medication.

    C. INCORRECT: Excitation and insomnia are adverse effects of this medication, not sedation.

    D. INCORRECT: Diarrhea is an adverse effect of this medication, not constipation.

    E. **CORRECT:** Virilization is an adverse effect of testosterone. The nurse should tell the client that the development of facial hair is an adverse effect of testosterone.

    Ⓝ NCLEX® Connection: Pharmacological Therapies, Adverse Effects/Contraindications/ Side Effects/Interactions

4.   A. INCORRECT: Rash is not an adverse effect of this medication.

     B. INCORRECT: Edema is not an adverse effect of this mediation.

     C. **CORRECT:** Alfuzosin relaxes muscle tone in veins and cardiac output decreases, which leads to hypotension. Clients taking this medication are advised to rise slowly from a sitting or lying position.

     D. INCORRECT: Jaundice is not an adverse effect of this medication.

     (N) NCLEX® Connection: Pharmacological Therapies, Adverse Effects/Contraindications/ Side Effects/Interactions

5.   A. INCORRECT: Some medications increase plasma levels of ranolazine, and concurrent use is avoided, but there are no contradictions for concurrent use of sildenafil.

     B. **CORRECT:** Isosorbide is an organic nitrate that manages pain from angina. Concurrent use of it is contraindicated because fatal hypotension can occur. The client should avoid taking a nitrate medication for 24 hr after taking isosorbide.

     C. INCORRECT: There are no contradictions for concurrent use of clopidogrel and sildenafil.

     D. INCORRECT: There are no contradictions for concurrent use of lisinopril and sildenafil.

     (N) NCLEX® Connection: Pharmacological Therapies, Adverse Effects/Contraindications/ Side Effects/Interactions

6.   *Using the ATI Active Learning Template: Medication*

     A. Expected Pharmacology
        • Finasteride slows the production of testosterone, which reduces the size of the prostate and subsequently promotes urinary elimination.

     B. Adverse Effects
        • Decreased libido
        • Decreased ejaculate volume
        • Gynecomastia
        • Orthostatic hypotension

     (N) NCLEX® Connection: Pharmacological Therapies, Expected Actions/Outcomes

UNIT 8   Medications for Joint and Bone Conditions

CHAPTERS

› Rheumatoid Arthritis
› Bone Disorders

NCLEX® CONNECTIONS

When reviewing the chapters in this unit, keep in mind the relevant sections of the NCLEX® outline, in particular:

Client Needs: Pharmacological Therapies

› Relevant topics/tasks include:

  » Adverse Effects/Contraindications/Side Effects/Interactions

    › Monitor for anticipated interactions among the client's prescribed medications and fluids (oral, IV, subcutaneous, IM, topical prescriptions).

  » Expected Actions/Outcomes

    › Monitor the client's use of medications over time (prescription, over-the-counter, home remedies).

  » Medication Administration

    › Reconcile and maintain a medication list or medication administration record (prescribed medications, herbal supplements, over-the-counter medications).

chapter 28

Overview

- Rheumatoid arthritis (RA) is a chronic disorder with autoimmune and inflammatory components. Pharmacological management provides symptomatic relief and some delay in progression of the disorder without resulting in cure.

- The American College of Rheumatology (ACR) provides recommendations for management of RA. These guidelines can be found at www.rheumatology.org.

- Categories of medications in this section include disease-modifying antirheumatic medications (DMARDs), glucocorticoids, immunosuppressants, and NSAIDs, which may be used individually or in combination to manage RA.

MEDICATION CLASSIFICATION: DISEASE-MODIFYING ANTIRHEUMATIC DRUGS (DMARDs)

- DMARDs I – Major Nonbiologic DMARDs

  - Immunosuppressant medications: methotrexate, leflunomide (Arava)

  - Antimalarial agents: hydroxychloroquine (Plaquenil)

  - Anti-inflammatory medication: sulfasalazine (Azulfidine)

  - Tetracycline antibiotic: minocycline (Minocin)

- DMARDs II – Major Biologic DMARDs

  - Tumor necrosis factor antagonists

    - Etanercept (Enbrel)

    - Infliximab (Remicade)

    - Adalimumab (Humira)

  - ß-lymphocyte-depleting agent

    - Rituximab (Rituxan)

  - Interleukin-1 receptor antagonist

    - Abatacept (Orencia)

- DMARDs III – Minor Nonbiologic and Biologic DMARDs

  - Gold salts: auranofin (Ridaura)

  - Penicillamine (Cuprimine, Depen)

  - Immunosuppressant medications: azathioprine (Imuran), cyclosporine (Sandimmune, Gengraf, Neoral)

Medication Classification: Glucocorticoids

- Prednisone, prednisolone (Prelone)

Medication Classification: Nonsteroidal Anti-Inflammatory Drugs (NSAIDs)

- Aspirin
- Ibuprofen (Motrin, Advil)
- Diclofenac (Voltaren)
- Indomethacin (Indocin)
- Meloxicam (Mobic)
- Naproxen (Naprosyn)
- Celecoxib (Celebrex)

Purpose

- Expected Pharmacological Action
  - DMARDs slow joint degeneration and progression of rheumatoid arthritis.
  - Glucocorticoids provide symptomatic relief of inflammation and pain.
  - NSAIDs provide rapid, symptomatic relief of inflammation and pain.
- Therapeutic Uses
  - Analgesia for pain, swelling, and joint stiffness
  - Maintenance of joint function
  - Slow/delay the worsening of the disease (DMARDs, glucocorticoids)
  - Short-term therapy until long-acting DMARDs take effect (NSAIDs, glucocorticoids)
  - Prevention of organ rejection in transplant clients such as kidney, liver, and heart transplants (glucocorticoids, immunosuppressants).
  - Management of inflammatory bowel disease (glucocorticoids, immunosuppressants, DMARDs)

Complications

CYTOTOXIC AGENT: METHOTREXATE	
Adverse Effects	Nursing Interventions/Client Education
› Increased risk of infection	› Advise clients to notify the provider immediately for manifestations of infection, such as sore throat.
› Hepatic fibrosis	› Monitor liver function test. › Advise clients to observe for anorexia, abdominal fullness, and jaundice, and to notify the provider if manifestations occur.
› Bone marrow suppression	› Obtain the client's baseline CBC, including platelet counts. Repeat every 3 to 6 months.
› Ulcerative stomatitis/ other GI ulcerations (early finding with toxicity)	› Inspect mouth, gums, and throat daily for ulcerations, bleeding, or color changes. › Advise clients to take the medication with food or a full glass of water. › Stop the medication if manifestations occur.
› Fetal death/congenital abnormalities	› Avoid use during pregnancy. › Use adequate contraception during therapy.

GOLD SALTS: AURANOFIN	
Adverse Effects	Nursing Interventions/Client Education
› Toxicity (severe pruritus, rashes, stomatitis)	› Stop medication. › Notify the provider if manifestations occur.
› Renal toxicity, such as proteinuria	› Stop medication. › Monitor I&O, BUN, creatinine, and UA.
› Blood dyscrasias (thrombocytopenia, leukopenia, agranulocytosis, aplastic anemia)	› Monitor CBC, WBC, and platelet counts periodically. › Advise clients to observe for bruising and gum bleeding and to notify the provider if these occur.
› Hepatitis	› Monitor liver function tests.
› GI discomfort (nausea, vomiting, abdominal pain)	› Observe for manifestations, and notify the provider if they occur.

SULFASALAZINE	
Adverse Effects	Nursing Interventions/Client Education
› Gastrointestinal discomfort (nausea, vomiting, diarrhea, abdominal pain)	› Use an enteric-coated preparation, and divide dosage daily.
› Hepatic dysfunction	› Monitor liver function tests.
› Bone marrow suppression	› Monitor CBC, including platelet counts.

ANTIMALARIAL AGENT: HYDROXYCHLOROQUINE

Adverse Effects	Nursing Interventions/Client Education
› Retinal damage (blindness)	› Advise clients to have baseline eye examination and follow-up eye exams every 6 months with an ophthalmologist. › Stop the medication and notify the provider if blurred vision occurs.

TUMOR NECROSIS FACTOR ANTAGONISTS: ETANERCEPT, INFLIXIMAB

Adverse Effects	Nursing Interventions/Client Education
› Subcutaneous injection-site irritation (redness, swelling, pain, itching)	› Monitor the injection site, and stop the medication if manifestations of irritation occur.
› IV infusion reactions (infliximab) including influenza-like findings, hypotension, possible anaphylaxis	› Assist with pretreatment with an antihistamine, acetaminophen, or a glucocorticoid. › Stop infusion and notify provider immediately for severe reaction. › Continue to monitor for reaction 2 hr after IV infusion.
› Risk of infection, especially TB and reactivation of hepatitis B	› Instruct client to monitor for infection (fever, sore throat, inflammation) and notify the provider if manifestations occur. Medication should be discontinued. › Test for hepatitis B, and perform TB testing.
› Severe skin reactions (including Stevens-Johnson syndrome)	› Instruct clients to monitor for adverse skin reactions and notify the provider if they occur. Medication should be discontinued.
› Heart failure	› Monitor for development or worsening of heart failure (distended neck veins, crackles in lungs, dyspnea). Medication should be discontinued.
› Blood dyscrasias	› Monitor for signs of bleeding, bruising, or fever. Medication should be discontinued.

PENICILLAMINE

Adverse Effects	Nursing Interventions/Client Education
› Bone marrow suppression	› Obtain the client's baseline CBC including platelet counts, and repeat every 3 to 6 months.
› Toxicity (severe pruritus, rashes)	› Stop the medication. › Notify the provider if manifestations occur.

CYCLOSPORINE

Adverse Effects	Nursing Interventions/Client Education
› Risk of infection (fever, sore throat)	› Advise clients to notify the provider immediately if manifestations occur.
› Hepatotoxicity (jaundice)	› Monitor liver function and adjust dosage.
› Nephrotoxicity	› Monitor BUN and creatinine. › Measure I&O.
› Hirsutism	› This effect is reversible with discontinuation of the medication.

GLUCOCORTICOIDS: PREDNISONE	
Adverse Effects	Nursing Interventions/Client Education
› Risk of infection (fever and/or sore throat)	› Advise clients to notify the provider immediately if manifestations occur.
› Osteoporosis	› Advise clients to take calcium supplements, vitamin D, and/or bisphosphonate (etidronate).
› Adrenal suppression	› Advise clients to observe for manifestations, and to notify the provider if they occur. › Administer fluids, such as 0.9% sodium chloride and hydrocortisone IV. Advise clients not to discontinue the medication suddenly.
› Fluid retention	› Monitor for manifestations of fluid excess, such as crackles, weight gain, and edema.
› GI discomfort	› Advise clients to observe for manifestations and to notify the provider if symptoms occur. › H_2-receptor antagonists can be used prophylactically. › Advise client to report manifestations of GI bleeding (coffee-ground emesis or black, tarry stools).
› Hyperglycemia	› Monitor blood glucose level. Clients who have diabetes mellitus may need to adjust hypoglycemic agent.
› Hypokalemia	› Monitor serum potassium levels. › Advise clients to eat potassium-rich foods. › Administer potassium supplements.

Contraindications/Precautions

- Methotrexate
  - This medication is Pregnancy Risk Category X.
  - Methotrexate is contraindicated in clients who have liver failure, alcohol use disorder, or blood dyscrasias.
  - Use with caution in clients who have liver or kidney dysfunction, cancer and suppressed bone marrow function, peptic ulcer disease, ulcerative colitis, impaired nutritional status, or infections.

  - Use cautiously with children or older adult clients.
- Etanercept (Enbrel)
  - Etanercept is contraindicated in clients who have malignancies, active infection, hematologic disorder, or during lactation. Use caution in clients who have heart failure, CNS demyelinating disorders such as multiple sclerosis, or blood dyscrasias.
- Cyclosporine is contraindicated in pregnancy, recent vaccination with live virus vaccines, and recent contact with or active infection of chickenpox or herpes zoster.
- Glucocorticoids are contraindicated in systemic fungal infections and live virus vaccines.
- Warn the client against abrupt discontinuation of glucocorticoids. Dosage of glucocorticoids always is adjusted and withdrawn gradually.

Interactions

MEDICATION/FOOD INTERACTIONS	NURSING INTERVENTIONS/CLIENT EDUCATION
Methotrexate	
› Salicylates, other NSAIDs, sulfonamides, penicillin, and tetracyclines can cause methotrexate toxicity.	› Monitor for toxic effects.
› Folic acid changes the body's response to methotrexate, decreasing its effect.	› Avoid folic acid supplements or vitamins containing folic acid.
Etanercept	
› Concurrent use of etanercept with a live vaccine increases the risk of getting or transmitting infection.	› Avoid live vaccines.
› Concurrent use with immunosuppressants increases the client's chance of serious infection.	› Use precautions against illness if taking immunosuppressants.
Cyclosporine	
› Concurrent use of phenytoin, phenobarbital, rifampin, carbamazepine, and trimethoprim-sulfamethoxazole decreases cyclosporine level, which can lead to organ rejection.	› Monitor the client's cyclosporine levels, and adjust dosage accordingly.
› Concurrent use of ketoconazole, erythromycin, and amphotericin B can increase cyclosporine level, leading to toxicity.	› Monitor cyclosporine dosage, and adjust accordingly to prevent toxicity.
› Amphotericin B, aminoglycoside, and NSAIDs are nephrotoxic. Concurrent use with cyclosporine increases the risk for kidney dysfunction.	› Monitor BUN, creatinine, and I&O.
› Consumption of grapefruit juice increases cyclosporine levels by 50%, which poses an increased risk of toxicity.	› Advise clients to avoid drinking grapefruit juice.
Glucocorticoids	
› Diuretics that promote potassium loss increase the risk of hypokalemia.	› Monitor the client's potassium level, and administer supplements as needed.
› Because of the risk for hypokalemia, concurrent use of glucocorticoids with digoxin increases the risk of digoxin-induced dysrhythmias.	› Monitor for digoxin-induced dysrhythmias. Monitor potassium levels.
› NSAIDs increase the risk of GI ulceration.	› Advise clients to avoid use of NSAIDs. Instruct clients to notify the provider if GI distress occurs.
› Glucocorticoids promote hyperglycemia, thereby counteracting the effects of insulin and oral hypoglycemics.	› The dose of hypoglycemic medications may need to be increased.

Nursing Administration

- Advise clients that effects of DMARDs are delayed and can take 3 to 6 weeks, with full therapeutic effect taking several months.

- Administer adalimumab subcutaneously every other week.

- Administer etanercept by subcutaneous injection two times a week. Ensure the solution is clear without particles present.

- Glucocorticoids may be used as oral agents or as intra-articular injections. Short-term therapy may be used to control exacerbations of manifestations and while waiting for the effects of DMARDs to develop.

- Cyclosporine
  - Administer the initial IV dose of cyclosporine over 2 to 6 hr.
  - Monitor clients for hypersensitivity reactions. Stay with clients for 30 min after administration of cyclosporine.
  - Mix oral cyclosporine with milk or orange juice right before ingestion to increase palatability.
  - Instruct clients regarding the importance of lifelong therapy if used to prevent organ rejection.

Nursing Evaluation of Medication Effectiveness

- Depending on the therapeutic intent, effectiveness can be evidenced by:
  - Improvement of manifestations of RA (reduced swelling of joints, absence of joint stiffness, ability to maintain joint function, absence of pain).
  - Decrease in systemic complications, such as weight loss and fatigue.
  - Prevention of organ rejection.

APPLICATION EXERCISES

1. A nurse is preparing to administer auranofin (Ridaura) for a client who has rheumatoid arthritis. The nurse should monitor the client for which of the following adverse effects of this medication? (Select all that apply.)

_____ A. Insomnia

_____ B. Stomatitis

_____ C. Visual changes

_____ D. Bruising

_____ E. Pruritus

2. A nurse is reinforcing teaching with a client who has rheumatoid arthritis and is beginning a prescription for methotrexate. Which of the following statements by the client indicates understanding of the teaching?

    A. "I will be sure to return to the clinic at least once a year to have my blood drawn while I'm taking methotrexate."

    B. "I will take this medication on an empty stomach."

    C. "I'll let the doctor know if I develop sores in my mouth while taking this medication.

    D. "I should stop taking oral contraceptives while I'm taking methotrexate."

3. A nurse is caring for a client who is beginning a new prescription for adalimumab (Humira) for rheumatoid arthritis. Based on the route of administration of adalimumab, which of the following should the nurse plan to monitor?

    A. The client's vein for thrombophlebitis during IV administration

    B. The client's subcutaneous site for redness following injection

    C. The client's oral mucosa for ulceration after oral administration

    D. The client's skin for irritation following removal of transdermal patch

4. A nurse is caring for a client who has a prescription for cyclosporine (Sandimmune) to treat rheumatoid arthritis. Which of the following medications taken concurrently with cyclosporine is a risk for cyclosporine toxicity?

    A. Phenytoin (Dilantin)

    B. Isoniazid (INH)

    C. Carbamazepine (Tegretol)

    D. Erythromycin (Erythrocin)

5. A nurse is reviewing medications with a client who has a new diagnosis of rheumatoid arthritis. The nurse should instruct the client that which of the following medications will relieve arthritis pain and inflammation but will not stop the disease from progressing?

    A. Indomethacin (Indocin)

    B. Methotrexate

    C. Infliximab (Remicade)

    D. Abatacept (Orencia)

6. A nurse is reinforcing teaching with a client who has rheumatoid arthritis (RA) about his new prescription for etanercept (Enbrel). What should the nurse instruct the client about this medication? Use the ATI Remediation Template: Medication to complete this item to include the following:

    A. Therapeutic Use: Describe the therapeutic use for etanercept in this client.

    B. Adverse Effects: Describe at least three adverse effects the client should monitor for.

    C. Nursing Interventions: Describe one for each of the adverse effects above.

    D. Medication Administration: Describe at least three important factors.

APPLICATION EXERCISES KEY

1. A. INCORRECT: Insomnia is not an adverse reaction caused by auranofin.

    B. **CORRECT:** Stomatitis is an adverse effect of auranofin. The nurse should hold the medication and notify the provider if the client reports stomatitis.

    C. INCORRECT: Visual changes are not an adverse effect of auranofin.

    D. **CORRECT:** Thrombocytopenia is an adverse effect of auranofin, and bruising is a common finding in thrombocytopenia. The nurse should hold the medication and notify the provider if frequent bruising occurs.

    E. **CORRECT:** Pruritus is an adverse effect of auranofin. The nurse should hold the medication and notify the provider if pruritus occurs.

    Ⓝ NCLEX® Connection: Pharmacological Therapies, Adverse Effects/Contraindications/ Side Effects/Interactions

2. A. INCORRECT: CBC including platelet count, and liver and kidney function tests will be monitored at baseline and frequently during treatment with methotrexate to check for adverse effects.

    B. INCORRECT: Methotrexate should be taken with food to decrease gastrointestinal distress.

    C. **CORRECT:** Ulcerations in the mouth, tongue, or throat are often the first manifestations of methotrexate toxicity and should be reported to the provider immediately.

    D. INCORRECT: Methotrexate is a Pregnancy Category X medication and can cause severe fetal damage. The client should have a pregnancy test before starting the medication and should use a reliable form of birth control during methotrexate therapy. Oral contraceptives are not contraindicated with methotrexate therapy.

    Ⓝ NCLEX® Connection: Pharmacological Therapies, Adverse Effects/Contraindications/ Side Effects/Interactions

3. A. INCORRECT: Adalimumab is not administered intravenously. Therefore, monitoring for thrombophlebitis during administration is not necessary.

    B. **CORRECT:** Adalimumab is administered subcutaneously, and injection-site redness and swelling are common. Therefore, it is appropriate for the nurse to check the site for redness following injection.

    C. INCORRECT: Adalimumab is not administered orally. Therefore, monitoring oral mucosa for ulceration following administration is not necessary.

    D. INCORRECT: Adalimumab is not administered transdermally. Therefore, inspecting the skin for irritation is not necessary.

    Ⓝ NCLEX® Connection: Pharmacological Therapies, Adverse Effects/Contraindications/ Side Effects/Interactions

4. A. INCORRECT: Phenytoin can decrease cyclosporine levels and would not cause cyclosporine toxicity.

    B. INCORRECT: Isoniazid can decrease cyclosporine levels and would not cause cyclosporine toxicity.

    C. INCORRECT: Carbamazepine can decrease cyclosporine levels and would not cause cyclosporine toxicity.

    D. **CORRECT:** Erythromycin increases cyclosporine levels. Cyclosporine toxicity can result when the two medications are taken concurrently.

    (N) NCLEX® Connection: Pharmacological Therapies, Adverse Effects/Contraindications/ Side Effects/Interactions

5. A. **CORRECT:** Indomethacin and other NSAIDs have a rapid onset and work well to decrease joint pain and inflammation. However, NSAIDs do not stop the progression of the disease.

    B. INCORRECT: Methotrexate is a nonbiologic DMARD that can halt progression of rheumatoid arthritis. Therapeutic effects take 3 to 6 weeks to occur.

    C. INCORRECT: Infliximab is a tumor necrosis factor antagonist that can slow progression rheumatoid arthritis.

    D. INCORRECT: Abatacept is a T-cell activation inhibitor, which slows progression of rheumatoid arthritis.

    (N) NCLEX® Connection: Pharmacological Therapies, Expected Actions/Outcomes

6. *Using the ATI Remediation Template: Medication*

    A. Therapeutic Use
      • Etanercept is a biologic DMARD classified as a tumor necrosis factor antagonist. It suppresses manifestations of moderate to severe RA and slows the progression of the disorder.

    B. Adverse Effects
      • Severe infections, including tuberculosis or reactivation of hepatitis B
      • Heart failure
      • Severe skin reactions, such as Stevens-Johnson syndrome
      • Hematologic disorders

    C. Nursing Interventions
      • Instruct the client to monitor for infection, and to report sore throat and other manifestations.
      • Discuss reasons for TB testing and possible hepatitis B testing.
      • Instruct the client to notify the provider for edema, shortness of breath, and other manifestations of heart failure.
      • Report skin rash to provider.
      • Report easy bruising, bleeding, or unusual fatigue to provider.

    D. Medication Administration
      • Instruct the client to administer appropriately by subcutaneous injection twice weekly.
      • Discard solutions that are discolored or that contain particulate matter.
      • Monitor for injection-site reactions and report to provider.
      • Rotate injection sites.
      • Avoid skin areas that are bruised or reddened when injecting.

    (N) NCLEX® Connection: Pharmacological Therapies, Expected Actions/Outcomes

chapter 29

Overview

- Calcium is necessary for the proper functioning of bones, nerves, muscles, the heart, and blood coagulation.
- Calcium may be given as a supplement when dietary intake is insufficient. Uses for other medications that affect the bones include prevention and treatment of osteoporosis and prevention of fractures.
- Medication classifications include calcium supplements, selective estrogen receptor modulators (also known as estrogen agonist/antagonists), bisphosphonates, and calcitonin.

MEDICATION CLASSIFICATION: CALCIUM SUPPLEMENTS

- Select Prototype Medication: calcium citrate (Citracal)
- Other Medications
  - Calcium carbonate (Tums, Rolaids)
  - Calcium acetate (PhosLo)
  - For IV administration
    - Calcium chloride
    - Calcium gluconate

Purpose

- Expected Pharmacological Action – maintenance of normal musculoskeletal, neurological, and cardiovascular function
- Therapeutic Uses
  - Oral calcium supplements are used for clients with hypocalcemia or deficiencies of parathyroid hormone, vitamin D, or dietary calcium.

  - Oral dietary supplements are used for adolescents, older adults, and women who are postmenopausal, pregnant, or breastfeeding.
  - Intravenous medications are used for clients who have critically low levels of calcium.

Complications

ADVERSE EFFECTS	NURSING INTERVENTIONS/CLIENT EDUCATION
› Hypercalcemia (calcium level greater than 10.5 mg/dL) › Findings include tachycardia and elevated blood pressure, leading to bradycardia, hypotension, muscle weakness, hypotonia, constipation, nausea, vomiting, abdominal pain, lethargy, and confusion.	› Instruct clients to monitor for symptoms and report to the provider. › Monitor serum calcium levels to maintain between 9.0 to 10.5 mg/dL. › Medications used to reverse hypercalcemia include IV furosemide (Lasix); IV glucocorticoids; gallium (Ganite); bisphosphonates, such as alendronate (Fosamax); and oral inorganic phosphates.

Contraindications/Precautions

- Calcium supplements are contraindicated in clients who have hypercalcemia, bone tumors, and hyperparathyroidism.
- Use cautiously in clients who have kidney disease or a decrease in GI function.

Interactions

MEDICATION/FOOD INTERACTIONS	NURSING INTERVENTIONS/CLIENT EDUCATION
› Concurrent use of glucocorticoids reduces absorption of calcium.	› Give medications at least 1 hr apart.
› Concurrent use of calcium decreases absorption of tetracyclines and thyroid hormone.	› Ensure 1 hr between administration of medications.
› Concurrent administration of thiazide diuretics increases risk of hypercalcemia.	› Check clients for hypercalcemia. › Avoid concurrent use.
› Spinach, rhubarb, bran, and whole grains can decrease calcium absorption.	› Do not administer calcium with foods that decrease absorption. › Instruct clients to avoid consuming these foods at the same time as taking calcium.
› IV calcium precipitates with phosphates, carbonates, sulfates, and tartrates.	› Do not mix parenteral calcium with compounds that cause precipitation.
› Concurrent use of digoxin and parenteral calcium can lead to severe bradycardia.	› IV injection of calcium must be given slowly with careful monitoring of client status.

Nursing Administration

- Instruct clients to take a calcium supplement with a meal at least 1 hr apart from glucocorticoids, tetracyclines, or thyroid hormone.
- Chewable tablets provide more consistent bioavailability.
- Recommended doses of oral calcium vary widely depending on the specific calcium preparation. Instruct client to follow provider prescription.
- Prior to administration, warm IV infusions of calcium to body temperature.
- Administer IV injections at 0.5 to 2 mL/min.

Nursing Evaluation of Medication Effectiveness

- Depending on therapeutic intent, effectiveness can be evidenced by serum calcium level within expected reference range (9.0 to 10.5 mg/dL).

MEDICATION CLASSIFICATION:
SELECTIVE ESTROGEN RECEPTOR MODULATOR (AGONIST/ANTAGONIST)

- Select Prototype Medication: raloxifene (Evista)

Purpose

- Expected Pharmacological Action
  - Works as endogenous estrogen in bone, lipid metabolism, and blood coagulation
  - Decreases bone resorption, which results in slowing down of bone loss and preservation of bone mineral density
  - Works as an antagonist to estrogen on breast and endometrial tissue
  - Can decrease plasma levels of cholesterol
- Therapeutic Uses
  - Prevent and treat postmenopausal osteoporosis and prevent spinal fractures in female clients
  - Reduces the risk of invasive breast cancer in high-risk postmenopausal women

Complications

ADVERSE EFFECTS	NURSING INTERVENTIONS/CLIENT EDUCATION
› Increases the risk for pulmonary embolism and deep-vein thrombosis (DVT)	› Medication should be stopped prior to scheduled immobilization, such as surgery. Medication can be resumed when the client is fully mobile.
	› Discourage long periods of sitting and inactivity.
› Hot flashes	› Inform clients that the medication can exacerbate, rather than reduce, hot flashes.

Contraindications/Precautions

- Raloxifene is Pregnancy Risk Category X.
- This medication is contraindicated in clients who have a history of venous thrombosis. The medication should be stopped 3 days before periods in which risk of DVT is high (such as before surgical procedures).

Interactions

- Concurrent use with estrogen hormone therapy (HT) is discouraged.

Nursing Administration

- For maximum benefit of the medication, encourage clients to consume adequate amounts of calcium (such as from dairy products) and vitamin D (such as from egg yolks). Inadequate amounts of dietary calcium and vitamin D cause release of parathyroid hormone, which stimulates calcium release from the bone.
- Medication may be taken with or without food once a day.
- Monitor the client's bone density. Clients should undergo a bone density scan every 12 to 18 months.
- Monitor the client's serum calcium. Expected reference range is 9 to 10.5 mg/dL.
- Monitor liver function tests. Raloxifene levels may be increased in clients who have hepatic impairment.
- Encourage clients to perform weight-bearing exercises daily, such as walking 30 to 40 min each day.

Nursing Evaluation of Medication Effectiveness

- Depending on therapeutic intent, effectiveness can be evidenced by:
  - Increase in bone density.
  - No fractures.

MEDICATION CLASSIFICATION: BISPHOSPHONATES

- Select Prototype Medications: alendronate (Fosamax)
- Other Medications
  - Ibandronate (Boniva)
  - Risedronate (Actonel)
  - For IV infusion – zoledronic (Reclast, Zometa)

Purpose

- Expected Pharmacological Action
  - Bisphosphonates decrease the number and action of osteoclasts, which thereby inhibits bone resorption.
- Therapeutic Uses
  - Prevents and treats of postmenopausal osteoporosis
  - Treats osteoporosis in men
  - Prevents and treats osteoporosis produced by long-term glucocorticoid use
  - Treats Paget's disease of the bone and hypercalcemia of malignancy

Complications

ADVERSE EFFECTS	NURSING INTERVENTIONS/CLIENT EDUCATION
› Esophagitis, esophageal ulceration (oral formulations)	› Instruct client to sit upright or ambulate for 30 min (60 min with ibandronate sodium) after taking this medication orally.
	› Clients taking ibandronate (Boniva) must remain upright and not ingest food or other medications for 1 hr after taking the medication orally.
	› Instruct client to take tablets with at least 8 oz water and liquid formulation with at least 2 oz.
› GI disturbances, such as abdominal pain, nausea, diarrhea, constipation (all bisphosphonates)	› Notify provider for GI problems that prevent adequate intake.
› Musculoskeletal pain	› Advise client to take a mild analgesic.
	› Instruct client to notify the provider if pain persists. Alternate medication may be prescribed.
› Visual disturbances such as blurred vision and eye pain	› Instruct clients to watch for symptoms and report to the provider. Medication should be discontinued.
› Bisphosphonate-related osteonecrosis of the jaw (IV infusion)	› See dentist prior to beginning treatment. Avoid dental work during administration of medication.
› Risk for hyperparathyroidism at higher dose used for Paget's disease	› Monitor parathyroid hormone (PTH) levels.

Contraindications/Precautions

- Most bisphosphonates are Pregnancy Risk Category C. Zoledronic acid (Reclast, Zometa) is Pregnancy Risk Category D.

- These medications are contraindicated for women who are lactating.

- These medications are contraindicated in clients who have esophageal stricture or difficulty swallowing, esophageal disorders, serious renal impairment, and hypocalcemia. Oral bisphosphonates also are contraindicated for clients who cannot sit upright or stand for at least 30 min after taking the medication.

- Use cautiously in clients with upper GI disorders, infection, and liver impairment.

- Older adults are a slight risk for femoral fractures, which can occur without trauma while taking bisphosphonates.

Interactions

MEDICATION/FOOD INTERACTIONS	NURSING INTERVENTIONS/CLIENT EDUCATION
› Alendronate absorption decreases when taken with calcium supplements, antacids, orange juice, and caffeine.	› Advise clients to take the medication on an empty stomach with at least 8 oz water.
	› Wait 30 min (60 min with ibandronate sodium) after administration to take antacids or calcium.

Nursing Administration

- Instructions for clients
  - Take the medication first thing in the morning after getting out of bed.
  - Take oral medication on an empty stomach, drinking at least 8 oz water with tablets and at least 2 oz water with liquid formulation.
  - Sit or ambulate for 30 min after taking the medication.
  - Wait 30 min (60 min with ibandronate sodium) before eating or drinking after taking the medication.
  - Avoid all calcium-containing foods and liquids or any medications within 30 min of taking alendronate.
  - Avoid chewing or sucking on the tablet.
  - Perform weight-bearing exercises daily, such as walking 30 to 40 min each day.
  - Notify the provider of difficulty swallowing, painful swallowing, or new or worsening heartburn.
  - If a dose is skipped, wait until the next day 30 min before eating breakfast to take the dose. Do not take two tablets on the same day.
  - For maximum benefit of the medication, consume adequate amounts of calcium and vitamin D.
- Tablets are prescribed once daily or once a week. Liquid form is prescribed once a week.
- Monitor the client's bone density. Clients should have a bone density scan every 12 to 18 months.
- Monitor the client's serum calcium; expected reference range 9 to 10.5 mg/dL.

Nursing Evaluation of Medication Effectiveness

- Depending on therapeutic intent, effectiveness can be evidenced by:
  - Increase in bone density
  - No fractures

MEDICATION CLASSIFICATION: CALCITONIN

- Select Prototype Medication: calcitonin-salmon (Fortical, Miacalcin)

Purpose

- Expected Pharmacological Action
  - Decreases bone resorption by inhibiting the activity of osteoclasts in osteoporosis
  - Increases renal calcium excretion by inhibiting tubular resorption
- Therapeutic Uses
  - Treats (but does not prevent) postmenopausal osteoporosis, and treats moderate to severe Paget's disease
  - Hypercalcemia caused by hyperparathyroidism and cancer

Complications

ADVERSE EFFECTS	NURSING INTERVENTIONS/CLIENT EDUCATION
› Nausea	› Advise clients that nausea is usually self-limiting.
› Nasal dryness and irritation with intranasal route	› Instruct clients to alternate nostrils daily. › Inspect nasal mucosa periodically for ulceration.

Contraindications/Precautions

- This medication is Pregnancy Risk Category C.
- The medication is contraindicated in clients who have hypersensitivity to the medication and fish protein. Perform an allergy skin test prior to administration if the client is at risk.
- Use cautiously with chidlren, women who are lactating, and clients who have kidney disease.

Interactions

- Concurrent use with lithium can decrease serum lithium levels. Monitor lithium levels closely.

Nursing Administration

- Calcitonin-salmon is most commonly given by nasal spray. It also can be given IM or SC. Rotate injection sites to prevent inflammation.
- Keep the container in an upright position.
- Teach clients to alternate nostrils daily.
- Check for Chvostek's or Trousseau's signs to monitor for hypocalcemia.
- Monitor the client's bone density scans periodically.
- Encourage clients to consume a diet high in calcium and vitamin D.

Nursing Evaluation of Medication Effectiveness

- Depending on therapeutic intent, effectiveness can be evidenced by:
  - Increase in bone density.
  - Serum calcium level within expected reference range of 9 to 10.5 mg/dL.

APPLICATION EXERCISES

1. A nurse is reinforcing teaching to a client who is taking raloxifene (Evista) to prevent postmenopausal osteoporosis. The nurse should advise the client that which of the following are adverse effects of this medication? (Select all that apply.)

_____ A. Hot flashes

_____ B. Lump in breast

_____ C. Swelling or redness in calf

_____ D. Shortness of breath

_____ E. Difficulty swallowing

2. A nurse is caring for a client who has osteoporosis and a new prescription for alendronate (Fosamax). Which of the following instructions should the nurse provide for the client? (Select all that apply.)

_____ A. Take medication in the morning before eating.

_____ B. Chew tablets to increase bioavailability.

_____ C. Drink a full glass of water with each tablet.

_____ D. Take alendronate with an antacid if heartburn occurs.

_____ E. Avoid lying down after taking this medication.

3. A nurse is caring for a client who has a new prescription for calcitonin-salmon for osteoporosis. Which of the following tests should the nurse tell the client to expect before beginning this medication?

A. Skin test for allergy to the medication

B. ECG to rule out cardiac dysrhythmias

C. Mantoux test to rule out exposure to tuberculosis

D. Liver function tests to determine risk for medication toxicity

4. A nurse is caring for a young adult client whose serum calcium is 8.8 mg/dL. Which of the following medications should the nurse anticipate administering to this client?

A. Calcitonin-salmon (Miacalcin)

B. Calcium carbonate (Tums)

C. Zoledronic (Reclast)

D. Ibandronate (Boniva)

5. A nurse is reinforcing teaching with a client who has a new prescription for calcitonin-salmon (Miacalcin) for postmenopausal osteoporosis. Which of the following should the nurse instruct the client regarding self-administration of this medication?

    A. Swallow tablets on an empty stomach with plenty of water.

    B. Watch for skin rash and redness when applying calcitonin-salmon topically.

    C. Mix the liquid medication with juice and take it after meals.

    D. Alternate nostrils each time calcitonin-salmon is inhaled.

6. A nurse in an outpatient facility is reinforcing teaching with a postmenopausal client who is at high risk for osteoporosis about her new prescription for alendronate (Fosamax). What should the nurse instruct the client about this medication? Use the ATI Active Learning Template: Medication to complete this item to include the following:

    A. Therapeutic Use: Identify the therapeutic use for alendronate.

    B. Adverse Effects: List two adverse effects of this medication.

    C. Nursing Interventions:
        • Describe two diagnostic tests to monitor.
        • Describe two nursing actions.

APPLICATION EXERCISES KEY

1. A. **CORRECT:** Raloxifene can cause hot flashes or increase existing hot flashes.

    B. INCORRECT: Raloxifene does not cause breast lumps and is used therapeutically to protect against breast and endometrial cancer.

    C. **CORRECT:** Raloxifene increases the risk for thrombophlebitis, which can cause swelling or redness in the calf.

    D. **CORRECT:** Raloxifene increases the risk for pulmonary embolism, which can cause shortness of breath.

    E. INCORRECT: Difficulty swallowing is not an adverse effect of taking raloxifene.

    Ⓝ NCLEX® Connection: Pharmacological Therapies, Medication Administration

2. A. **CORRECT:** To prevent esophagitis, alendronate should be taking first thing in the morning before eating.

    B. INCORRECT: Chewing alendronate tablets can cause esophageal ulcers. The tablets should be swallowed whole.

    C. **CORRECT:** Clients should drink at least 8 oz water with alendronate tablets.

    D. INCORRECT: Alendronate should not be taken within 2 hr of an antacid.

    E. **CORRECT:** Clients should sit upright or stand for at least 30 min after taking alendronate.

    Ⓝ NCLEX® Connection: Pharmacological Therapies, Medication Administration

3. A. **CORRECT:** Anaphylaxis can occur if the client is allergic to calcitonin-salmon. A skin test to determine allergy may be done before starting this medication. The nurse also should ask the client about previous allergies to fish.

    B. INCORRECT: An ECG to rule out cardiac dysrhythmias is not necessary before beginning calcitonin-salmon. This medication does not affect heart rhythm.

    C. INCORRECT: A Mantoux test to rule out exposure to tuberculosis is not necessary before beginning calcitonin-salmon. This medication does not affect resistance to TB.

    D. INCORRECT: Liver function tests are not necessary before beginning calcitonin-salmon. This medication is metabolized in the kidneys and does not affect the liver.

    Ⓝ NCLEX® Connection: Pharmacological Therapies, Medication Administration

4. A. INCORRECT: Calcitonin-salmon increases excretion of calcium and is not appropriate for a client who has a serum calcium of 8.8 mg/dL.

    B. **CORRECT:** The client's serum calcium level is below the expected reference range. Calcium carbonate is an oral form of calcium used to increase serum calcium to the expected reference range.

    C. INCORRECT: Zoledronic acid (Reclast) is an IV bisphosphonate used to treat osteoporosis. This medication can decrease serum calcium levels by inhibiting bone resorption of calcium, and would not be prescribed for a client who has a serum calcium of 8.8 mg/dL.

    D. INCORRECT: Ibandronate is a bisphosphonate used to treat osteoporosis. This medication can decrease serum calcium levels by inhibiting bone reabsorption of calcium, and would not be prescribed for a client who has a serum calcium of 8.8 mg/dL.

    Ⓝ NCLEX® Connection: Pharmacological Therapies, Expected Actions/Outcomes

5. A. INCORRECT: Calcitonin-salmon is not supplied in tablet form.

    B. INCORRECT: Calcitonin-salmon is not supplied as a topical preparation.

    C. INCORRECT: Calcitonin-salmon is not supplied as a liquid preparation.

    D. **CORRECT:** Calcitonin-salmon may be injected, but is commonly administered intranasally for postmenopausal osteoporosis. The client should use alternate nostrils daily.

    Ⓝ NCLEX® Connection: Pharmacological Therapies, Medication Administration

6. *Using the ATI Active Learning Template: Medication*

    A. Therapeutic Use
    -   In the client who is at high risk for osteoporosis, the purpose of alendronate is to prevent osteoporosis from occurring by decreasing resorption of bone. The medication also is used to treat existing osteoporosis and Paget's disease.

    B. Adverse Effects
    -   Alendronate can cause esophagitis and esophageal ulceration; other GI effects, such as nausea, diarrhea, and constipation; muscle pain; and visual disturbances. Rarely, it can cause atraumatic femoral fracture.

    C. Nursing Interventions
    -   Diagnostic tests to monitor: serum calcium, bone density scans.
    -   Check the client's ability to follow administration directions (must be able to sit upright or stand for at least 30 min after taking alendronate and 60 min after taking ibandronate sodium).
    -   Instruct the client to take this medication first thing in the morning with at least 8 oz water and wait 30 min before eating or drinking anything else or taking any other medications or supplements.
    -   Instruct the client other ways to help prevent osteoporosis, such as performing weight-bearing exercises daily and obtaining adequate amounts of calcium and vitamin D.

    Ⓝ NCLEX® Connection: Pharmacological Therapies, Expected Actions/Outcomes

UNIT 9   Medications for Pain and Inflammation

CHAPTERS

› Nonopioid Analgesics
› Opioid Agonists and Antagonists
› Adjuvant Medications for Pain
› Miscellaneous Pain Medications

NCLEX® CONNECTIONS

When reviewing the chapters in this unit, keep in mind the relevant sections of the NCLEX® outline, in particular:

Client Needs: Pharmacological Therapies

› Relevant topics/tasks include:
  » Medication Administration
    › Identify the client's need for PRN medications.
  » Pharmacological Pain Management
    › Administer pharmacological pain medication
    › Monitor and document the client's response to pharmacological interventions (pain rating scale, verbal reports).
    › > Maintain pain control devices (epidural, patient-controlled analgesia, peripheral nerve catheter).

chapter 30

Overview

- Nonopioid analgesics can have anti-inflammatory, antipyretic, and analgesic action. These medications include nonsteroidal anti-inflammatory drugs (NSAIDs) and acetaminophen.

MEDICATION CLASSIFICATION: NONSTEROIDAL ANTI-INFLAMMATORY DRUGS

- First-generation NSAIDs (COX-1 and COX-2 inhibitors)

  ○ Aspirin

  ○ Ibuprofen (oral – Motrin, Advil; IV – Caldolor, NeoProfen)

  ○ Naproxen (Naprosyn); naproxen sodium (Aleve)

  ○ Indomethacin (Indocin)

  ○ Diclofenac (oral – Voltaren, Cataflam, Cambia, Zipsor; intradermal – Flector patch, Pennsaid, Voltaren gel)

  ○ Ketorolac (generic; Sprix – intranasal)

  ○ Meloxicam (Mobic)

- Second-generation NSAIDs (selective COX-2 inhibitor)

  ○ Celecoxib (Celebrex)

Purpose

- Expected Pharmacological Action

  ○ Inhibition of cyclooxygenase – Inhibition of COX-1 can result in decreased platelet aggregation and kidney damage. Inhibition of COX-2 results in decreased inflammation, fever, and pain.

- Therapeutic Uses

  ○ Inflammation suppression

  ○ Analgesia for mild to moderate pain, such as with osteoarthritis and rheumatoid arthritis

  ○ Fever reduction

  ○ Dysmenorrhea

  ○ Inhibition of platelet aggregation, which protects against ischemic stroke and myocardial infarction (aspirin)

Complications

ADVERSE EFFECTS	NURSING INTERVENTIONS/CLIENT EDUCATION
› Gastrointestinal discomfort (dyspepsia, abdominal pain, heartburn, nausea). › Damage to gastric mucosa can lead to GI bleeding and perforation, especially with long-term use. › Risk is increased in older adults, clients who smoke or abuse alcohol, and those who have a history of peptic ulcers or previous inability to tolerate NSAIDS.	› Advise clients to take medication with food, a full glass of water, or milk. › Advise clients to avoid alcohol. › Observe for manifestations of bleeding (passage of black or dark-colored stools, severe abdominal pain, nausea, vomiting). › Administer a proton pump inhibitor, such as omeprazole (Prilosec), or an H_2-receptor antagonist, such as ranitidine (Zantac), to decrease the risk of ulcer formation. › Use prophylaxis agents such as misoprostol (Cytotec).
› Renal dysfunction (decreased urine output, weight gain from fluid retention, increased BUN and creatinine levels).	› Use cautiously with older adults and clients who have heart failure. › Monitor I&O and kidney function (BUN, creatinine).
› Increased risk of heart attack and stroke (nonaspirin NSAIDs).	› Use the smallest effective dose for clients who have known cardiovascular disease.
› Salicylism can occur with aspirin. Clinical manifestations include tinnitus, sweating, headache and dizziness, and respiratory alkalosis.	› Advise clients to notify the provider and to stop taking aspirin if manifestations occur.
› Reye syndrome is a rare but serious complication. This occurs when aspirin is used for fever reduction in children and adolescents who have a viral illness, such as chickenpox or influenza.	› Advise clients to avoid giving aspirin when a child or adolescent has a viral illness, such as chickenpox or influenza.
› Aspirin toxicity (progresses from the mild findings in salicylism to sweating, high fever, acidosis, dehydration, electrolyte imbalances, coma, respiratory depression).	› Aspirin toxicity should be managed as a medical emergency in the hospital. › Therapy » Cooling with tepid water » Correction of dehydration and electrolyte imbalance with IV fluids » Reversal of acidosis and promotion of salicylate excretion with bicarbonate » Gastric lavage › Activated charcoal also may be given to decrease absorption. › Hemodialysis may be indicated.

Contraindications/Precautions

- Contraindications for aspirin and other first-generation NSAIDs
  - Pregnancy (Pregnancy Risk Category D)
  - Peptic ulcer disease
  - Bleeding disorders, such as hemophilia and vitamin K deficiency
  - Hypersensitivity to aspirin and other NSAIDs
  - Children and adolescents who have chickenpox or influenza (aspirin)

- Use NSAIDs cautiously in older adults, clients who smoke cigarettes, and in clients who have *Helicobacter pylori* infection, hypovolemia, asthma, chronic urticaria, and/or a history of alcohol use disorder.
- Celecoxib is contraindicated in clients who have an allergy to sulfonamides.
- Ketorolac is contraindicated in clients who have advanced renal dysfunction. Use should be no longer than 5 days because of the risk for kidney damage.
- Second-generation NSAIDs should be used cautiously in clients who have known cardiovascular disease.

Interactions

MEDICATION/FOOD INTERACTIONS	NURSING INTERVENTIONS/CLIENT EDUCATION
› Anticoagulants, such as heparin and warfarin, increase the risk of bleeding.	› Monitor PTT, PT, and INR. › Advise clients about the potential risk of bleeding when an NSAID is combined with an anticoagulant. Instruct clients to report manifestations of bleeding.
› Glucocorticoids increase the risk of gastric bleeding.	› Instruct clients to take antiulcer prophylaxis, such as misoprostol (Cytotec), to decrease the risk for gastric ulcer.
› Alcohol increases the risk of bleeding.	› Instruct clients to avoid consuming alcoholic beverages to decrease the risk of GI bleeding.
› Ibuprofen decreases the antiplatelet effects of low-dose aspirin used to prevent MI.	› Instruct clients not to take ibuprofen concurrently with aspirin.
› Ketorolac and concurrent use of other NSAIDs increase the risk of known adverse effects.	› Ketorolac should not be used concurrently with other NSAIDs.

Nursing Administration

- Instruct clients to stop aspirin 1 week before an elective surgery or expected date of childbirth.
- Instruct clients to take NSAIDs with food, milk, or a full glass of water to reduce gastric discomfort.
- Instruct clients not to chew or crush enteric-coated or sustained-release aspirin tablets.
- Advise clients to notify the provider if manifestations of gastric discomfort or ulceration occur.

- Advise clients to notify the provider if manifestations of salicylism occur. Medication should be discontinued until manifestations are resolved. Medication can be restarted at a lower dose.
- Ketorolac may be used for short-term treatment of moderate to severe pain, such as that associated with postoperative recovery.
  - Concurrent use with opioids allows for lower dosages of opioids and thus minimizes adverse effects such as constipation and respiratory depression.
  - Ketorolac is usually first administered parenterally and then switched to oral doses. Use should not be longer than 5 days because of the risk for kidney damage.

Nursing Evaluation of Medication Effectiveness

- Depending on therapeutic intent, effectiveness can be evidenced by the following.
  - Reduction in inflammation
  - Reduction of fever
  - Relief from mild to moderate pain
  - Absence of injury

MEDICATION CLASSIFICATION: ACETAMINOPHEN

- Select Prototype Medication: acetaminophen (Tylenol)

Purpose

- Expected Pharmacological Action
  - Acetaminophen slows the production of prostaglandins in the central nervous system.
- Therapeutic Uses
  - Analgesic (relief of pain) effect
  - Antipyretic (reduction of fever) effects

Complications

ADVERSE EFFECTS	NURSING INTERVENTIONS/CLIENT EDUCATION
› Adverse effects are rare at therapeutic dosages, but acute toxicity results in liver damage with early manifestations of nausea, vomiting, diarrhea, sweating, and abdominal discomfort progressing to hepatic failure, coma, and death.	› Advise clients to take acetaminophen as prescribed and not to exceed 4 g/day. Parents should carefully follow providers' advice regarding administration of acetaminophen to children. › Administer the antidote, acetylcysteine (Mucomyst).

Contraindications/Precautions

- Use cautiously in clients who consume three or more alcoholic drinks per day and those taking warfarin (interferes with metabolism), thus increasing the risk of bleeding.

Interactions

MEDICATION/FOOD INTERACTIONS	NURSING INTERVENTIONS/CLIENT EDUCATION
› Alcohol increases the risk of liver damage.	› Advise clients about the potential risk of liver damage with consumption of alcohol.
› Acetaminophen slows the metabolism of warfarin (Coumadin) leading to increased levels of warfarin. This places clients at risk for bleeding.	› Instruct clients to observe for signs of bleeding (bruising, petechiae, hematuria). › Monitor prothrombin time and INR levels, and adjust dosages of warfarin accordingly.

Nursing Administration

- Acetaminophen is a component of multiple prescribed and over-the-counter medications. Keep a running total of daily acetaminophen intake, and follow recommended dosages as prescribed by the provider to prevent toxicity, not to exceed 4 g/day.

- The U.S. Food and Drug Administration recommends that clients take only one product containing acetaminophen at a given time. Teach clients to read medication labels carefully to determine the amount of medication contained in each dose.

- In the event of an overdose, administer acetylcysteine (Mucomyst; the antidote for acetaminophen) to prevent liver damage. Administer via an oroduodenal tube to prevent emesis and subsequent aspiration.

Nursing Evaluation of Medication Effectiveness

- Depending on therapeutic intent, effectiveness can be evidenced by the following.
  - Relief of pain
  - Reduction of fever

APPLICATION EXERCISES

1. A nurse is caring for a client who is diagnosed with salicylism. Which of the following findings should the nurse expect? (Select all that apply.)

_____ A. Dizziness

_____ B. Diarrhea

_____ C. Jaundice

_____ D. Tinnitus

_____ E. Headache

2. A nurse is assisting with the admission of a toddler to the hospital following an acetaminophen overdose. Which of the following medications should the nurse anticipate being administered to this client?

A. Acetylcysteine (Mucomyst)

B. Pegfilgrastim (Neulasta)

C. Misoprostol (Cytotec)

D. Naltrexone (ReVia)

3. A nurse is preparing to administer acetaminophen (Tylenol) 10 mg/kg PO to a toddler who weighs 9 kg (19.8 lb). Available is acetaminophen liquid 160 mg/5 mL. How many mL should the nurse plan to administer? (Round the answer to the nearest tenth.)

4. A nurse is checking a client who has severe aspirin toxicity. Which of the following findings should the nurse expect?

A. Body temperature 35° C (95° F)

B. Lung crackles

C. Cool, dry skin

D. Respiratory depression

5. A nurse is taking a history from a client who reports that he is taking aspirin about four times daily for a sprained wrist. Which of the prescribed medications taken by the client is contraindicated with aspirin?

    A. Digoxin (Lanoxin)

    B. Metformin (Glucophage)

    C. Warfarin (Coumadin)

    D. Nitroglycerin (Nitro-Dur)

6. A nurse in an outpatient facility is reinforcing teaching with a client who has osteoarthritis and is starting long-term therapy with naproxen sodium (Aleve) 500 mg twice daily. What should the nurse instruct the client about this medication? Use the ATI Active Learning Template: Medication to complete this item to include the following:

    A. Therapeutic Use

    B. Adverse Effects: Describe two.

    C. Nursing Interventions:
- Describe two laboratory values the nurse should monitor.
- Describe two nursing actions.

APPLICATION EXERCISES KEY

1. A. **CORRECT:** Dizziness is a common finding in the client who has salicylism.

    B. INCORRECT: Diarrhea is not a finding in salicylism.

    C. INCORRECT: Jaundice is not a finding in salicylism.

    D. **CORRECT:** Tinnitus is a common finding in the client who has salicylism.

    E. **CORRECT:** Headache is a common finding in the client who has salicylism.

    Ⓝ NCLEX® Connection: Pharmacological Therapies, Adverse Effects/Contraindications/
    Side Effects/Interactions

2. A. **CORRECT:** Acetylcysteine is the antidote for acetaminophen overdose.

    B. INCORRECT: Pegfilgrastim is a long-acting medication used to increase the body's production
    of neutrophils.

    C. INCORRECT: Misoprostol is a prostaglandin hormone used to prevent the formation of gastric ulcers.

    D. INCORRECT: Naltrexone is an opioid antagonist used to prevent alcohol craving.

    Ⓝ NCLEX® Connection: Pharmacological Therapies, Adverse Effects/Contraindications/
    Side Effects/Interactions

3. **2.8** mL

Using Ratio and Proportion		
STEP 1: *What is the unit of measurement to calculate?* mg	STEP 6: *What is the dose available? Dose available = Have.* 160 mg	STEP 10: *Round if necessary.* 2.8125 = 2.8
STEP 2: *Set up an equation and solve for X.* mg x kg/dose = X 10 mg x 9 kg = 90 mg	STEP 7: *Should the nurse convert the units of measurement?* No	STEP 11: *Reassess to determine whether the amount to give makes sense.* If there are 160 mg/5 mL and the prescribed amount is 90 mg, it makes sense to give 2.8 mL. The nurse should administer acetaminophen liquid 2.8 mL PO.
STEP 3: *Round if necessary.*	STEP 8: *What is the quantity of the dose available?* 5 mL	
STEP 4: *Reassess to determine whether the amount makes sense.* If the prescribed amount is 10 mg/kg and the toddler weighs 9 kg, it makes sense to give 90 mg.	STEP 9: *Set up an equation and solve for X.* $\dfrac{\text{Have}}{\text{Quantity}} = \dfrac{\text{Desired}}{X}$ $\dfrac{160 \text{ mg}}{5 \text{ mL}} = \dfrac{90 \text{ mg}}{X \text{ mL}}$ X = 2.8125	
STEP 5: *What is the unit of measurement to calculate?* mL		

Using Desired Over Have

STEP 1: *What is the unit of measurement to calculate?*
mg

STEP 2: *Set up an equation and solve for X.*
mg x kg/dose = X
10 mg x 9 kg = 90 mg

STEP 3: *Round if necessary.*

STEP 4: *Reassess to determine whether the amount makes sense.*
If the prescribed amount is 10 mg/kg and the toddler weighs 9 kg, it makes sense to give 90 mg.

STEP 5: *What is the unit of measurement to calculate?*
mL

STEP 6: *What is the dose available? Dose available = Have*
160 mg

STEP 7: *Should the nurse convert the units of measurement?*
No

STEP 8: *What is the quantity of the dose available?*
5 mL

STEP 9: *Set up an equation and solve for X.*

$$\frac{\text{Desired x Quantity}}{\text{Have}} = X$$

$$\frac{90 \text{ mg x } 5 \text{ mL}}{160 \text{ mg}} = X \text{ mL}$$

2.8125 = X

STEP 10: *Round if necessary.*
2.8125 = 2.8

STEP 11: *Reassess to determine whether the amount to give makes sense.*
If there are 160 mg/5 mL and the prescribed amount is 90 mg, it makes sense to give 2.8 mL. The nurse should administer acetaminophen liquid 2.8 mL PO.

Using Dimensional Analysis

STEP 1: *What is the unit of measurement to calculate?*
mg

STEP 2: *Set up an equation and solve for X.*
mg x kg/dose = X
10 mg x 9 kg = 90 mg

STEP 3: *Round if necessary.*

STEP 4: *Reassess to determine whether the amount makes sense.*
If the prescribed amount is 10 mg/kg and the toddler weighs 9 kg, it makes sense to give 90 mg.

STEP 5: *What is the unit of measurement to calculate?*
mL

STEP 6: *What quantity of the dose is available?*
5 mL

STEP 7: *What is the dose available? Dose available = Have*
160 mg

STEP 8: *What is the dose needed? Dose needed = Desired*
90 mg

STEP 9: *Should the nurse convert the units of measurement?*
No

STEP 10: *Set up an equation of factors and solve for X.*

$$X = \frac{\text{Quantity}}{\text{Have}} \times \frac{\text{Conversion (Have)}}{\text{Conversion (Desired)}} \times \frac{\text{Desired}}{}$$

$$X \text{ mL} = \frac{5 \text{ mL}}{160 \text{ mg}} \times \frac{90 \text{ mg}}{160 \text{ mg}}$$

X = 2.8125

STEP 11: *Round if necessary.*
2.8125 = 2.8

STEP 12: *Reassess to determine whether the amount to give makes sense.*
If there are 160 mg/5 mL and the prescribed amount is 90 mg, it makes sense to give 2.8 mL. The nurse should administer acetaminophen liquid 2.8 mL PO.

 NCLEX® Connection: Pharmacological Therapies, Dosage Calculation

4. A. INCORRECT: A clinical manifestation of severe aspirin toxicity is hyperthermia.

    B. INCORRECT: A clinical manifestation of severe aspirin toxicity is dehydration. Lung crackles are not an expected finding.

    C. INCORRECT: A clinical manifestation of severe aspirin toxicity is diaphoresis. Cool, dry skin is not an expected finding.

    D. **CORRECT:** Respiratory depression due to increasing respiratory acidosis is an expected clinical manifestation of severe aspirin toxicity.

    Ⓝ NCLEX® Connection: Pharmacological Therapies, Adverse Effects/Contraindications/ Side Effects/Interactions

5. A. INCORRECT: Digoxin does not interact with aspirin and therefore is not contraindicated.

    B. INCORRECT: Metformin does not interact with aspirin and therefore is not contraindicated.

    C. **CORRECT:** The effect of warfarin and other anticoagulants is increased by aspirin, which inhibits platelet aggregation. This client would have an increased risk for bleeding. Use of aspirin generally is contraindicated for clients who take warfarin.

    D. INCORRECT: Nitroglycerin does not interact with aspirin and therefore is not contraindicated.

    Ⓝ NCLEX® Connection: Pharmacological Therapies, Adverse Effects/Contraindications/ Side Effects/Interactions

6. *Using ATI Active Learning Template: Medication*

    A. Therapeutic Use
    - Naproxen sodium is an NSAID. It will treat mild to moderate joint pain and stiffness, and decrease inflammation in the client who has osteoarthritis.

    B. Adverse Effects
    - Gastrointestinal effects can occur, including anorexia, abdominal pain, nausea, vomiting, and heartburn.
    - GI bleeding can occur because naproxen sodium affects platelet function.
    - Nephrotoxicity can occur.
    - Naproxen sodium and other NSAIDS can cause the CNS effects of dizziness, headache, blurred vision, and tinnitus.
    - Allergy can occur, including cross allergy with other NSAIDS, such as aspirin.

    C. Nursing Interventions
    - Diagnostic tests to monitor: Hgb/Hct and kidney function tests. Naproxen sodium is metabolized in the liver, so the nurse should also be prepared to monitor liver function.
    - Check the client for previous allergy to NSAIDs.
    - Check the GI system, and ask about any history of GI bleed or peptic ulcer disease.
    - Advise the client to take the medication with food or prescribed antacid if GI distress occurs.
    - Advise the client to tell provider about any over-the-counter medications, vitamins, or herbals before taking them.

    Ⓝ NCLEX® Connection: Pharmacological Therapies, Expected Actions/Outcomes

chapter 31

Overview

- Opioid analgesics are medications used to treat moderate to severe pain. Most opioid analgesics reduce pain by attaching to a receptor in the central nervous system, altering perception and response to pain.
- Opioids are classified as agonists, agonist-antagonists, and antagonists.
    - An agonist attaches to a receptor and produces a response.
    - An agonist-antagonist binds to one receptor, causing a response, and binds to another receptor, which prevents a response.
    - An antagonist attaches to a receptor site and prevents a response.
- The desired outcome is to reduce pain and increase activity with few adverse effects.

OPIOID AGONISTS

- Select Prototype Medication: morphine
- Other Medications
    - Fentanyl (Sublimaze, Duragesic)
    - Meperidine (Demerol)
    - Methadone (Dolophine)
    - Codeine
    - Oxycodone (OxyContin)

Purpose

- Expected Pharmacological Action
    - Opioid agonists, such as morphine, codeine, meperidine, and other morphine-like medications (fentanyl), act on the mu receptors, and to a lesser degree on kappa receptors. Activation of mu receptors produces analgesia, respiratory depression, euphoria, and sedation, whereas kappa receptor activation produces analgesia, sedation, and decreased GI motility.
- Therapeutic Uses
    - Relief of moderate to severe pain (postoperative, myocardial infarction, cancer)
    - Sedation
    - Reduction of bowel motility
    - Codeine — cough suppression

- Route of administration
  - ○ Morphine – oral, subcutaneous, IM, rectal, IV, epidural, intrathecal
  - ○ Other Medications
    - Fentanyl – IV, IM, transmucosal, transdermal
    - Meperidine – oral, subcutaneous, IM, IV
    - Codeine – oral, subcutaneous, IM, IV
    - Methadone – oral, subcutaneous, IM
    - Oxycodone – oral
    - Hydromorphone – oral, subcutaneous, rectal, IM, IV

Complications

ADVERSE EFFECTS	NURSING INTERVENTIONS/CLIENT EDUCATION
› Respiratory depression	› Monitor vital signs. › Stop opioids for respiratory rate less than 12/min, and notify the provider. › Have naloxone and resuscitation equipment available. › Avoid use of opioids with CNS depressant medications (barbiturates, benzodiazepines, consumption of alcohol).
› Constipation	› Advise the client to increase fluid/fiber intake and physical activity. › Administer a stimulant laxative such as bisacodyl (Dulcolax) to counteract decreased bowel motility, or a stool softener such as docusate sodium (Colace) to prevent constipation. › For clients who have end-stage disorders, such as cancer or AIDS, administer an opioid antagonist, such as methylnaltrexone (Relistor), designed to treat severe constipation in opioid-dependent clients.
› Orthostatic hypotension	› Advise clients to sit or lie down if lightheadedness or dizziness occur. › Avoid sudden changes in position by slowly moving clients from a lying to a sitting or standing position. › Provide assistance with ambulation as needed.
› Urinary retention	› Advise clients to void every 4 hr. › Monitor I&O. › Monitor the bladder for distention by palpating the lower abdomen area every 4 to 6 hr.
› Cough suppression	› Advise clients to cough at regular intervals to prevent accumulation of secretions in the airway. › Auscultate the lungs for crackles, and instruct clients to increase intake of fluid to liquefy secretions.

ADVERSE EFFECTS	NURSING INTERVENTIONS/CLIENT EDUCATION
› Sedation	› Advise clients to avoid hazardous activities, such as driving or operating heavy machinery.
› Biliary colic	› Avoid giving morphine to clients who have a history of biliary colic. Use meperidine as an alternative.
› Nausea/vomiting	› Administer an antiemetic such as promethazine.
› Opioid overdose triad of coma, respiratory depression, and pinpoint pupils	› Monitor vital signs. › Provide mechanical ventilation. › Administer naloxone, an opioid antagonist that reverses respiratory depression and other overdose manifestations.

Contraindications/Precautions

- Morphine is contraindicated after biliary tract surgery.
- Morphine is contraindicated for premature infants during and after delivery because of respiratory depressant effects.
- Meperidine is contraindicated for clients who have kidney failure because of the accumulation of normeperidine, which can result in seizures and neurotoxicity.
- Use cautiously with:
  - Clients who have asthma, emphysema, and/or head injuries; infants; and older adult clients (risk of respiratory depression).
  - Clients who are pregnant (risk of physical dependence of the fetus).
  - Clients in labor (risk of respiratory depression in the newborn and inhibition of labor by decreasing uterine contractions).
  - Clients who are extremely obese (greater risk for prolonged adverse effects because of the accumulation of medication that is metabolized at a slower rate).
  - Clients who have inflammatory bowel disease (risk of megacolon or paralytic ileus).
  - Clients who have an enlarged prostate (risk of acute urinary retention).
  - Clients who have hepatic or renal disease.

Interactions

MEDICATION/FOOD INTERACTIONS	NURSING INTERVENTIONS/CLIENT EDUCATION
› CNS depressants (barbiturates, phenobarbital, benzodiazepines, alcohol) have additive CNS depression action.	› Warn clients about the use of these medications in conjunction with opioid agonists. › Advise clients to avoid consumption of alcohol.
› Anticholinergic agents (atropine or scopolamine), antihistamines (diphenhydramine), and tricyclic antidepressants (amitriptyline) have additive anticholinergic effects (constipation, urinary retention).	› Advise clients to increase fluids and dietary fiber to prevent constipation.
› Meperidine can interact with monoamine oxidase inhibitors (MAOIs) and cause hyperpyrexic coma, characterized by excitation, seizures, and respiratory depression.	› Avoid the use of meperidine with MAOIs to prevent occurrence of this syndrome.
› Antihypertensives have additive hypotensive effects.	› Warn clients to refrain from using opioids with antihypertensive agents.

Nursing Administration

- Monitor the client's pain level on a regular basis. Document the client's response.
- Take the client's baseline vital signs. If the respiratory rate is less than 12/min, notify the provider and withhold the medication.
- Follow controlled substance procedures.
- Double check opioid doses with another nurse prior to administration.
- Assist the nurse in the administration of opioids IV slowly over a period of 4 to 5 min. Have naloxone and resuscitation equipment available.
- Warn clients not to increase dosage without consulting the provider.
- For clients who have cancer, administer opioids on a fixed schedule around the clock. Administer supplemental doses as needed.
- Advise clients who have physical dependence not to discontinue opioids abruptly. Opioids should be withdrawn slowly, and the dosage should be tapered over a period of 3 days.
- Closely monitor patient-controlled analgesia (PCA) pump settings (dose, lockout interval, 4-hr limit). Reassure clients regarding safety measures that safeguard against self-administration of excessive doses. Encourage clients to use PCA prophylactically prior to activities likely to augment pain levels.
- When switching clients from PCA to oral doses of opioids, make sure the client receives adequate PCA dosing until the onset of oral medication takes place.
- The first administration of a transdermal fentanyl patch will take several hours to achieve the desired therapeutic effect. Administer short-acting opioids prior to onset of therapeutic effects and for breakthrough pain.

Nursing Evaluation of Medication Effectiveness

- Depending on the therapeutic intent, effectiveness may be evidenced by:
  - Relief of moderate to severe pain (postoperative pain, cancer pain, myocardial pain)
  - Cough suppression
  - Resolution of diarrhea

MEDICATION CLASSIFICATION: AGONIST-ANTAGONIST OPIOIDS

- Select Prototype Medication: pentazocine (Talwin)
- Other Medications
  - Nalbuphine
  - Buprenorphine (Buprenex)
  - Butorphanol (Stadol)

Purpose

- Expected Pharmacological Action
  - These medications act as antagonists on mu receptors and agonists on kappa receptors, except for buprenorphine, whose agonist-antagonist activity is on opposite receptors.
  - Compared to pure opioid agonists, agonist-antagonists have:
    - A low potential for abuse causing little euphoria. In fact, high doses can cause adverse effects (anxiety, restlessness, mental confusion).
    - Less respiratory depression.
    - Less analgesic effect.
- Therapeutic Uses
  - Relief of moderate to severe pain
  - Treatment of opioid dependence (buprenorphine)
  - Adjunct to balanced anesthesia
  - Relief of labor pain (butorphanol)
- Route of administration
  - Butorphanol – IV, IM, intranasal
  - Nalbuphine – IV, IM, subcutaneous
  - Buprenorphine – IV, IM, sublingual, transdermal patch
  - Pentazocine – IV, IM, subcutaneous, oral

Complications

ADVERSE EFFECTS	NURSING INTERVENTIONS/CLIENT EDUCATION
› Abstinence syndrome (cramping, hypertension, vomiting, fever, and anxiety)	› This syndrome may be precipitated when these medications are given to clients who are physically dependent on opioid agonists. › Advise clients to stop opioid agonists, such as morphine, before using agonist-antagonist medications, such as pentazocine. › Avoid giving to clients if undisclosed opioid use is suspected.
› Sedation, respiratory depression	› Have naloxone and resuscitation equipment available. Monitor for respiratory depression.
› Dizziness	› Instruct the client to use caution in standing up and to avoid driving or using heavy machinery.
› Headache	› Monitor for headache. Determine level of consciousness.

Contraindications/Precautions

- Use cautiously in clients who have a history of myocardial infarction, kidney or liver disease, respiratory depression, or head injury, and clients who are physically dependent on opioids.

Interactions

MEDICATION/FOOD INTERACTIONS	NURSING INTERVENTIONS/CLIENT EDUCATION
› CNS depressants and alcohol can cause additive effects.	› Use together cautiously. › Monitor respirations.
› Opioid agonists can antagonize and reduce analgesic effects of the opioid.	› Do not use concurrently.

Nursing Administration

- Obtain the client's baseline vital signs. If the respiratory rate is less than 12/min, withhold the medication and notify the provider.

- Have naloxone and resuscitation equipment available.

- Determine client opioid dependence prior to administration. Agonist-antagonists may trigger withdrawal symptoms.

- Warn clients not to increase dosage without consulting the provider.

- Advise clients to use caution when getting out of bed or standing. Clients should not operate heavy machinery or drive until CNS effects are known.

- Warn clients not to increase dosage without consulting the provider.

Nursing Evaluation of Medication Effectiveness

- Monitor for improvement of symptoms, such as relief of pain.

MEDICATION CLASSIFICATION: OPIOID ANTAGONISTS

- Select Prototype Medication: naloxone
- Other Medications
  - Naltrexone (ReVia, Vivitrol)
  - Methylnaltrexone (Relistor)

Purpose

- Expected Pharmacological Action – Opioid antagonists interfere with the action of opioids by competing for opioid receptors. Opioid antagonists have no effect in the absence of opioids.
- Therapeutic Uses
  - Treatment of opioid overdose
  - Reversal of effects of opioids, such as respiratory depression
  - Reversal of respiratory depression in an infant
  - Reversal of severe opioid-caused constipation in clients who have late-stage cancer or other disorders (methylnaltrexone)
- Route of administration
  - Naloxone – IV, IM, subcutaneous
  - Naltrexone – oral, IM
  - Methylnaltrexone – subcutaneous

Complications

ADVERSE EFFECTS	NURSING INTERVENTIONS/CLIENT EDUCATION
› Tachycardia and tachypnea	› Monitor heart rhythm (risk of ventricular tachycardia) and respiratory function. › Have resuscitative equipment, including oxygen, on standby during administration.
› Abstinence syndrome (cramping, hypertension, vomiting, and reversal of analgesia)	› These manifestations can occur when given to clients physically dependent on opioid agonists.

Contraindications/Precautions

- Opioid antagonists are Pregnancy Risk Category C.
- These medications are contraindicated in clients who have opioid dependency.
- Naltrexone is contraindicated for clients who have acute hepatitis or liver failure and during lactation.

Interactions

- None noted

Nursing Administration

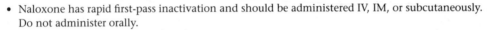

- Naloxone has rapid first-pass inactivation and should be administered IV, IM, or subcutaneously. Do not administer orally.
- Observe clients for withdrawal symptoms or abrupt onset of pain. Be prepared to address the client's need for analgesia (if given for postoperative opioid-related respiratory depression).
- Titrate dosage to achieve reversal of respiratory depression without full reversal of pain management effects.
- Rapid infusion of naloxone can cause hypertension, tachycardia, nausea, and vomiting.
- Half-life of opioid analgesic can exceed the half-life of naloxone (60 to 90 min).
- Monitor respirations for up to 2 hr after use for reoccurrence of respiratory depression and the need for repeat dosage of naloxone.

Nursing Evaluation of Medication Effectiveness

- Reversal of respiratory depression (respirations are regular, client is without shortness of breath, respiratory rate is 16 to 20/min in adults and 40 to 60/min in newborns)
- Reduced euphoria in alcohol dependency and decreased craving for alcohol in alcohol dependency (naltrexone)
- Severe opioid-caused constipation relieved (methylnaltrexone)

APPLICATION EXERCISES

1. A nurse is assisting with the preparation of morphine 12 mg IV for a client who has severe cancer pain. Available is 15 mg/mL morphine for injection. How many mL should the nurse anticipate for administration? (Round the answer to the nearest tenth.)

2. A nurse is planning to assist with the administration of meperidine (Demerol) IV to a client who is postoperative. Which of the following is an appropriate nursing action when administering meperidine?

    A. Monitor for seizures and confusion with repeated doses.

    B. Protect client's skin from the severe diarrhea that occurs with meperidine.

    C. Stop administering this medication if client's respiratory rate is less than 15/min.

    D. Monitor the administration of meperidine via IV push over 30 seconds or less.

3. A nurse is reinforcing teaching the daughter of a client who has end-stage lung cancer and is receiving large doses of morphine for pain. The client has a new prescription for methylnaltrexone (Relistor), and the daughter asks why the nurse is administering this medication. Which of the following replies by the nurse is appropriate?

    A. "The medication will increase your mother's respirations."

    B. "The medication will prevent dependence on the morphine."

    C. "The medication will relieve your mother's constipation."

    D. "The medication works with the morphine to increase pain relief."

4. A nurse is preparing to administer butorphanol (Stadol) to a newly admitted client who has a history of substance use disorder. Which of the following is true regarding butorphanol?

    A. Butorphanol has a greater risk for abuse than morphine.

    B. Butorphanol causes a higher incidence of respiratory depression than morphine.

    C. Butorphanol cannot be reversed with an opioid antagonist.

    D. Butorphanol can cause abstinence syndrome in opioid-dependent clients.

5. A nurse is caring for a hospitalized client who is receiving intradermal fentanyl (Duragesic) for severe pain. Which of the following medications should the nurse expect to cause an adverse effect when administered concurrently with fentanyl?

   A. Ampicillin (Principen)

   B. Diazepam (Valium)

   C. Furosemide (Lasix)

   D. Prednisone

6. A nurse is reinforcing discharge teaching for a postoperative client who is to take oxycodone (OxyContin) 20 mg twice daily PO for the next 3 days. What should the nurse include in the instructions? Use the ATI Active Learning Template: Medication to complete this item to include the following:

   A. Therapeutic Use: Describe for oxycodone.

   B. Adverse Effects: List three for oxycodone.

   C. Nursing Interventions: List three.

APPLICATION EXERCISES KEY

1. **0.8** mL

Using Ratio and Proportion

STEP 1: *What is the unit of measurement to calculate?*
mL

STEP 2: *What is the dose needed? Dose needed = Desired.*
12 mg

STEP 3: *What is the dose available? Dose available = Have.*
15 mg

STEP 4: *Should the nurse convert the units of measurement?*
No

STEP 5: *What is the quantity of the dose available?*
1 mL

STEP 6: *Set up an equation and solve for X.*

$$\frac{Have}{Quantity} = \frac{Desired}{X}$$

$$\frac{15\ mg}{1\ mL} = \frac{12\ mg}{X\ mL}$$

$$X = 0.8$$

STEP 7: *Round if necessary.*

STEP 8: *Reassess to determine whether the amount to give makes sense.*
If there is 15 mg/mL and the prescribed amount is 12 mg, it makes sense to give 0.8 mL. The nurse should monitor the administration of morphine injection 0.8 mL IV bolus.

Using Desired Over Have

STEP 1: *What is the unit of measurement to calculate?*
mL

STEP 2: *What is the dose needed? Dose needed = Desired.*
12 mg

STEP 3: *What is the dose available? Dose available = Have.*
15 mg

STEP 4: *Should the nurse convert the units of measurement?*
No

STEP 5: *What is the quantity of the dose available?*
1 mL

STEP 6: *Set up an equation and solve for X.*

$$\frac{Desired \times Quantity}{Have} = X$$

$$\frac{12\ mg \times 1\ mL}{15\ mg} = X\ mL$$

$$0.8 = X$$

STEP 7: *Round if necessary.*

STEP 8: *Reassess to determine whether the amount to give makes sense.*
If there is 15 mg/mL and the prescribed amount is 12 mg, it makes sense to give 0.8 mL. The nurse should monitor the administration of morphine injection 0.8 mL IV bolus.

Using Dimensional Analysis

STEP 1: *What is the unit of measurement to calculate?*
mL

STEP 2: *What quantity of the dose is available?*
1 mL

STEP 3: *What is the dose available? Dose available = Have.*
15 mg

STEP 4: *What is the dose needed? Dose needed = Desired.*
12 mg

STEP 5: *Should the nurse convert the units of measurement?*
No

STEP 6: *Set up an equation of factors and solve for X.*

$$X = \frac{Quantity}{Have} \times \frac{Conversion\ (Have)}{Conversion\ (Desired)} \times \frac{Desired}{}$$

$$X\ mL = \frac{1\ mL}{15\ mg} \times \frac{12\ mg}{}$$

$$X = 0.8$$

STEP 7: *Round if necessary.*

STEP 8: *Reassess to determine whether the amount to give makes sense.*
If there is 15 mg/mL and the prescribed amount is 12 mg, it makes sense to give 0.8 mL. The nurse should monitor the administration of morphine injection 0.8 mL IV bolus.

 NCLEX® Connection: Pharmacological Therapies, Dosage Calculation

2.   A. **CORRECT:** With repeated doses of meperidine, a toxic metabolite can build up and cause severe CNS effects such as agitation, confusion, and seizures.

   B. INCORRECT: Constipation, rather than diarrhea, is an expected effect of administering opioids, such as meperidine.

   C. INCORRECT: Opioids should be stopped and the provider notified for a respiratory rate of 12/min or less.

   D. INCORRECT: Monitor the administration of meperidine IV bolus slowly over 3 to 5 min.

   Ⓝ NCLEX® Connection: Pharmacological Therapies, Adverse Effects/Contraindications/ Side Effects/Interactions

3.   A. INCORRECT: Methylnaltrexone does not decrease analgesia or increase a depressed respiratory rate.

   B. INCORRECT: Methylnaltrexone does not prevent dependence on opioids, such as morphine.

   C. **CORRECT:** Methylnaltrexone is an opioid antagonist used for treating severe constipation that is unrelieved by laxatives in opioid-dependent clients.

   D. INCORRECT: Methylnaltrexone is not an adjunct to opioids for pain relief.

   Ⓝ NCLEX® Connection: Pharmacological Therapies, Adverse Effects/Contraindications/ Side Effects/Interactions

4.   A. INCORRECT: Butorphanol has less risk for abuse than morphine.

   B. INCORRECT: Butorphanol is less likely to cause respiratory depression than morphine.

   C. INCORRECT: Manifestations of butorphanol overdose can be reversed with an opioid antagonist if necessary.

   D. **CORRECT:** Opioid agonist-antagonist medications, such as butorphanol, can cause abstinence syndrome in opioid-dependent clients. Manifestations include abdominal pain, fever, and anxiety.

   Ⓝ NCLEX® Connection: Pharmacological Therapies, Adverse Effects/Contraindications/ Side Effects/Interactions

5. A. INCORRECT: Ampicillin, an antibiotic, does not interact with fentanyl and should not cause an adverse effect.

    B. **CORRECT:** Diazepam, a benzodiazepine, is a CNS depressant, which can interact to cause severe sedation when administered concurrently with an opioid agonist or agonist-antagonist.

    C. INCORRECT: Furosemide, a loop diuretic, does not interact with fentanyl and should not cause an adverse effect.

    D. INCORRECT: Prednisone, a glucocorticoid, does not interact with fentanyl and should not cause an adverse effect.

    Ⓝ NCLEX® Connection: Pharmacological Therapies, Adverse Effects/Contraindications/ Side Effects/Interactions

6. *Using the ATI Active Learning Template: Medication*

    A. Therapeutic Use
    *   Oxycodone is indicated for relief of moderate to severe pain.

    B. Adverse Effects
    *   Sedation
    *   Nausea/vomiting
    *   Constipation
    *   Orthostatic hypotension
    *   Urinary retention

    C. Nursing Interventions
    *   Instruct the client not to drive or perform other hazardous activities while using this medication.
    *   Notify the provider for severe nausea/vomiting.
    *   Prevent constipation by increasing intake of liquids and foods with fiber. Consider use of a stool softener or laxatives if necessary.
    *   Move slowly from lying or sitting to standing to minimize effects of orthostatic hypotension.
    *   Void every 4 hr. Contact provider for dysuria manifestations.

    Ⓝ NCLEX® Connection: Pharmacological Therapies, Expected Actions/Outcomes

chapter 32

Overview

- Adjuvant medications for pain are used with a primary pain medication, usually an opioid agonist, to increase pain relief while reducing the dosage of the opioid agonist.

- Reduced dosage of the opioid results in reduced adverse reactions, such as respiratory depression, sedation, and constipation. Targeting pain stimulus using different types of medications often provides improved pain reduction.

- Categories of medications in this section include tricyclic antidepressants, anticonvulsants, CNS stimulants, antihistamines, glucocorticoids, bisphosphonates, and nonsteroidal anti-inflammatory drugs (NSAIDs).

MEDICATION CLASSIFICATION: ADJUVANT MEDICATIONS FOR PAIN

- Select Prototype Medications
  - Tricyclic antidepressants: amitriptyline – oral/IM
  - Anticonvulsants: carbamazepine (Tegretol), gabapentin (Neurontin) – oral
  - CNS stimulants: methylphenidate (Ritalin) – oral
  - Antihistamines: hydroxyzine (Vistaril) – oral, IM
  - Glucocorticoids: dexamethasone – oral, IV, IM
  - Bisphosphonates: etidronate (Didronel) – oral
  - NSAIDs: ibuprofen (Motrin) – oral
- Other Medications
  - Tricyclic antidepressants: imipramine (Tofranil) – oral
  - Anticonvulsants: phenytoin (Dilantin) – oral, IV, IM
  - CNS stimulants: dextroamphetamine (Dexedrine) – oral
  - Glucocorticoids: prednisone – oral
  - Bisphosphonates: pamidronate (Aredia) – IV
  - NSAIDs: ketorolac – oral, IM, IV, intranasal

Purpose

- Expected Pharmacological Action
  - ○ Adjuvant medications for pain enhance the effects of opioids.
- Therapeutic Uses
  - ○ These medications are used in combination with opioids and cannot be used as a substitute for opioids.
  - ○ NSAIDs are used to treat inflammation.
  - ○ Tricyclic antidepressants are used to treat depression and neuropathic pain, such as cramping, aching, burning, darting, and lancinating pain.
  - ○ Anticonvulsants are used to relieve neuropathic pain.
  - ○ CNS stimulants augment analgesia and decrease sedation.
  - ○ Antihistamines decrease anxiety, prevent insomnia, and relieve nausea.
  - ○ Glucocorticoids decrease pain from intracranial pressure and spinal cord compression.
  - ○ Bisphosphonates manage hypercalcemia and bone pain.

Complications

ADVERSE EFFECTS	NURSING INTERVENTIONS/CLIENT EDUCATION
Tricyclic antidepressants: amitriptyline	
› Orthostatic hypotension	› Advise clients to sit or lie down if lightheadedness or dizziness occur, and to change positions slowly. › Provide assistance with ambulation as needed. › Monitor the client's blood pressure while the client is lying down, sitting, and standing.
› Sedation	› Advise clients to avoid hazardous activities, such as driving or operating heavy machinery.
› Anticholinergic effects, such as dry mouth, urinary retention, constipation, and blurred vision	› Advise clients to increase fluid intake, sip fluids throughout the day, chew gum, or suck on hard candy. › Instruct clients to increase physical activity by engaging in a regular exercise routine. › Administer a stimulant laxative, such as bisacodyl (Dulcolax), to counteract decreased bowel motility, and a stool softener, such as docusate sodium (Colace), to prevent constipation. › Advise clients to void every 4 hr and to report urinary retention. › Advise clients to report blurred vision. › Monitor I&O, and check the client's bladder for distention by palpating the lower abdomen area every 4 to 6 hr.

ADVERSE EFFECTS	NURSING INTERVENTIONS/CLIENT EDUCATION
Anticonvulsants: carbamazepine, gabapentin	
› Bone marrow suppression	› Periodically monitor complete blood count, including platelets.
	› Advise clients to observe for indications of bone marrow suppression, such as easy bruising and bleeding, fever, or sore throat, and to notify the provider if they occur.
› Gastrointestinal distress (nausea, vomiting, and diarrhea)	› Advise clients to take the medication with food.
CNS stimulants: methylphenidate	
› Weight loss	› Monitor the client's weight. Encourage good nutrition.
› Insomnia	› Instruct clients to take the last dose of the day no later than 4 p.m.
Antihistamines: hydroxyzine	
› Sedation	› Advise clients to avoid hazardous activities, such as driving or operating heavy machinery. Reduce dosage in older adult clients.
› Dry mouth	› Advise clients to increase fluid intake, sip fluids throughout the day, chew gum, or suck on hard candy.
Glucocorticoids: dexamethasone	
› Adrenal insufficiency (hypotension, dehydration, weakness, lethargy, vomiting, diarrhea associated with prolonged use)	› Advise clients to observe for indications and to notify the provider if they occur.
› Osteoporosis	› Advise clients to take calcium supplements, vitamin D, and/or bisphosphonate (alendronate [Fosamax]).
› Hypokalemia	› Monitor potassium levels, and administer potassium supplements as needed.
› Glucose intolerance	› Monitor blood glucose levels.
› Peptic ulcer disease	› Advise clients to take the medication with meals.
	› Encourage prophylactic use of an H_2 antagonist, such as ranitidine (Zantac).
Bisphosphonates: etidronate, pamidronate	
› Transient flulike symptoms	› Monitor for fever. Advise clients to notify the provider if symptoms occur.
› Venous irritation at injection site (pamidronate)	› Monitor the injection site and monitor that medication is infused with sufficient IV fluids.
› Hypocalcemia	› Monitor calcium, magnesium, potassium, and phosphate levels. Instruct client to report numbness/tingling around the mouth, spasms, or seizures to provider

ADVERSE EFFECTS	NURSING INTERVENTIONS/CLIENT EDUCATION
NSAIDs: ibuprofen	
› Bone marrow suppression	› Periodically monitor the client's complete blood count including platelets. › Advise clients to observe for indications of easy bruising and bleeding, fever, or sore throat, and to notify the provider if they occur.
› Gastrointestinal distress, such as nausea, vomiting, and diarrhea, or ulceration	› Advise client to take with food or meals. › Monitor for GI bleed (coffee-ground emesis; bloody, tarry stools; abdominal pain).

Contraindications/Precautions

MEDICATION	CONTRAINDICATIONS
Tricyclic antidepressants: amitriptyline	› These medications are contraindicated in clients recovering from an MI and within 14 days of taking a MAOI. › Use caution with clients who have a seizure disorder, urinary retention, prostatic hyperplasia, angle-closure glaucoma, hyperthyroidism, and liver or kidney disease.
Anticonvulsants: carbamazepine, gabapentin	› These medications are contraindicated in clients who have bone marrow suppression and within 14 days of taking a MAOI. › Use caution with clients who have a seizure disorder. › Pregnancy Risk Category D. Avoid use in pregnancy.
CNS stimulants: methylphenidate	› Methylphenidate is contraindicated in clients who have hyperthyroidism and hypertension and within 14 days of taking a MAOI. › Use caution with clients who have agitation or tics.
Antihistamines: hydroxyzine	› Hydroxyzine is contraindicated in clients who are hypersensitive to this medication. › Use caution with older adults.
Glucocorticoids: dexamethasone	› Dexamethasone is contraindicated in clients who have fungal infection. › Use caution with clients who have a seizure disorder, peptic ulcer disease, hypertension, hypothyroidism, diabetes mellitus, or liver disease.
Bisphosphonate: etidronate	› Etidronate is contraindicated in clients who are hypersensitive to this medication. › Use caution with clients who have kidney disease.
NSAIDs: ibuprofen	› Ibuprofen is contraindicated in clients who have a history of bronchospasms with aspirin or NSAIDs. › Use caution with clients who have peptic ulcers, hypertension, and liver or kidney disease.

Interactions

MEDICATION/FOOD INTERACTIONS	NURSING INTERVENTIONS/CLIENT EDUCATION
Tricyclic antidepressants: amitriptyline	
› Barbiturates, CNS depressants, and alcohol can cause additive CNS depression.	› Do not use together.
Anticonvulsants: carbamazepine, gabapentin	
› Carbamazepine causes a decrease in the effects of oral contraceptives and warfarin (Coumadin) because of the stimulation of hepatic drug-metabolizing enzymes.	› Advise client to discuss possible contraceptive changes with provider. › Monitor for therapeutic effects of warfarin with PT and INR. › Warfarin dosage may need to be adjusted.
› Grapefruit juice inhibits metabolism, and thus increases carbamazepine levels.	› Advise clients to avoid intake of grapefruit juice.
› Phenytoin and phenobarbital decrease the effects of carbamazepine.	› Concurrent use is not recommended.
CNS stimulants: methylphenidate	
› Alkalizing medications can cause increase in reabsorption.	› Monitor for increase in amphetamine effects.
› Acidifying medications can increase excretion of amphetamine.	› Monitor for decrease in amphetamine effects.
› Insulin and oral antidiabetic medications can decrease glucose level.	› Monitor glucose level.
› MAOIs can cause severe hypertension.	› Avoid concurrent use.
› Caffeine may increase stimulant effect.	› Advise clients to avoid caffeine.
› OTC medications with sympathomimetic action can lead to increased CNS stimulation.	› Instruct clients to avoid use of OTC medications.
Antihistamines: hydroxyzine	
› Barbiturates, CNS depressants, and alcohol can cause additive CNS depression.	› Do not use together.
Glucocorticoids: dexamethasone	
› Glucocorticoids promote hyperglycemia, thereby counteracting the effects of insulin and oral hypoglycemics.	› The dose of hypoglycemic medications may need to be increased.
› Concurrent use of salicylates and NSAIDs can increase the risk for GI bleed.	› Monitor for GI bleed. Use together cautiously.
› Because of the risk for hypokalemia, there is an increased risk of dysrhythmias caused by digoxin.	› Monitor potassium and cardiac rhythm. › Administer potassium supplements.
› Diuretics that promote potassium loss increase the risk for hypokalemia.	› Monitor serum potassium level. › Encourage clients to eat potassium-rich foods. › Administer potassium supplements.

MEDICATION/FOOD INTERACTIONS	NURSING INTERVENTIONS/CLIENT EDUCATION
Bisphosphonates: etidronate, pamidronate	
› Decreased absorption with calcium or iron supplements and high-calcium foods.	› Advise clients to take etidronate on an empty stomach 2 hr before meals with a full glass of water.
NSAIDs: ibuprofen	
› NSAIDs can reduce effectiveness of antihypertensives, furosemide, and thiazide diuretics.	› Monitor for medication effectiveness.
› Aspirin and corticosteroids may increase GI effects.	› Do not use together.
› NSAIDs can increase levels of oral anticoagulants and lithium.	› Monitor medication levels.

Nursing Administration

- Contribute to the client's pain management plan.
- Encourage clients who have cancer to voice fears and concerns about cancer, cancer pain, and pain treatment.

- Advise clients that pain medications should be given on a fixed schedule around the clock, and not as-needed.
- Advise clients that physical dependence is not considered addiction.

Nursing Evaluation of Medication Effectiveness

- Depending on the therapeutic intent, effectiveness can be evidenced by:
  - Relief of depression, seizures, dysrhythmias, and other symptoms that aggravate the client's pain level.
  - Decreased opioid adverse effects.
  - Relief of neuropathic pain.
  - Decreased cancer bone pain.

APPLICATION EXERCISES

1. A nurse is caring for a client who takes oral morphine and carbamazepine (Tegretol) for cancer pain. Which of the following effects can occur when both medications are administered to this client? (Select all that apply.)

_____ A. Dosage of the opioid is reduced.

_____ B. Adverse effects of the opioid are reduced.

_____ C. Analgesic effects are increased.

_____ D. CNS stimulation is enhanced.

_____ E. Opioid tolerance is increased.

2. A nurse is contributing to the plan of care for a client who has brain cancer and experiences headache caused by cerebral edema. Which of the following adjuvant medications may be indicated for this client?

A. Dexamethasone

B. Methylphenidate (Ritalin)

C. Hydroxyzine (Vistaril)

D. Amitriptyline

3. A nurse is caring for a client who has cancer and is taking a glucocorticoid as an adjuvant for pain control. The nurse should plan to perform which of the following interventions? (Select all that apply.)

_____ A. Monitor for urinary retention.

_____ B. Monitor serum glucose.

_____ C. Monitor serum potassium level.

_____ D. Monitor for gastric bleeding.

_____ E. Monitor for respiratory depression.

4. A nurse is assisting with the administration of pamidronate (Aredia) to a client who has bone pain caused by cancer. Which of the following precautions should the nurse take when assisting with the administration of pamidronate?

A. Inspect skin for redness and irritation when changing the client's intradermal patch.

B. Check IV site for thrombophlebitis frequently during administration.

C. Instruct the client to sit upright or stand for 30 min following oral administration.

D. Watch for manifestations of anaphylaxis for 20 min after IM administration.

5. A nurse is administering amitriptyline to a client who has pain caused by a malignant tumor. Which of the following is an adverse effect of amitriptyline that should be monitored by the nurse?

    A. Decreased appetite

    B. Explosive diarrhea

    C. Decreased pulse rate

    D. Orthostatic hypotension

6. A nurse in an acute care facility is reinforcing teaching for a client who has metastatic cancer and is receiving morphine and carbamazepine (Tegretol) for pain. What should the nurse instruct the client about the medications? Use the ATI Remediation Template: Medication to complete this item to include the following:

    A. Therapeutic Use: Describe the therapeutic use for carbamazepine in this client.

    B. Adverse Effects: Describe two adverse effects the client should monitor for.

    C. Food/Medication Interactions: Describe two interactions with carbamazepine.

    D. Nursing Interventions: Describe two.

APPLICATION EXERCISES KEY

1. A. **CORRECT:** Dosage of the opioid may be reduced when adjuvant medications are added for pain.

    B. **CORRECT:** Adverse effects of the opioid can be reduced when adjuvant medications are added for pain.

    C. **CORRECT:** Analgesic effects are increased when adjuvant medications are added for pain.

    D. INCORRECT: CNS stimulation is not enhanced when morphine and carbamazepine are used together for pain relief.

    E. INCORRECT: Opioid tolerance can be decreased, rather than increased, when an adjuvant medication is added for pain.

    Ⓝ NCLEX® Connection: Pharmacological Therapies, Adverse Effects/Contraindications/ Side Effects/Interactions

2. A. **CORRECT:** Dexamethasone, a glucocorticoid, decreases inflammation and swelling. It is used to reduce cerebral edema and relieve pressure from the tumor.

    B. INCORRECT: Methylphenidate's use as an adjuvant is to elevate mood and increase pain relief. It does not reduce cerebral edema.

    C. INCORRECT: Hydroxyzine's use as an adjuvant is to decrease anxiety and help the client sleep. It does not reduce cerebral edema.

    D. INCORRECT: Amitriptyline's use as an adjuvant is to relieve neuropathic pain and elevate the client's mood. It does not reduce cerebral edema.

    Ⓝ NCLEX® Connection: Pharmacological Therapies, Expected Actions/Outcomes

3. A. INCORRECT: Monitoring for urinary retention is not necessary because glucocorticoids do not cause this effect.

    B. **CORRECT:** Monitoring serum glucose is important because glucocorticoids raise the glucose level, especially in clients who have diabetes mellitus.

    C. **CORRECT:** Monitoring serum potassium level is important because glucocorticoids can cause hypokalemia.

    D. **CORRECT:** Monitoring for gastric bleeding is important because glucocorticoids irritate the gastric mucosa and put the client at risk for a peptic ulcer.

    E. INCORRECT: Monitoring for respiratory depression is not necessary because glucocorticoids do not depress respirations.

    Ⓝ NCLEX® Connection: Pharmacological Therapies, Adverse Effects/Contraindications/ Side Effects/Interactions

4. A. INCORRECT: This medication is not administered by the intradermal route.

    B. **CORRECT:** Pamidronate is administered by IV infusion. This medication is irritating to veins, and the nurse should check for thrombophlebitis during administration.

    C. INCORRECT: This medication is not administered orally.

    D. INCORRECT: This medication is not administered by the IM route.

    Ⓝ NCLEX® Connection: Pharmacological Therapies, Medication Administration

5. A. INCORRECT: Amitriptyline can cause increased appetite and weight gain rather than decreased appetite.

    B. INCORRECT: Amitriptyline can cause constipation rather than explosive diarrhea.

    C. INCORRECT: Amitriptyline can cause increased, rather than decreased, pulse rate.

    D. **CORRECT:** Amitriptyline can cause orthostatic hypotension. The nurse should monitor the client for this effect and should instruct the client to move slowly from lying down or sitting after taking this medication.

    Ⓝ NCLEX® Connection: Pharmacological Therapies, Adverse Effects/Contraindications/ Side Effects/Interactions

6. *Using the ATI Remediation Template: Medication*

    A. Therapeutic Use
    - Carbamazepine relieves neuropathic (nerve) pain, which can be described as sharp, burning, or aching.

    B. Adverse Effects
    - Adverse effects of carbamazepine include GI manifestations such as abdominal pain, nausea, and vomiting. It also can cause bone marrow suppression, including all blood cell types.

    C. Food/Medication Interactions
    - The medication may cause hypertensive crisis if taken within 14 days of an MAOI antidepressant.
    - Toxicity may result if the client drinks grapefruit juice while taking carbamazepine.

    D. Nursing Interventions
    - Monitor client's CBC, including platelet counts.
    - Check client for abnormal bleeding, bruising, or infection.
    - Monitor for GI manifestations, and advise client to take the medication with food.

    Ⓝ NCLEX® Connection: Pharmacological Therapies, Expected Actions/Outcomes

chapter 33

Overview

- Pain is subjective and can be indicative of tissue injury or impending tissue injury.

- Pain can result from the release of chemical mediators, inflammation, or pressure.

- Gout is caused by elevated levels of uric acid, which can accumulate and cause localized inflammation in synovial areas. Antigout medications act either by reducing inflammation or decreasing serum uric acid levels.

- Migraine headaches can be caused by the inflammation and vasodilation of cerebral blood vessels. Medications used to control migraine headaches may be used as needed to stop an oncoming migraine or to prevent a migraine from occurring.

- Local anesthetics block motor and sensory neurons to a specific area. They may be given topically; injected directly into an area; or given regionally, epidurally, or into the subarachnoid (spinal) space.

MEDICATION CLASSIFICATION: ANTIGOUT MEDICATIONS

MEDICATIONS	EXPECTED PHARMACOLOGICAL ACTION	THERAPEUTIC USES
Anti-inflammatory agents		
› Select Prototype Medication: colchicine (Colcrys) › Other Medications » NSAIDs: indomethacin (Indocin), naproxen (Naprosyn), diclofenac (Voltaren)	› Colchicine is only effective for inflammation of gout. › These medications decrease inflammation.	› Abort an acute gout attack in response to precursor symptoms › Treatment of acute attacks › Decrease incidence of acute attacks for clients who have chronic gout
» Glucocorticoids: prednisone		› Prednisone is used for clients with acute gout who are unable to take or unresponsive to NSAIDs.
Agents for hyperuricemia		
› Select Prototype Medication: allopurinol (Zyloprim) › Other Medications: febuxostat (Uloric), probenecid	› Allopurinol and febuxostat inhibit uric acid production. › Probenecid inhibits uric acid reabsorption by renal tubules.	› Hyperuricemia due to chronic gout or secondary to cancer chemotherapy

Route of Administration

- Colchicine – oral
- Allopurinol – oral, IV

Complications

ADVERSE EFFECTS	NURSING INTERVENTIONS/CLIENT EDUCATION
Colchicine	
› Mild GI distress, which can progress to GI toxicity (abdominal pain, diarrhea, nausea, vomiting)	› Advise clients to take oral medications with food. › Provide antidiarrheal agents as prescribed. › If severe GI distress occurs, stop colchicine and notify provider.
› Thrombocytopenia, suppressed bone marrow	› Advise clients to notify the provider of bleeding, bruising or sore throat.
› Sudden onset of muscle pain, tenderness (rhabdomyolysis)	› Advise clients to notify provider for new onset of these findings.
Probenecid	
› Renal calculi (occur with higher excretion of uric acid)	› Advise clients to drink 3 L fluid daily to decrease risk.
Allopurinol	
› Hypersensitivity reaction, fever, and rash	› If giving IV, stop infusion. Severe reaction can require hemodialysis or glucocorticoids.
› Kidney injury	› Alkalinize the urine and encourage intake of 2 to 3 L of fluids/day. Monitor I&O, BUN, and creatinine.
› Hepatitis	› Monitor liver enzymes.
› GI distress (nausea and vomiting)	› Give with food.

Contraindications/Precautions

- Colchicine
  - Pregnancy Risk Category C

  - Use cautiously in older adults; clients who are debilitated; and clients who have renal, cardiac, hepatic, or gastrointestinal dysfunction.
- Probenecid
  - Can precipitate acute gout. Do not give within 2 to 3 weeks of an acute attack.
- Allopurinol
  - Pregnancy Risk Category C
  - This medication is contraindicated in clients who have medication hypersensitivity or idiopathic hemochromatosis.
  - Rhabdomyolysis is most likely with long-term use. Risk is higher in clients taking statins for high cholesterol and those who have impaired kidneys or liver.

Interactions

MEDICATION/FOOD INTERACTIONS	NURSING INTERVENTIONS/CLIENT EDUCATION
Colchicine	
› Grapefruit juice may increase adverse effects.	› Advise clients to avoid drinking grapefruit juice when taking colchicine.
Probenecid	
› Salicylates can lessen the effectiveness of probenecid and can precipitate gout.	› Advise clients not to use salicylates during colchicine/probenecid therapy.
› Salicylates, such as aspirin, interfere with probenecid's therapeutic effect.	› Avoid concurrent use of salicylates with probenecid.
Allopurinol	
› Allopurinol slows the metabolism of warfarin within the liver, which places clients at risk for bleeding.	› Instruct clients to observe for manifestations of bleeding (bruising, petechiae, hematuria). › Monitor prothrombin time and INR levels, and adjust warfarin dosages accordingly.

Nursing Administration

- When clients are taking medications for gout, monitor uric acid levels, CBC, urinalysis, and liver and kidney function tests.
- Monitor administration of allopurinol IV. It should be well diluted and administered as an infusion over 30 to 60 min.
- Advise clients to take oral gout medication with food or after meals to minimize GI distress.
- Allopurinol and probenecid – If a rash develops, advise clients to stop the medication and report the occurrence to the provider.

- Instruct clients to concurrently take preventive measures, such as avoiding alcohol and foods high in purine (red meat, scallops, cream sauces). Clients should ensure an adequate intake of water, exercise regularly, and maintain an appropriate body weight.

Nursing Evaluation of Medication Effectiveness

- Depending on the therapeutic intent, effectiveness can be evidenced by:
  - Improvement of pain caused by a gout attack (decrease in joint swelling, redness, uric acid levels).
  - Decrease in number of gout attacks.
  - Decrease in uric acid levels.

MEDICATION CLASSIFICATION: MIGRAINE MEDICATIONS

- Select Prototype Medications
  - Acetaminophen, NSAIDs (aspirin, naproxen (Naprosyn), and others
  - Ergot alkaloids: ergotamine (Ergomar), dihydroergotamine (Migranal)
  - Serotonin receptor agonists (triptans): sumatriptan (Imitrex)
  - Beta-blockers: propranolol (Inderal)
  - Anticonvulsants: divalproex (Depakote ER), topiramate (Topamax)
  - Tricyclic antidepressants: amitriptyline
  - Calcium channel blockers: verapamil (Calan)
  - Estrogens: estrogen gel and estrogen patches (Alora, Climara, Estraderm)
- Other Medications:
  - Ergot alkaloids: ergotamine and caffeine (Cafergot)
  - Triptans: almotriptan (Axert), frovatriptan (Frova), naratriptan (Amerge), zolmitriptan (Zomig)
  - Combination OTC analgesics: acetaminophen, aspirin, caffeine (Excedrin Migraine)
  - Other combinations: isometheptene, dichloralphenazone/acetaminophen (Midrin). Isometheptene relieves headaches through vasoconstriction of arterioles; dichloralphenazone has sedative properties; acetaminophen is a mild analgesic.

Purpose

- Expected Pharmacological Action
  - Migraine medications prevent the inflammation and dilation of the intracranial blood vessels, thereby relieving migraine pain.
- Therapeutic Uses
  - Some medications are used to stop a migraine after it begins or after prodromal manifestations start. These include NSAIDs and combination anti-inflammatory medications, ergotamine, and triptans.
  - Other medications help to prevent a migraine headache. Preventive agents include beta-blockers, anticonvulsants, amitriptyline, calcium channel blockers, and estrogens.
- Route of Administration
  - Ergotamine – oral, sublingual, rectal
  - Dihydroergotamine – IV, IM, subcutaneous, intranasal
  - Sumatriptan – oral, subcutaneous, inhalation
  - Propranolol, divalproex, verapamil – oral
  - Amitriptyline – oral

Complications

ADVERSE EFFECTS	NURSING INTERVENTIONS/CLIENT EDUCATION
Ergot alkaloids: ergotamine and dihydroergotamine	
› Gastrointestinal discomfort such as nausea and vomiting	› Administer metoclopramide (Reglan).
› Ergotism (muscle pain; paresthesias in fingers and toes; cold, pale extremities)	› Stop medication, and immediately notify the provider if manifestations occur.
› Physical dependence	› Advise clients not to exceed the prescribed dose. › Inform clients regarding manifestations of withdrawal (headache, nausea, vomiting, restlessness). › Instruct clients to notify the provider if manifestations occur.
› Fetal abortion	› Avoid using this medication during pregnancy. › Use adequate contraception during therapy.
Serotonin receptor antagonists (triptans): sumatriptan	
› Chest pressure (heavy arms or chest tightness)	› Warn clients about manifestations, and reassure clients that effects are self-limiting and not dangerous. › Advise clients to notify the provider for continuous or severe chest pain.
› Coronary artery vasospasm/angina	› Do not administer to a client who has or is at risk for coronary artery disease (CAD).
› Dizziness or vertigo	› Advise client to avoid driving or operating machinery until medication effects are known.
Beta-blockers: propranolol	
› Extreme tiredness, fatigue, depression, and asthma exacerbation	› Advise clients to observe for manifestations and notify the provider if they occur.
› Bradycardia, hypotension	› Monitor heart rate and blood pressure. Instruct client to take apical pulse prior to dosage. Notify the provider of significant change.
Anticonvulsants: divalproex	
› Neural tube defects	› Avoid use during pregnancy. › Use adequate contraception during therapy.
› Liver toxicity	› Monitor liver enzymes. Notify the provider of lethargy or fever.
› Pancreatitis	› Instruct clients to report abdominal pain, nausea, vomiting, and anorexia. Medication should be discontinued.

ADVERSE EFFECTS	NURSING INTERVENTIONS/CLIENT EDUCATION
Tricyclic antidepressants: amitriptyline	
› Anticholinergic effects (dry mouth, constipation, urinary retention, blurred vision, tachycardia)	› Increase fluid intake. › Increase physical activity by engaging in regular exercise. › Administer stimulant laxatives (such as bisacodyl [Dulcolax]) to counteract reduced bowel motility, or stool softeners (such as docusate sodium [Colace]) to prevent constipation. › Advise clients to void every 4 hr and to report urinary retention. › Advise clients to report blurred vision.
› Drowsiness or dizziness	› Advise clients to avoid driving or operating machinery until medication effects are known.
Calcium channel blockers: verapamil	
› Orthostatic hypotension or bradycardia	› Advise clients to sit or lie down if lightheadedness or dizziness occur and to change positions slowly. › Provide assistance with ambulation as needed. › Monitor heart rate.
› Constipation	› Increase fluid intake. › Increase physical activity by engaging in regular exercise. › Administer stimulant laxatives (such as bisacodyl [Dulcolax]) to counteract reduced bowel motility, or stool softeners (such as docusate sodium [Colace]) to prevent constipation.

Contraindications/Precautions

- Ergotamine is contraindicated in clients who have kidney or liver dysfunction, sepsis, hypertension, history of myocardial infarction, and CAD, as well as during pregnancy.
  - Pregnancy Risk Category X
- Triptans are contraindicated in clients who have liver failure, ischemic heart disease, a history of myocardial infarction, uncontrolled hypertension, and other heart diseases.
  - Pregnancy Risk Category C
- Propranolol is contraindicated in clients who have greater than first-degree heart block, bradycardia, bronchial asthma, cardiogenic shock, or heart failure.
  - Use with caution in clients taking other antihypertensives or who have liver or kidney impairment, diabetes mellitus, or Wolff-Parkinson-White syndrome.
  - Pregnancy Risk Category C
- Divalproex sodium (Depakote) is contraindicated in clients who have liver disease.
  - Pregnancy Risk Category D

- Amitriptyline is contraindicated in clients who have recent MI or within 14 days of a MAOI. Use with caution in clients who have seizure history, urinary retention, prostatic hyperplasia, angle-closure glaucoma, hyperthyroidism, and others.
  - Pregnancy Risk Category C
- Verapamil (Calan) is contraindicated in clients who have greater than first degree heart block, bradycardia, hypotension, left ventricle disease, atrial fibrillation or flutter, or heart failure.
  - Use with caution in clients who have liver or renal impairment or increased intracranial pressure.
  - Pregnancy Risk Category C

Interactions

MEDICATION/FOOD INTERACTIONS	NURSING INTERVENTIONS/CLIENT EDUCATION
Ergotamine and dihydroergotamine	
› Concurrent use with any of the triptans can cause cardiac ischemia.	› Triptans should be taken at least 24 hr apart from an ergotamine medication.
› Some HIV protease inhibitors, antifungal medications, and macrolide antibiotics can increase ergotamine levels, causing increased vasospasm.	› Do not use together.
Sumatriptan	
› Concurrent use of MAOIs can lead to MAO toxicity.	› Do not give triptans within 2 weeks of stopping MAOIs.
› Concurrent use with ergotamine or another triptan can cause vasoconstriction and cardiac ischemia.	› Avoid concurrent use of these medications.
› SSRIs taken with triptans may cause serotonin syndrome (confusion, hyperthermia, diaphoresis, possible death).	› Monitor carefully.
Propranolol	
› Verapamil (Calan) and diltiazem (Cardizem) have additive cardiosuppression effects.	› Monitor ECG, heart rate, and blood pressure.
› Diuretics and antihypertensive medications have additive hypotensive effects.	› Monitor blood pressure.
› Propranolol use can mask the hypoglycemic effect of insulin and prevent the breakdown of fat in response to hypoglycemia.	› Use with caution.
Divalproex	
› Aspirin, chlorpromazine, and cimetidine can cause divalproex sodium toxicity.	› Monitor medication levels.
› Benzodiazepines can cause CNS depression.	› Do not use together.
› Divalproex can increase levels of phenobarbital and phenytoin.	› Monitor medication levels.

MEDICATION/FOOD INTERACTIONS	NURSING INTERVENTIONS/CLIENT EDUCATION
Amitriptyline	
› Barbiturates can cause increased CNS depression.	› Do not use together.
› Cimetidine can increase amitriptyline levels.	› Monitor medication effects.
› MAOIs can increase CNS excitation or cause seizures.	› Do not give amitriptyline within 2 weeks of stopping MAOIs.
Verapamil	
› Carbamazepine and digoxin can increase medication levels.	› Monitor medication levels.
› Atenolol, esmolol, propranolol, and timolol can potentiate medication effects.	› Monitor medication effects. › Adjust dosage.

Nursing Administration

- Advise clients who have migraines to avoid trigger factors that cause stress and fatigue, such as consumption of alcohol and tyramine-containing foods (wine, aged cheese).
- Advise clients that lying down in a dark, quiet place can help ease symptoms.
- Advise clients to check apical pulse before dosage (propranolol).
- Clients may take medication with food to reduce GI distress (divalproex sodium, verapamil) and increase absorption (propranolol).
- Advise clients to protect skin from sun (amitriptyline) and avoid driving or operating machinery until medication effects are known (amitriptyline, verapamil).
- Use caution in case of orthostatic hypotension (amitriptyline).

Nursing Evaluation of Medication Effectiveness

- Depending on the therapeutic intent, effectiveness can be evidenced by:
  - Reduction in intensity and frequency of migraine attacks.
  - Prophylaxis against migraine attacks.
  - Termination of migraine headaches.

MEDICATION CLASSIFICATION: LOCAL ANESTHETICS

- Select Prototype Medications
  - Amide type: lidocaine (Xylocaine)
- Other Medications
  - Ester type: tetracaine (Pontocaine), procaine (Novocain)
  - Amide type: eutectic mixture of 2.5% lidocaine/2.5% prilocaine (EMLA cream)

Purpose

- Expected Pharmacological Action
    - These medications decrease pain by blocking conduction of pain impulses in a circumscribed area. Loss of consciousness does not occur.
- Therapeutic Uses
    - Parenteral administration
        - Pain management for dental procedures, minor surgical procedures, labor and delivery, and diagnostic procedures
        - Regional anesthesia (spinal, epidural)
    - Topical administration
        - Skin and mucous membrane disorders
        - Minor procedures, such as IV insertion, injection (pediatric), and wart removal

Complications

ADVERSE EFFECTS	NURSING INTERVENTIONS/CLIENT EDUCATION
› CNS excitation (seizures, followed by respiratory depression, leading to unconsciousness)	› Monitor for manifestations of seizure activity, sedation, and change in mental status (decrease in level of consciousness). › Monitor vital signs and respiratory status. › Have equipment ready for resuscitation. › Monitor the administration of benzodiazepines, such as midazolam (Versed) or diazepam (Valium), to treat seizures.
› Hypotension, cardiosuppression as evidenced by bradycardia, heart block, and cardiac arrest (common in spinal anesthesia because of sympathetic block)	› Monitor vital signs and ECG. › If manifestations occur, administer treatment accordingly as prescribed.
› Allergic reactions (more likely with ester-type agents, such as procaine)	› Amide-type agents are less likely to cause allergic reactions, and therefore are used for injection. › Observe for manifestations of allergy to anesthetics, such as allergic dermatitis or anaphylaxis. › Treat with antihistamines or agency protocol.
› Labor and delivery » Labor can be prolonged due to a decrease in uterine contractility. » Local anesthetics can cross the placenta and result in fetal bradycardia and CNS depression.	› Use cautiously in women who are in labor. › Monitor uterine activity for effectiveness. › Monitor fetal heart rate (FHR) for bradycardia and decreased variability.
› Spinal headache	› Monitor manifestations of severe headache. › Advise clients to remain flat in bed for 12 hr postprocedure.
› Urinary retention (can occur with spinal anesthesia)	› Monitor urinary output. › Notify the provider if the client has not voided within 8 hr.

Contraindications/Precautions

- Local anesthetics are Pregnancy Risk Category B.
- Supraventricular dysrhythmias or heart block.
- Use cautiously in clients who have liver and kidney dysfunction, heart failure, and myasthenia gravis.
- Epinephrine added to the local anesthetic is contraindicated for use in fingers, nose, and other body parts with end arteries. Gangrene can result due to vasoconstriction.

Interactions

MEDICATION/FOOD INTERACTIONS	NURSING INTERVENTIONS/CLIENT EDUCATION
› Antihypertensive medications have additive hypotensive effects with parenteral administration of local anesthetics.	› Monitor heart rate and blood pressure.

Nursing Administration

- Advise clients to avoid hazardous activities when recovering from anesthesia.
- Maintain clients in a comfortable position during recovery.
- Injection of local anesthetic
  - Vasoconstrictors, such as epinephrine (adrenaline), often are used in combination with local anesthetics to prevent the spread of the local anesthetic. Keeping the anesthetic contained prolongs the anesthesia and decreases the chance of systemic toxicity. Epinephrine added to the local anesthetic is contraindicated for use in fingers, nose, and other body parts with end arteries. Gangrene can result due to vasoconstriction.
  - Prepare injection site for local anesthetic.
  - Maintain IV access for administration of emergency medications if necessary.
  - Have equipment ready for resuscitation.
  - For regional block, protect the area of numbness from injury.

- Spinal or epidural nerve blocks
  - Monitor during insertion for hypotension, anaphylaxis, seizure, and dura puncture.
  - Monitor for respiratory depression and sedation.
  - Monitor insertion site for hematoma and indications of an infection.
  - Check level of sensory block. Evaluate leg strength prior to ambulating.
  - Assist with the preparation of IV fluids to administer to compensate for the sympathetic blocking effects of regional anesthetics.

- Client Education
  - Advise clients to notify the provider for manifestations of infection, such as fever, swelling, and redness; increase in pain or severe headache; sudden weakness to lower extremities; or decrease in bowel or bladder control.
  - Notify the provider for manifestations of systemic infusion, such as a metallic taste, ringing in ears, perioral numbness, and seizures.
- Topical cream: eutectic mixture of lidocaine and prilocaine (EMLA)
  - Apply a thick layer to intact skin 1 hr before routine procedures or superficial puncture and 2 hr before more extensive procedures or deep puncture. Cover with occlusive dressing.
  - Prior to the procedure, remove the dressing and clean the skin with aseptic solution.
  - EMLA may be applied at home prior to coming to a health care facility for a procedure.

Nursing Evaluation of Medication Effectiveness

- Depending on the therapeutic intent, effectiveness may be evidenced by the following.
  - Client undergoes procedure without experiencing pain.
  - Pain is relieved.

APPLICATION EXERCISES

1. A nurse is reinforcing teaching with a client who is starting colchicine (Colcrys) for an acute attack of gout. Which of the following interventions should the nurse reinforce in the teaching?

    A. Avoid aspirin and other NSAIDs while taking colchicine.

    B. Take colchicine on an empty stomach an hour before or 2 hr after food.

    C. Decrease daily fluid intake to prevent adverse effects.

    D. Report sore throat and easy bruising while taking colchicine.

2. A nurse is reinforcing teaching with a client who experiences migraine headaches. Which of the following instructions should the nurse give this client? (Select all that apply.)

    _____ A. Take ergotamine as a prophylaxis to prevent a migraine headache.

    _____ B. Identify and avoid trigger factors.

    _____ C. Lie down in a dark quiet room at the onset of a migraine.

    _____ D. Avoid foods that contain tyramine.

    _____ E. Avoid exercise that may increase heart rate.

3. A nurse is caring for a client who has a local anesthetic of lidocaine with epinephrine for the removal of a skin lesion. Epinephrine is used with the lidocaine for which of the following reasons?

    A. Reduce risk of systemic toxicity

    B. Reduce the occurrence of tachycardia

    C. Produce localized vasodilation

    D. Speed absorption of anesthesia

4. A nurse is caring for a client who receives a local anesthetic of lidocaine during the repair of a skin laceration. For which of the following adverse reactions should the nurse monitor the client?

    A. Seizures

    B. Tachycardia

    C. Hypertension

    D. Fever

5. A nurse is reinforcing teaching with a client who has a new prescription for ergotamine (Ergomar) to treat migraine headaches. For which of the following should the nurse instruct the client to stop taking the medication and notify the provider? (Select all that apply.)

_____ A. Nausea

_____ B. Visual disturbances

_____ C. Positive home pregnancy test

_____ D. Numbness and tingling in fingers

_____ E. Muscle pain

6. A nurse is reinforcing teaching with a client who has frequent migraine headaches about her new prescription for sumatriptan (Imitrex). What should the nurse instruct the client about this medication? Use the ATI Remediation Template: Medication to complete this item to include the following:

A. Therapeutic Use: Describe the therapeutic use for sumatriptan in this client.

B. Adverse Effects: Describe two adverse effects the client should monitor for.

C. Medication/Food Interactions: Describe two the nurse should teach the client about.

D. Nursing Interventions/Client Education: Describe two for this client.

APPLICATION EXERCISES KEY

1. A. INCORRECT: Aspirin and other NSAIDs do not interact negatively with colchicines and may be taken concurrently.

    B. INCORRECT: Colchicines have numerous adverse GI effects. Taking the medication with food reduces gastrointestinal distress.

    C. INCORRECT: The daily fluid intake should be increased for clients who have gout to promote excretion of uric acid and to prevent development of kidney stones.

    D. **CORRECT:** Colchicine can cause bone marrow depression, so the client should report signs of infection, such as sore throat, and manifestations of myelosuppression, such as easy bruising, fatigue, and bleeding.

    Ⓝ NCLEX® Connection: Pharmacological Therapies, Adverse Effects/Contraindications/ Side Effects/Interactions

2. A. INCORRECT: Ergotamine is used at the onset of a migraine to abort headache manifestations. It should not be used regularly because it can cause physical dependence and toxicity.

    B. **CORRECT:** Identifying and avoiding trigger factors is an important action that can help to prevent some migraines.

    C. **CORRECT:** Lying down in a dark, quiet room at the onset of a migraine may prevent the onset of more severe manifestations.

    D. **CORRECT:** Foods that contain tyramine can be a trigger for some migraines and should be avoided.

    E. INCORRECT: Exercise should be encouraged between migraines because it can relieve stress, which can trigger headaches.

    Ⓝ NCLEX® Connection: Pharmacological Therapies, Expected Actions/Outcomes

3. A. **CORRECT:** Epinephrine added to the local anesthetic reduces the risk of systemic toxicity because a reduced amount of anesthetic may be used.

    B. INCORRECT: Epinephrine, by itself, can produce tachycardia, anxiety, and hypertension. The nurse should monitor for these adverse effects.

    C. INCORRECT: Epinephrine causes localized vasoconstriction rather than vasodilation.

    D. INCORRECT: Epinephrine slows absorption of the local anesthetic rather than speeding its absorption. This effect is beneficial because it prolongs anesthesia and allows less anesthetic to be administered.

    Ⓝ NCLEX® Connection: Pharmacological Therapies, Expected Actions/Outcomes

4.   A. **CORRECT:** Seizure activity is an adverse effect that can occur as a result of local anesthetic injection.

     B. INCORRECT: Bradycardia, rather than tachycardia, can occur as a result of local anesthetic injection.

     C. INCORRECT: Hypotension, rather than hypertension, can occur as a result of local anesthetic injection.

     D. INCORRECT: Fever is not an adverse effect of local anesthetic injection.

     (N) NCLEX® Connection: Pharmacological Therapies, Adverse Effects/Contraindications/
     Side Effects/Interactions

5.   A. INCORRECT: Nausea that occurs with a migraine is a common associated finding and does not
     warrant stopping the medication and notifying the provider. Nausea and vomiting also are
     common adverse effects of ergotamine, and the provider may prescribe an antiemetic.

     B. INCORRECT: Visual disturbances, such as flashing lights, are common findings associated with
     migraine and do not warrant stopping the medication and notifying the provider.

     C. **CORRECT:** A client who has a positive home pregnancy test should stop taking ergotamine and notify
     the provider. Ergotamine is classified as Pregnancy Risk Category X and can cause fetal abortion.

     D. **CORRECT:** Numbness and tingling in fingers or toes can be a finding in ergotamine overdose. The
     medication should be stopped and the provider notified.

     E. **CORRECT:** Unexplained muscle pain can be a finding in ergotamine overdose. The medication
     should be stopped and the provider notified.

     (N) NCLEX® Connection: Pharmacological Therapies, Adverse Effects/Contraindications/
     Side Effects/Interactions

6.   *Using the ATI Remediation Template: Medication*
     A. Therapeutic Use
         • Sumatriptan is used to abort a migraine
            headache and associated manifestations,
            such as nausea and vomiting, after it begins
            by causing cranial artery vasoconstriction.
     B. Adverse Effects
         • The nurse should monitor for chest and
            arm heaviness/pressure, angina caused by
            coronary vasospasm, dizziness, and vertigo.
     C. Medication/Food Interactions
         • Toxicity can result if sumatriptan is given
            concurrently or within 2 weeks of an
            MAOI antidepressant. Sumatriptan should
            not be given concurrently with other
            triptan medications or within 24 hr of
            ergotamine or dihydroergotamine.

     D. Nursing Interventions/Client Education
         • Instruct the client to take sumatriptan at
            first sign of migraine manifestations.
         • Instruct the client how to administer
            sumatriptan if it is prescribed intranasally
            or by subcutaneous injection.
         • Monitor cardiovascular risk factors
            and vital signs while the client takes
            this medication.
         • Advise the client to notify the provider
            immediately for onset of angina pain.
            Instruct the client to distinguish transient
            chest or arm heaviness caused by
            sumatriptan from angina pain.

     (N) NCLEX® Connection: Pharmacological Therapies, Expected Actions/Outcomes

UNIT 10   Medications Affecting the Endocrine System

CHAPTERS
› Diabetes Mellitus
› Endocrine Disorders

NCLEX® CONNECTIONS

When reviewing the chapters in this unit, keep in mind the relevant sections of the NCLEX® outline, in particular:

Client Needs: Pharmacological Therapies

› Relevant topics/tasks include:
  » Adverse Effects/Contraindications/Side Effects/Interactions
    › Identify potential and actual incompatibilities of the client's medications.
  » Dosage Calculation
    › Use clinical decision making when calculating dosages.
  » Medication Administration
    › Mix medications from two vials when necessary.
    › Reinforce client teaching on self-administration of medications (insulin, subcutaneous insulin pump).

chapter 34

Overview

- Diabetes mellitus is a chronic illness that results from an absolute or relative deficiency of insulin, often combined with a cellular resistance to insulin's actions.

  - Various insulins are available to manage diabetes. These medications differ in their onset, peak, and duration.

  - Oral antidiabetic medications work in various ways to increase available insulin or modify carbohydrate metabolism.

  - Newer injectable medications are used to supplement insulin or oral agents to manage glucose control.

MEDICATION CLASSIFICATION: INSULIN

- Select Prototype Medications

CLASSIFICATION	GENERIC (TRADE NAME)	ONSET	PEAK	DURATION
Rapid-acting	› Lispro insulin (Humalog)	15 to 30 min	0.5 to 2.5 hr	3 to 6 hr
Short-acting	› Regular insulin (Humulin R)	0.5 to 1 hr	1 to 5 hr	6 to 10 hr
Intermediate-acting	› NPH insulin (Humulin N)	1 to 2 hr	6 to 14 hr	16 to 24 hr
Long-acting	› Insulin glargine (Lantus)	70 min	None	24 hr

- Other Medications

CLASSIFICATION	GENERIC (TRADE NAME)
Rapid-acting	› Insulin aspart (NovoLog) › Insulin glulisine (Apidra)
Short-acting	› Regular insulin (Novolin R)
Intermediate-acting	› Insulin detemir (Levemir)

- Premixed insulins

  - 70% NPH and 30% regular (Humulin 70/30) – mixture of intermediate-acting and short-acting insulin

  - 75% insulin lispro protamine and 25% insulin lispro (Humalog 75/25) – mixture of intermediate-acting and rapid-acting insulin

Purpose

- Expected Pharmacological Actions
  - Promotes cellular uptake of glucose (decreases glucose levels)
  - Converts glucose into glycogen
  - Moves potassium into cells (along with glucose)
- Therapeutic Uses
  - Insulin is used for glycemic control of diabetes mellitus (type 1, type 2, gestational) to prevent complications.
  - Clients who have type 2 diabetes mellitus can require insulin when:
    - Oral antidiabetic medications, diet, and exercise are unable to control blood glucose levels.
    - Severe kidney or liver disease is present.
    - Painful neuropathy is present.
    - Undergoing surgery or diagnostic tests.
    - Experiencing severe stress, such as infection and trauma.
    - Undergoing emergency treatment of diabetes ketoacidosis (DKA) and hyperosmolar hyperglycemic nonketotic syndrome (HHNS).
    - Requiring treatment of hyperkalemia.

Complications

ADVERSE EFFECTS	NURSING INTERVENTIONS/CLIENT EDUCATION
› Risk for hypoglycemia (too much insulin)	› Monitor clients for hypoglycemia. If abrupt onset, client will experience sympathetic nervous system (SNS) effects (tachycardia, palpitations, diaphoresis, shakiness). If gradual onset, client will experience parasympathetic nervous system (PNS) manifestations (headache, tremors, drowsiness, weakness).
	› Administer glucose. For clients who are conscious, administer a snack of 15 g of carbohydrate (4 oz orange juice, 2 oz grape juice, 8 oz milk, glucose tablets per manufacturer's suggestion to equal 15 g).
	› If the client is not fully conscious, do not risk aspiration. Administer glucose parenterally, such as IV glucose, or subcutaneous/IM glucagon.
	› Encourage clients to wear a medical alert bracelet.
› Lipohypertrophy	› Instruct clients to systematically rotate injection sites and to allow 1 inch between injection sites.

Interactions

MEDICATION/FOOD INTERACTIONS	NURSING INTERVENTIONS/CLIENT EDUCATION
› Sulfonylureas, meglitinides, beta blockers, and alcohol have additive hypoglycemic effects with concurrent use.	› Monitor serum glucose levels for hypoglycemia (less than 50 mg/dL), and adjust insulin or oral antidiabetic dosages accordingly.
› Concurrent use of thiazide diuretics and glucocorticoids can raise blood glucose levels and thereby counteract the effects of insulin.	› Monitor serum glucose levels for hyperglycemia, and adjust insulin doses accordingly. Higher insulin doses may be indicated.
› Beta blockers can mask SNS response to hypoglycemia (tachycardia, tremors), making it difficult for clients to identify hypoglycemia	› Advise clients of the importance of monitoring glucose levels and not relying on SNS symptoms as an alert to developing hypoglycemia. › Instruct clients to maintain a regular eating schedule to ensure adequate glucose during times of hypoglycemic action.

Nursing Administration

- Adjust insulin dosage to meet insulin needs.
  - The client's dosage may need to be increased in response to increase in caloric intake, infection, stress, growth spurts, and in the second and third trimesters of pregnancy.
  - The dosage may need to be decreased in response to level of exercise or first trimester of pregnancy.
- Ensure adequate glucose is available at the time of onset of insulin and during all peak times.
- When mixing short-acting insulin with longer-acting insulin, draw the short-acting insulin up into the syringe first, then the longer-acting insulin. This prevents the possibility of accidentally injecting some of the longer-acting insulin into the shorter-acting insulin vial. (This can pose a risk for unexpected insulin effects with subsequent uses of the vial.)
- For insulin suspensions, gently rotate the vial between the palms to disperse the particles throughout the vial prior to withdrawing insulin.
- Do not administer short-acting insulins if they appear cloudy or discolored.
- Insulin glargine and insulin detemir are both clear in color, not administered IV, and should not be mixed in a syringe with any other insulin.
- Administer lispro, aspart, glulisine, and regular insulin by subcutaneous injection, continuous subcutaneous infusion, and IV route.
- Administer NPH by subcutaneous route.
- Instruct clients to administer subcutaneous insulin in one general area to have consistent rates of absorption. Absorption rates from subcutaneous tissue increase from thigh to upper arm to abdomen.
- Use only insulin-specific syringes that correspond to the concentration of insulin being administered. Administer U-100 insulin with a U-100 syringe. Administer U-500 insulin with a U-500 syringe.
- Select an appropriate needle length to ensure insulin is injected into subcutaneous tissue vs. intradermal (too short) or intramuscular (too long).
- Encourage clients to enhance diabetes medication therapy with a proper diet and consistent activity.

- Ensure proper storage of insulin.
  - ○ Unopened vials of a single type of insulin may be stored in the refrigerator until their expiration date.
  - ○ Vials of premixed insulins may be stored for up to 3 months.
  - ○ Insulins premixed in syringes may be kept for 1 to 2 weeks under refrigeration. Keep the syringes in a vertical position, with the needles pointing up. Prior to administration, the insulin should be resuspended by gently moving the syringe.
  - ○ Store the vial that is in use at room temperature, avoiding proximity to sunlight and intense heat. Discard after 1 month.

MEDICATION CLASSIFICATION: ORAL ANTIDIABETICS

MEDICATIONS	EXPECTED PHARMACOLOGICAL ACTION
› Sulfonylureas » Select Prototype Medications 　› 1st generation – chlorpropamide 　› 2nd generation – glipizide (Glucotrol, Glucotrol XL) » Other Medications 　› 1st generation – tolazamide 　› 2nd generation – glyburide (DiaBeta), glimepiride (Amaryl)	› Insulin release from the pancreas
› Meglitinides » Select Prototype Medication: repaglinide (Prandin) » Other Medication: nateglinide (Starlix)	› Insulin release from the pancreas
› Biguanides » Select Prototype Medication: metformin (Glucophage)	› Reduces the production of glucose within the liver through suppression of gluconeogenesis › Increases muscles' glucose uptake and use
› Thiazolidinediones (Glitazones) » Select Prototype Medication: pioglitazone (Actos)	› Increases cellular response to insulin by decreasing insulin resistance › Increased glucose uptake and decreased glucose production
› Alpha glucosidase inhibitors » Select Prototype Medication: acarbose (Precose) » Other Medications: miglitol (Glyset)	› Slows carbohydrate absorption and digestion
› Gliptins » Sitagliptin (Januvia)	› Augments naturally occurring incretin hormones, which promote release of insulin and decrease secretion of glucagon › Lowers fasting and postprandial blood glucose levels

- Therapeutic Uses
  - All classifications of antidiabetic agents control blood glucose levels in clients who have type 2 diabetes mellitus and are used in conjunction with diet and exercise lifestyle changes.
  - Metformin is used to treat polycystic ovary syndrome (PCOS).

Complications

ADVERSE EFFECTS	NURSING INTERVENTIONS/CLIENT EDUCATION
Glipizide and repaglinide	
› Hypoglycemia	› Monitor for signs of hypoglycemia. If abrupt onset, the client will experience SNS manifestations, such as tachycardia, palpitations, diaphoresis, and shakiness. If gradual onset, the client will experience PNS manifestations, such as headache, tremors, and weakness. › Instruct clients to self-administer a snack of 15 g of carbohydrate (4 oz orange juice, 2 oz grape juice, 8 oz milk, glucose tablets per manufacturer's suggestion to equal 15 g). › Instruct clients to notify the provider if there is a recurrent problem. › If severe hypoglycemia occurs, IV glucose may be needed. › Encourage clients to wear a medical alert bracelet.
Metformin	
› Gastrointestinal effects (anorexia, nausea, and vomiting, which frequently result in weight loss of 3 to 4 kg [6.6 to 8.8 lb])	› Monitor for severity of these effects. › Discontinue the medication if necessary.
› Vitamin B_{12} and folic acid deficiency caused by altered absorption	› Provide supplements as needed.
› Lactic acidosis (hyperventilation, myalgia, sluggishness, somnolence) » 50% mortality rate	› Instruct clients to withhold medication if these manifestations occur, and to inform the provider immediately. › Severe lactic acidosis can be treated with hemodialysis.
Pioglitazone	
› Fluid retention	› Monitor for edema, weight gain, and indications of heart failure.
› Elevations in low density lipoproteins (LDL) cholesterol	› Monitor cholesterol levels.
› Hepatotoxicity	› Perform baseline and periodic liver function tests. › Instruct clients to report any hepatotoxicity manifestations, such as jaundice or dark urine.

ADVERSE EFFECTS	NURSING INTERVENTIONS/CLIENT EDUCATION
Acarbose	
› Intestinal effects (abdominal distention and cramping, hyperactive bowel sounds, diarrhea, excessive gas)	› Monitor impact of these effects on the client. › Discontinue the medication if necessary.
› Anemia due to the decrease of iron absorption	› Monitor hemoglobin and iron levels. › Discontinue the medication if necessary.
› Hepatotoxicity with long-term use	› Check baseline liver function and perform periodic liver function tests. › Discontinue the medication if elevations occur. › Liver function will return to normal after the medication is discontinued.
Sitagliptin	
› Generally well tolerated › Rare occurrence of respiratory tract infection and pancreatitis	

Contraindications/Precautions

- Glipizide, repaglinide, and pioglitazone are Pregnancy Risk Category C medications.
- Metformin (Glucophage), acarbose (Precose), and sitagliptin (Januvia) are Pregnancy Risk Category B medications.
  - These oral agents generally are avoided in pregnancy and lactation, but the provider may decide to prescribe them.
- Use cautiously in clients who have kidney failure, hepatic dysfunction, or heart failure because of the risk of medication accumulation and resulting hypoglycemia. Severity of disease can indicate contraindication.
- Contraindicated in the treatment of diabetic ketoacidosis (DKA).
- Metformin is contraindicated for clients who have severe infection, shock, and any hypoxic condition.
- Acarbose is contraindicated for clients who have gastrointestinal disorders, such as inflammatory disease, ulceration, or obstruction.

- Pioglitazone is contraindicated for clients who have severe heart failure, history of bladder cancer, and active hepatic disease. Use cautiously in clients who have mild heart failure and in older adults.

Interactions

MEDICATION/FOOD INTERACTIONS	NURSING INTERVENTIONS/CLIENT EDUCATION
Glipizide	
› Use of alcohol can result in disulfiram-like reaction (intense nausea and vomiting, flushing, palpitations).	› Inform clients about the risk, and encourage them to avoid alcohol.
› Alcohol, NSAIDs, sulfonamide antibiotics, ranitidine (Zantac), and cimetidine (Tagamet) have additive hypoglycemic effect.	› Inform clients about the risk, and encourage them to avoid alcohol. › Instruct clients to closely monitor glucose levels when these other agents are used concurrently. › Dosage adjustment of the oral antidiabetic medication may be indicated.
› Beta blockers can mask SNS response to hypoglycemia (tachycardia, tremors, palpitations, diaphoresis), making it difficult for clients to identify hypoglycemia.	› Advise clients of the importance of monitoring glucose levels and not relying on SNS symptoms as an alert to developing hypoglycemia. › Instruct clients to maintain a regular eating schedule to ensure adequate glucose during times of hypoglycemic action.
Repaglinide and pioglitazone	
› Concurrent use of gemfibrozil (Lopid) results in inhibition of repaglinide metabolism, leading to an increased risk for hypoglycemia.	› Avoid concurrent use of repaglinide or pioglitazone and gemfibrozil. › Closely monitor for signs of hypoglycemia.
Metformin HCl	
› Alcohol increases the risk of lactic acidosis with concurrent use.	› Inform clients of the risks, and encourage them to avoid consuming alcohol.
› Concurrent use of iodine-containing contrast media can result in acute kidney failure.	› Clients taking metformin should discontinue the medication 24 to 48 hr prior to procedure. They can resume medication 48 hr after test if lab results indicate normal kidney function.
Acarbose	
› Concurrent use of acarbose with sulfonylureas or insulin increase the risk for hypoglycemia.	› Monitor carefully for hypoglycemia.
› Concurrent use of metformin causes additive gastrointestinal effects and risk for hypoglycemia.	› Monitor carefully for gastrointestinal effects and hypoglycemia.
Sitagliptin – no significant interactions	

Nursing Administration

- Encourage clients to exercise consistently and to follow appropriate dietary guidelines.
- Encourage clients to maintain a log of glucose levels and to note patterns that affect glucose levels (increased dietary intake, infection).
- Consider referring clients to a registered dietitian and/or diabetic nurse educator.
- Administer medications orally and at appropriate times.
    - Glipizide – Best taken 30 min prior to meal.
    - Repaglinide – Instruct clients to eat within 30 min of taking a dose of the medication, three times per day.
    - Metformin – Instruct clients to take immediate-release tablets two times per day with breakfast and dinner and to take sustained-release tablets once daily with dinner.
    - Pioglitazone – Instruct clients to take once per day, with or without food.
    - Acarbose – Instruct clients to take with the first bite of food, three times per day. If a dose is missed, take the dose at the next meal but do not take two doses.
    - Sitagliptin – Instruct clients to take once per day, with or without food.
- Instruct clients that formulations may combine two medications.
- Instruct clients who are also taking insulin to monitor for signs of hypoglycemia.

MEDICATION CLASSIFICATION: AMYLIN MIMETICS

- Select prototype medication: pramlintide (Symlin)

Purpose

- Expected Pharmacological Action
    - Pramlintide mimics the actions of the naturally occurring peptide hormone amylin, resulting in reduction of postprandial glucose levels from decreased gastric emptying time and inhibition of secretion of glucagon. There is also an increase in the sensation of satiety, which helps decrease caloric intake.
- Therapeutic Uses
    - Supplemental glucose control for clients who have type 1 or type 2 diabetes
    - May be used in conjunction with insulin or an oral antidiabetic medication, usually metformin or a sulfonylurea

Complications

ADVERSE EFFECTS	NURSING INTERVENTIONS/CLIENT EDUCATION
› Nausea	› Instruct clients to report symptom to the provider. Dose may be decreased.
› Hypoglycemia	› Instruct clients to report symptom to the provider.
› Reaction at injection sites	› Generally self-limiting.

Contraindications/Precautions

- Pregnancy Risk Category C.
- This medication is contraindicated for clients who have kidney failure or are receiving dialysis.
- Use cautiously in clients who have thyroid disease, osteoporosis, or alcohol use disorder.

Interactions

MEDICATION/FOOD INTERACTIONS	NURSING INTERVENTIONS/CLIENT EDUCATION
› Insulin increases risk for hypoglycemia.	› Concurrent use can require a decrease in insulin dose, usually 50% of rapid- or short-acting insulin. Avoid use in clients unable to self-monitor blood glucose levels.
› Concurrent use of pramlintide with medications that slow gastric emptying, such as opioids, or medications that delay food absorption, such as acarbose, can further slow gastric emptying time.	› Avoid concurrent use.
› Oral medication absorption is delayed.	› Administer oral medications 1 hr before or 2 hr after injection of pramlintide.

Nursing Administration

- Administer subcutaneously prior to meals, using the thigh or abdomen.
- Instruct clients to keep unopened vials in the refrigerator and not to freeze. Opened vials may be kept cool or at room temperature but should be discarded after 28 days. Keep vials out of direct sunlight.
- Instruct clients not to mix medication with insulin in the same syringe.

MEDICATION CLASSIFICATION: INCRETIN MIMETICS

- Select Prototype Medication: exenatide (Byetta)
- Other medication: liraglutide (Victoza)

Purpose

- Expected Pharmacological Action
  - Mimics the effects of naturally occurring glucagon-like peptide-1, and thereby promotes release of insulin, decreases secretion of glucagon, and slows gastric emptying. Fasting and postprandial blood glucose levels are lowered.
- Therapeutic Uses
  - Supplemental glucose control for clients who have type 2 diabetes
  - May be used in conjunction with an oral antidiabetic medication, usually metformin or a sulfonylurea

Complications

ADVERSE EFFECTS	NURSING INTERVENTIONS/CLIENT EDUCATION
› GI effects (nausea, vomiting, diarrhea)	› Instruct client to notify provider if manifestations are intolerable.
› Pancreatitis (severe and intolerable abdominal pain)	› Instruct client to withhold medication and to notify provider.

Contraindications/Precautions

- Pregnancy Risk Category C.
- Contraindicated for clients who have kidney failure, ulcerative colitis, or Crohn's disease.
- Use cautiously in older adult clients and clients who have kidney impairment or thyroid disease.

Interactions

MEDICATION/FOOD INTERACTIONS	NURSING INTERVENTIONS/CLIENT EDUCATION
› Oral medication absorption is delayed, especially oral contraceptives, antibiotics, and acetaminophen.	› Administer oral medications 1 hr before or 2 hr after injection of exenatide.
› Concurrent use of sulfonylurea increases risk of hypoglycemia.	› Clients can require a lower dose of sulfonylurea. Instruct clients to monitor blood glucose levels.

Nursing Administration

- This medication is supplied in prefilled injector pens.
- Administer subcutaneously in the thigh, abdomen, or upper arm.
- Give injection within 60 min before the morning and evening meal. Never administer after a meal.
- Instruct clients to keep the injection pen in the refrigerator and to discard after 30 days.

Nursing Evaluation of Medication Effectiveness

- Depending on therapeutic intent, effectiveness can be evidenced by the following.
  - Preprandial glucose levels 90 to 130 mg/dL and postprandial levels less than 180 mg/dL
  - HbA1c less than 7%

MEDICATION CLASSIFICATION: HYPERGLYCEMIC AGENT

- Select Prototype Medication: glucagon (GlucaGen)

Purpose

- Expected Pharmacological Action
  - Increases blood glucose levels by increasing the breakdown of glycogen into glucose, decreasing glycogen synthesis enhances the synthesis of glucose
- Therapeutic Uses
  - Emergency management of hypoglycemic reactions, such as insulin overdose in clients who are unable to take oral glucose
  - Decrease in gastrointestinal motility in clients undergoing radiological procedures of the stomach and intestines

Complications

ADVERSE EFFECTS	NURSING INTERVENTIONS/CLIENT EDUCATION
› GI distress (nausea, vomiting)	› Turn clients onto the left side following administration to reduce the risk of aspiration if emesis occurs.

Contraindications/Precautions

- Glucagon is ineffective for hypoglycemia resulting from inadequate glycogen stores (starvation).
- Pregnancy Risk Category B.
- Use cautiously in clients who have cardiovascular disease.

Nursing Administration

- Administer glucagon subcutaneously, IM, or IV immediately following reconstitution parameters.
- Provide food as soon as the client regains full consciousness and is able to swallow.
- Instruct the client to maintain access to a source of glucose and glucagon kit at all times.

Nursing Evaluation of Medication Effectiveness

- Depending on therapeutic intent, effectiveness can be evidenced by elevation in blood glucose level to greater than 50 mg/dL.

APPLICATION EXERCISES

1. A nurse is reinforcing teaching with clients in an outpatient facility about the use of insulin to treat type 1 diabetes mellitus. For which of the following types of insulin should the nurse tell the clients to expect a peak effect 1 to 5 hr after administration?

    A. Insulin glargine (Lantus)

    B. NPH insulin (Humulin N)

    C. Regular insulin (Humulin R)

    D. Insulin lispro (Humalog)

2. A nurse is reinforcing teaching with a client who has type 2 diabetes mellitus and is starting repaglinide (Prandin). Which of the following statements made by the client indicates understanding of the administration of this medication?

    A. "I'll take this medicine with my meals."

    B. "I'll take this medicine 30 minutes before I eat."

    C. "I'll take this medicine just before I go to bed."

    D. "I'll take this medicine as soon as I wake up in the morning."

3. A nurse is caring for a client who has a prescription for metformin (Glucophage). The nurse should monitor the client for which of the following adverse effects?

    A. Lactic acidosis

    B. Hypoglycemia

    C. Hyperlipidemia

    D. Respiratory alkalosis

4. A nurse is reinforcing teaching with a client who has a prescription for pramlintide (Symlin) for type 1 diabetes mellitus. Which of the following should the nurse reinforce in the teaching? (Select all that apply.)

    _____ A. "Take oral medications 1 hr before injection."

    _____ B. "Use upper arms as preferred injection sites."

    _____ C. "Mix pramlintide with breakfast dose of insulin."

    _____ D. "Inject pramlintide just before a meal."

    _____ E. "Discard open vials after 28 days."

5. A nurse in an outpatient facility is caring for a client who has been taking acarbose (Precose) for type 2 diabetes mellitus. Which of the following laboratory tests should the nurse plan to monitor?

    A. WBC

    B. Serum potassium

    C. Platelet count

    D. Liver function tests

6. A nurse in an acute care facility is reinforcing teaching with a client who has type 2 diabetes mellitus and is taking exenatide (Byetta) along with an oral antidiabetic agent. What should the nurse inform the client about this medication? Use the ATI Active Learning Template: Medication to complete this item to include the following:

    A. Therapeutic Use: Identify the therapeutic use for exenatide in this client.

    B. Adverse Effects: Identify two adverse effects the client should watch for.

    C. Nursing Interventions: Describe two laboratory tests the nurse should monitor.

    D. Client Teaching: Describe teaching points to give client taking exenatide.

APPLICATION EXERCISES KEY

1. A. INCORRECT: Insulin glargine, a long-acting insulin, does not have a peak effect time, but is fairly stable in effect after metabolized.

    B. INCORRECT: NPH insulin has a peak effect around 6 to 14 hr following administration.

    C. **CORRECT:** Regular insulin has a peak effect around 1 to 5 hr following administration.

    D. INCORRECT: Insulin lispro has a peak effect around 30 min to 2.5 hr following administration.

    Ⓝ NCLEX® Connection: Pharmacological Therapies, Expected Actions/Outcomes

2. A. INCORRECT: Repaglinide should not be taken with a meal.

    B. **CORRECT:** Repaglinide causes a rapid, short-lived release of insulin. The client should take this medication within 30 min before each meal so that insulin is available when food is digested.

    C. INCORRECT: Repaglinide should not be taken just before bedtime.

    D. INCORRECT: Repaglinide is not taken upon awakening in the morning.

    Ⓝ NCLEX® Connection: Pharmacological Therapies, Medication Administration

3. A. **CORRECT:** Lactic acidosis, manifested by extreme drowsiness, hyperventilation, and muscle pain, is a rare but very serious adverse effect caused by metformin.

    B. INCORRECT: Although many oral antidiabetic medications cause hypoglycemia, this is not an effect caused by metformin, which works by slowing glucose production in the liver.

    C. INCORRECT: Hyperlipidemia is not an adverse effect caused by metformin.

    D. INCORRECT: Respiratory alkalosis is not an adverse effect caused by metformin.

    Ⓝ NCLEX® Connection: Pharmacological Therapies, Adverse Effects/Contraindications/ Side Effects/Interactions

4. A. **CORRECT:** Pramlintide delays oral medication absorption, so oral medications should be taken 1 to 2 hr after pramlintide injection.

    B. INCORRECT: The thigh or abdomen, rather than the upper arms, are preferred sites for pramlintide injection.

    C. INCORRECT: Pramlintide should not be mixed in a syringe with any type of insulin.

    D. **CORRECT:** Pramlintide can cause hypoglycemia, especially when the client also takes insulin, so it is important to eat a meal after injecting this medication.

    E. **CORRECT:** Unused medication in the open pramlintide vial should be discarded after 28 days.

    Ⓝ NCLEX® Connection: Pharmacological Therapies, Medication Administration

5. A. INCORRECT: Infection is not an adverse effect of acarbose. It is not necessary to monitor the client's WBC while he is taking this medication.

    B. INCORRECT: Acarbose does not affect potassium levels. It is not necessary to monitor serum potassium while the client is taking this medication.

    C. INCORRECT: Acarbose does not affect the platelet levels. It is not necessary to monitor the platelet count while the client is taking this medication.

    D. **CORRECT:** Acarbose can cause liver toxicity when taken long-term. Liver function tests should be monitored periodically while the client takes this medication.

    (N) NCLEX® Connection: Pharmacological Therapies, Adverse Effects/Contraindications/ Side Effects/Interactions

6. *Using the ATI Active Learning Template: Medication*

    A. Therapeutic Use
    - Exenatide is prescribed along with an oral antidiabetic medication, such as metformin or a sulfonylurea medication, for clients who have type 2 diabetes mellitus to improve diabetes control. Exenatide improves insulin secretion by the pancreas, decreases secretion of glucagon, and slows gastric emptying.

    B. Adverse Effects
    - GI effects, such as nausea and vomiting
    - Pancreatitis manifested by acute abdominal pain and possibly severe vomiting
    - Hypoglycemia, especially when taken concurrently with a sulfonylurea medication, such as glipizide

    C. Nursing Interventions
    - The nurse should monitor daily blood glucose testing by the client, periodic HbA1c tests, and periodic kidney function testing. Exenatide should be used cautiously in clients who have any renal impairment.

    D. Client Teaching
    - Instruct the client how to inject exenatide subcutaneously.
    - Instruct the client to take exenatide within 60 min before the morning and evening meal but not following the meal.
    - Advise the client to withhold exenatide and notify the provider for severe abdominal pain.
    - Instruct the client how to recognize and treat hypoglycemia.
    - Instruct the client that exenatide should not be given within 1 hr of oral antibiotics, acetaminophen, or an oral contraceptive due to its ability to slow gastric emptying.

    (N) NCLEX® Connection: Pharmacological Therapies, Expected Actions/Outcomes

chapter 35

Overview

- The endocrine system is made up of glands that secrete hormones, which act on specific receptor sites. Hormones target receptor sites to regulate response to stress, growth, metabolism, and homeostasis.
- An endocrine disorder usually involves the oversecretion or undersecretion of hormones, or an altered response by the target area or receptor.
- Medications used to treat disorders of the thyroid, anterior and posterior pituitary, and adrenal glands are discussed in this chapter.

MEDICATION CLASSIFICATION: THYROID HORMONE

- Select Prototype Medication: levothyroxine (Synthroid, Levothroid)
- Other Medications
  - Liothyronine (Cytomel)
  - Liotrix (Thyrolar)
  - Thyroid (Thyroid USP)

Purpose

- Expected Pharmacological Action
  - Thyroid hormones are a synthetic form of thyroxine (T_4), a form of liothyronine (T_3), or a combination of T_3 and T_4, that increase metabolic rate, protein synthesis, cardiac output, renal perfusion, oxygen use, body temperature, blood volume, and growth processes.
- Therapeutic Uses
  - Thyroid hormone replacement is used for treatment of hypothyroidism (all ages, all forms).
  - Thyroid hormones are used for the emergency treatment of myxedema coma (IV route).
- Route of administration: oral, IV (myxedema coma)

Complications

ADVERSE EFFECTS	NURSING INTERVENTIONS/CLIENT EDUCATION
› Overmedication can result in indications of hyperthyroidism (anxiety, tachycardia, palpitations, altered appetite, abdominal cramping, heat intolerance, fever, diaphoresis, weight loss, menstrual irregularities).	› Instruct clients to report indications of overmedication to the provider.

Contraindications/Precautions

- Pregnancy Risk Category A.
- Use cautiously in pregnancy and lactation.
- Use is contraindicated for clients who have thyrotoxicosis.
- Because of cardiac stimulant effects, use is contraindicated following a MI.

- Use cautiously in clients who have cardiovascular problems (hypertension, angina pectoris, ischemic heart disease) because of cardiac stimulant effects, and in older adults.
- Thyroid hormone replacement is not for use in the treatment of obesity.

Interactions

MEDICATION/FOOD INTERACTIONS	NURSING INTERVENTIONS/CLIENT EDUCATION
› Binding agents (cholestyramine, antacids, iron and calcium supplements) and sucralfate (Carafate) reduce levothyroxine absorption with concurrent use.	› Allow at least 4 hr between medication administration.
› Many antiseizure and antidepressant medications, including carbamazepine (Tegretol), phenytoin (Dilantin), phenobarbital, and sertraline (Zoloft), can increase levothyroxine metabolism.	› Monitor clients for therapeutic effects of levothyroxine. The client's dosages of levothyroxine may need to be increased.
› Levothyroxine can increase the anticoagulant effects of warfarin (Coumadin) by breaking down vitamin K.	› Monitor prothrombin time (PT) and international normalized ratio (INR). › Instruct clients to report signs of bleeding (bruising, petechia). › Decreased dosages of warfarin may be needed.

Nursing Administration

- Obtain baseline vital signs, weight, and height, and monitor periodically throughout treatment.
- Monitor and report signs of cardiac excitability (angina, chest pain, palpitations, dysrhythmias).
- Daily therapy begins with a low dose that increases gradually over several weeks.
- Monitor T_4 and TSH levels.
- Instruct clients to take daily on an empty stomach (before breakfast daily).
- Reinforce client education regarding the importance of lifelong replacement (even after improvement of symptoms). Advise clients not to discontinue the medication without checking with the provider.

- Instruct clients to check with the provider before switching to another brand of levothyroxine because some concerns regarding interchangeability of brands have been raised, and dosage adjustments may be necessary.

Nursing Evaluation of Medication Effectiveness

- Depending on therapeutic intent, evidence of effectiveness can include:
  - Decreased TSH levels.
  - T_4 levels within expected reference range.
  - Absence of hypothyroidism clinical manifestations (depression, weight gain, bradycardia, anorexia, cold intolerance, dry skin, menorrhagia).

MEDICATION CLASSIFICATION: ANTITHYROID MEDICATIONS

- Select Prototype Medication: propylthiouracil (PTU)
- Other Medications: methimazole (Tapazole)

Purpose

- Expected Pharmacological Action
  - Blocks the synthesis of thyroid hormones
  - Prevents the oxidation of iodide
  - Blocks conversion of T_4 into T_3
- Therapeutic Uses
  - Treatment of Graves' disease
  - Produces a euthyroid state prior to thyroid removal surgery
  - As an adjunct to irradiation of the thyroid gland
  - In the emergency treatment of thyrotoxicosis
- Route of administration: Oral

Complications

ADVERSE EFFECTS	NURSING INTERVENTIONS/CLIENT EDUCATION
› Overmedication can result in indications of hypothyroidism (drowsiness, depression, weight gain, edema, bradycardia, anorexia, cold intolerance, dry skin, menorrhagia).	› Instruct clients to report signs of overmedication to the provider. › Reduced dosages and/or temporary administration of thyroid supplements may be needed.
› Agranulocytosis	› Monitor for early indications of agranulocytosis (sore throat, fever), and instruct clients to report them promptly to provider. › Monitor blood counts at baseline and periodically. › If agranulocytosis occurs, stop treatment and monitor for reversal of agranulocytosis. › Neupogen may be indicated to treat agranulocytosis.
› Liver injury, hepatitis	› Monitor for jaundice, dark urine, light-colored stools, and elevated liver function tests during treatment.

Contraindications/Precautions

- Use is contraindicated in pregnancy (Pregnancy Risk Category D) and during lactation because of the risk of neonatal hypothyroidism. Propylthiouracil is safer than methimazole during the first trimester of pregnancy and is considered safer during lactation if an antithyroid medication is necessary.

- Use cautiously in clients who have bone marrow depression and/or immunosuppression and in clients at risk for liver failure.

Interactions

MEDICATION/FOOD INTERACTIONS	NURSING INTERVENTIONS/CLIENT EDUCATION
› Concurrent use of antithyroid medications and anticoagulants can increase anticoagulation.	› Monitor PT, INR, and activated partial thromboplastin time (aPTT), and adjust dosages of anticoagulants accordingly.
› Concurrent use of antithyroid medications and digoxin (Lanoxin) can increase glycoside level.	› Monitor digoxin level and reduce digoxin dose as needed.

Nursing Administration

- Advise clients that therapeutic effects can take 1 to 2 weeks to be evident. Propylthiouracil does not destroy the thyroid hormone that is present, but rather prevents continued synthesis of TH.

- Monitor vital signs, weight, and I&O at baseline and periodically.

- Instruct clients to take medication at consistent times each day and with meals to maintain a consistent therapeutic level and decrease gastric distress.

- Instruct clients not to discontinue the medication abruptly (risk of thyroid crisis due to stress response).

- Monitor for manifestations of hyperthyroidism (indicating inadequate medication).

- Clients who have hyperthyroidism may be given a beta-adrenergic antagonist, such as propranolol (Inderal), to decrease tremors and tachycardia.

- Monitor for indications of hypothyroidism (indicating overmedication), such as drowsiness, depression, weight gain, edema, bradycardia, anorexia, cold intolerance, and dry skin.

- Monitor CBC for leukopenia or thrombocytopenia.

Nursing Evaluation of Medication Effectiveness

- Depending on therapeutic intent, evidence of effectiveness can include:
  - Weight gain.
  - Vital signs within expected reference range.
  - Decreased T_4 levels.
  - Absence of signs of hyperthyroidism (anxiety, tachycardia, palpitations, increased appetite, abdominal cramping, heat intolerance, fever, diaphoresis, weight loss, menstrual irregularities).

MEDICATION CLASSIFICATION: ANTITHYROID MEDICATIONS

- Select Prototype Medication: radioactive iodine (RAI) (^{131}I)

Purpose

- Expected Pharmacological Action
  - ○ Radioactive iodine is absorbed by the thyroid and destroys some of the thyroid-producing cells. At high doses, thyroid-radioactive iodine destroys thyroid cells.
- Therapeutic Uses
  - ○ At high doses, thyroid-radioactive iodine is used for:
    - ▪ Hyperthyroidism.
    - ▪ Thyroid cancer.
  - ○ At low doses, RAI (^{131}I) is used for:
    - ▪ Thyroid function studies (visualization of the degree of iodine uptake by the thyroid gland is helpful in the diagnosis of thyroid disorders).
- Route of administration: oral

Complications

ADVERSE EFFECTS	NURSING INTERVENTIONS/CLIENT EDUCATION
› Radiation sickness	› Monitor for manifestations of radiation sickness (hematemesis, epistaxis, intense nausea, vomiting). › Stop treatment and notify the provider.
› Bone marrow depression	› Monitor for anemia, leukopenia, and thrombocytopenia.
› Hypothyroidism (intolerance to cold, edema, bradycardia, increase in weight, depression)	› Instruct clients to report manifestations of hypothyroidism to the provider.

Contraindications/Precautions

- Due to irradiating effects, use is contraindicated in pregnancy (Pregnancy Risk Category X), clients of childbearing age/intent, and during lactation.

Interactions

MEDICATION/FOOD INTERACTIONS	NURSING INTERVENTIONS/CLIENT EDUCATION
› Concurrent use of other antithyroid medications reduces uptake of radioactive iodine.	› Discontinue use of other antithyroid medications for 1 week prior to therapy.

Nursing Administration

- Instruct clients regarding radioactivity precautions.
  - ○ Encourage clients to void frequently to avoid irradiation of gonads.
  - ○ Limit contact with clients to 30 min/day/person.
  - ○ Encourage clients to increase fluid intake, usually 2 to 3 L/day.
  - ○ Instruct clients to dispose of body wastes per protocol.
  - ○ Instruct clients to avoid coughing and expectoration (source of radioactive iodine).

MEDICATION CLASSIFICATION: ANTITHYROID MEDICATIONS

- Select Prototype Medication: strong iodine solution (Lugol's solution) – nonradioactive iodine
- Other Medications: sodium iodide, potassium iodide

Purpose

- Expected Pharmacological Action
  - ○ Thyroid-nonradioactive iodine creates high levels of iodide that will reduce iodine uptake (by the thyroid gland), inhibit thyroid hormone production, and block the release of thyroid hormones into the bloodstream.
- Therapeutic Uses
  - ○ Thyroid-nonradioactive iodine is used for the development of euthyroid state and reduction of thyroid gland size prior to thyroid removal surgery.
  - ○ Thyroid-nonradioactive iodine is used for the emergency treatment of thyrotoxicosis.
- Route of administration: oral

Complications

ADVERSE EFFECTS	NURSING INTERVENTIONS/CLIENT EDUCATION
› Iodism due to corrosive property (metallic taste, stomatitis, sore teeth and gums, frontal headache, skin rash). Iodism (early toxicity) can progress to overdose (severe GI distress and swelling of the glottis).	› Instruct clients to notify provider for any manifestations of overdose. › Prepare to administer sodium thiosulfate (to reverse findings). Assist with gastric lavage as needed.

Contraindications/Precautions

- Use in pregnancy is contraindicated (Pregnancy Risk Category D).

Interactions

MEDICATION/FOOD INTERACTIONS	NURSING INTERVENTIONS/CLIENT EDUCATION
› Concurrent intake of foods high in iodine (iodized salt, seafood) increases risk for iodism.	› Monitor for manifestations of iodism (brassy taste in mouth, burning sensation in mouth, sore teeth). › Instruct clients regarding foods high in iodine.

Nursing Administration

- Thyroid-nonradioactive iodine can be used in conjunction with other therapy because effects are not usually complete or permanent.
- Obtain baseline vital signs, weight, and I&O, and monitor periodically.
- Instruct clients to dilute strong iodine solution (Lugol's solution) with juice to improve taste.
- Instruct clients to take at the same time each day to maintain therapeutic levels.
- Encourage clients to increase fluid intake, unless contraindicated.

Nursing Evaluation of Medication Effectiveness

- Depending on therapeutic intent, effectiveness can be evidenced by:
  - Weight gain.
  - Vital signs within expected reference range.
  - Decreased T_4 levels.
  - Reduction in size of thyroid gland.
  - Client is able to get adequate sleep, achieve and maintain appropriate weight, maintain blood pressure and heart rate within expected reference range, and be free of complications of hyperthyroidism.

MEDICATION CLASSIFICATION: ANTERIOR PITUITARY HORMONES/GROWTH HORMONES

- Select Prototype Medication: somatropin (Genotropin, Nutropin)

Purpose

- Expected Pharmacological Action
  - Anterior pituitary hormones/growth hormones stimulate overall growth and the production of protein, and decrease the use of glucose.
- Therapeutic Uses
  - Anterior pituitary hormones/growth hormones are used to treat growth hormone deficiencies (pediatric and adult growth hormone deficiencies, Turner's syndrome, Prader-Willi syndrome).
- Routes of administration: IM or subcutaneous

Complications

ADVERSE EFFECTS	NURSING INTERVENTIONS/CLIENT EDUCATION
› Hyperglycemia	› Observe for indications of hyperglycemia (polyphagia, polydipsia, polyuria).
› Hypercalciuria and renal calculi	› Instruct the client to monitor for flank pain, fever, and dysuria, and report these to the provider.

Contraindications/Precautions

- These medications are Pregnancy Risk Category B or C (depending on the brand prescribed).
- Use is contraindicated in clients who have Prader-Willi syndrome and are severely obese or have severe respiratory impairment (sleep apnea) because of higher risk of fatality.
- Use cautiously in clients who have diabetes because of the risk of hyperglycemia.
- Treatment should be stopped prior to epiphyseal closure.

Interactions

MEDICATION/FOOD INTERACTIONS	NURSING INTERVENTIONS/CLIENT EDUCATION
› Concurrent use of glucocorticoids can counteract growth-promoting effects.	› Avoid concurrent use of glucocorticoids and somatrem if possible.

Nursing Administration

- Obtain baseline height and weight.
- Monitor growth patterns during medication administration, usually monthly.
- Reconstitute medication per directions. Mix gently and do not shake prior to administration.
- Rotate injection sites. Abdomen (subcutaneous) and thighs (subcutaneous, IM) are preferred.

Nursing Evaluation of Medication Effectiveness

- Depending on therapeutic intent, effectiveness can be evidenced by increased height and weight.

MEDICATION CLASSIFICATION: ANTIDIURETIC HORMONE (ADH)

- Select Prototype Medication: vasopressin
- Other Medication: desmopressin (DDAVP, Stimate)

Purpose

- Expected Pharmacological Action
  - Antidiuretic hormone (ADH), produced by the posterior pituitary, promotes reabsorption of water within the kidney.
  - Natural ADH causes vasoconstriction because of the contraction of vascular smooth muscle. Synthetic preparations (desmopressin) cause much less vasoconstriction.
- Therapeutic Uses
  - These hormones are used to treat diabetes insipidus.
  - Antidiuretic hormones are sometimes used during CPR to temporarily decrease blood flow to the periphery and increase flow to the brain and heart.
- Route of Administration
  - Desmopressin – oral, intranasal, subcutaneous, IV
  - Vasopressin – intranasal, subcutaneous, IM, IV

Complications

ADVERSE EFFECTS	NURSING INTERVENTIONS/CLIENT EDUCATION
› Reabsorption of too much water	› Monitor for indications of overhydration (sleepiness, pounding headache).
	› In general, clients should reduce fluid intake during therapy.
	› Clients should use the smallest effective dose of desmopressin.
› Myocardial ischemia from excessive vasoconstriction (vasopressin)	› Monitor ECG and blood pressure. Advise clients to notify the provider of chest pain, tightness, or diaphoresis.

Contraindications/Precautions

- Use of vasopressin is contraindicated in clients who have coronary artery disease (risk for angina, MI), peripheral circulation (risk for gangrene), or chronic nephritis.

Interactions

MEDICATION/FOOD INTERACTIONS	NURSING INTERVENTIONS/CLIENT EDUCATION
› Carbamazepine and tricyclic antidepressants can increase the antidiuretic action.	› Use cautiously together.
› Concurrent use of alcohol, heparin, lithium, and phenytoin can decrease antidiuretic effects.	› Establish baseline I&O and weight, and monitor frequently.

Nursing Administration

- Monitor vital signs, central venous pressure, I&O, specific gravity, and laboratory studies (potassium, sodium, BUN, creatinine, specific gravity, osmolality).
- Monitor blood pressure and heart rate.
- Monitor for headache, confusion, or other indications of water intoxication.
- With IV administration of vasopressin, monitor the client's IV site carefully because extravasation can lead to gangrene.
- Intranasal desmopressin starts with a bedtime dose. I&O is monitored. When nocturia is controlled, doses are given twice daily.

Nursing Evaluation of Medication Effectiveness

- Depending on therapeutic intent, evidence of effectiveness can include:
  - A reduction in the large volumes of urine output associated with diabetes insipidus to normal levels of urine output (1.5 to 2 L/24 hr).
  - Cardiac arrest survival.

MEDICATION CLASSIFICATION: ADRENAL HORMONE REPLACEMENT

- Select Prototype Medication: hydrocortisone (Solu-Cortef)
- Other Medications
  - Prednisone, dexamethasone
  - Mineral corticoids: fludrocortisone

Purpose

- Expected Pharmacological Action – mimic effect of natural hormones
- Therapeutic Uses
  - Acute and chronic replacement therapy for adrenocortical insufficiency (Addison's disease).
  - Nonendocrine disorders include cancer, inflammation, and allergic reactions.
- Route of administration: oral, IV

Complications

ADVERSE EFFECTS	NURSING INTERVENTIONS/CLIENT EDUCATION
Glucocorticoids: hydrocortisone	
› Osteoporosis	› Advise clients to take calcium supplements, vitamin D, and/or bisphosphonate (Etidronate).
› Adrenal suppression	› Advise clients to observe for manifestations, and to notify the provider if they occur. › Increase dose with stress. Do not stop the medication suddenly. Taper dose to discontinue.
› Peptic ulcer, GI discomfort	› Advise clients to observe for manifestations (coffee-ground emesis, bloody or tarry stools, abdominal pain), and to notify the provider if they occur. › Administer prophylactic H$_2$ antagonists.
› Infection	› Advise clients to avoid contact with people who have a communicable disease. Monitor for indications of infection, such as fever.
Mineralocorticoid: fludrocortisone	
› Retention of sodium and water, which can lead to hypertension, edema, heart failure, and hypokalemia	› Monitor weight, blood pressure, and serum potassium. Monitor breath sounds and urine output.

Contraindications/Precautions

- Pregnancy Risk Category
  - Hydrocortisone is Pregnancy Risk Category C.
  - Mineralocorticoid: Fludrocortisone is Pregnancy Risk Category C.
- Use is contraindicated in clients who have a viral or bacterial infection not controlled by antibiotics.
- Use with caution in clients who have a recent MI, gastric ulcer, hypertension, kidney disorder, osteoporosis, diabetes mellitus, hypothyroidism, myasthenia gravis, glaucoma, or seizure disorder.

Interactions

MEDICATION/FOOD INTERACTIONS	NURSING INTERVENTIONS/CLIENT EDUCATION
Glucocorticoids	
› NSAIDs or alcohol use can cause increased gastric distress or bleed.	› Use together with caution.
› Concurrent use with oral anticoagulants can increase or decrease anticoagulation.	› Monitor coagulations studies and drug levels.
› Concurrent use with potassium depleting agents can cause increased potassium loss.	› Monitor serum potassium and ECG.
› Concurrent use with vaccines and toxoids can reduce the antibody response.	› Do not use together.
Fludrocortisone	
› Barbiturates and phenytoin can reduce effects of fludrocortisone.	› Monitor for reduced medication effects.
› Antidiabetic effects of insulin and sulfonylureas decreases with concurrent use of fludrocortisone.	› Closely monitor blood glucose levels in clients who have diabetes mellitus.

Nursing Administration

- Monitor weight, blood pressure, and electrolytes.
- Give with food to reduce gastric distress.
- Advise clients to observe for indications of peptic ulcer (coffee-ground emesis, bloody or tarry stools, abdominal pain) and to notify the provider if they occur.
- Do not stop the medication suddenly. Taper off dosage if discontinuing.
- Instruct clients to notify the provider of indications of acute adrenal insufficiency (fever, muscle and joint pain, weakness, and fatigue).

Nursing Evaluation of Medication Effectiveness

- Depending on therapeutic intent, evidence of effectiveness can include relief of effects of adrenocortical deficiency, such as weakness, hypoglycemia, hyperkalemia, and fatigue, with minimal adverse effects.

APPLICATION EXERCISES

1. A nurse is caring for a client who is taking propylthiouracil (PTU). For which of the following adverse effects of this medication should the nurse monitor?

    A. Bradycardia

    B. Insomnia

    C. Heat intolerance

    D. Weight loss

2. A client asks a nurse why she is taking propranolol (Inderal) along with her therapy for hyperthyroidism. Which of the following replies by the nurse is appropriate?

    A. "Propranolol helps increase blood flow to your thyroid gland."

    B. "Propranolol is used to prevent excess glucose in your blood."

    C. "Propranolol will decrease your tremors and fast heart beat."

    D. "Propranolol promotes conversion of T_4 to T_3 in your body."

3. A nurse is caring for an older adult client in a long-term care facility who has hypothyroidism and is beginning levothyroxine (Synthroid). Which of the following dosage schedules should the nurse expect for this client?

    A. The client will start at a high dose, and the dose will be tapered down as needed.

    B. The client will remain on the initial dosage during the course of treatment.

    C. The client's dosage will be adjusted daily based on blood levels.

    D. The client will start on a low dose, which will be gradually increased.

4. A nurse is caring for a client who has a prescription for somatropin (Genotropin) to stimulate growth. The nurse should plan to monitor the client's urine for which of the following?

    A. Bilirubin

    B. Protein

    C. Potassium

    D. Calcium

5. A nurse is caring for a client who takes vasopressin for diabetes insipidus. For which of the following adverse effects should the nurse monitor?

    A. Hypovolemia

    B. Hypercalcemia

    C. Hypoglycemia

    D. Hypertension

6. A nurse is assisting with admitting a client to an acute care facility for a total hip arthroplasty. The client takes hydrocortisone for Addison's disease. Which of the following is the priority nursing action?

    A. Administering a supplemental dose of hydrocortisone

    B. Instructing the client about coughing and deep breathing

    C. Collecting addition information from the client about his history of Addison's disease

    D. Inserting an indwelling urinary catheter

7. A nurse in a provider's office is providing instructions to a client who has a new prescription for levothyroxine (Synthroid) to treat hypothyroidism. Use the ATI Active Learning Template: Medication to complete this item to include the following:

    A. Therapeutic Use: Describe the therapeutic use of levothyroxine in this client.

    B. Adverse Effects: Identify two adverse effects of this medication.

    C. Nursing Interventions: Describe two laboratory tests the nurse should monitor.

    D. Client Teaching: Describe teaching points for a client taking levothyroxine.

APPLICATION EXERCISES KEY

1. A. **CORRECT:** Bradycardia is an adverse effect of propylthiouracil. The nurse should monitor the client for bradycardia.

    B. INCORRECT: Drowsiness, rather than insomnia, is an adverse effect of propylthiouracil.

    C. INCORRECT: Cold intolerance, rather than heat intolerance, is an adverse effect of propylthiouracil.

    D. INCORRECT: Weight gain, rather than weight loss, is an adverse effect of propylthiouracil.

    Ⓝ NCLEX® Connection: Pharmacological Therapies, Adverse Effects/Contraindications/ Side Effects/Interactions

2. A. INCORRECT: Propranolol lowers blood pressure, but does not increase blood flow to the thyroid gland.

    B. INCORRECT: Propranolol does not help prevent hyperglycemia.

    C. **CORRECT:** Propranolol is a beta-adrenergic antagonist that decreases heart rate and controls tremors.

    D. INCORRECT: Propranolol does not promote conversion of T_4 to T_3.

    Ⓝ NCLEX® Connection: Pharmacological Therapies, Expected Actions/Outcomes

3. A. INCORRECT: The nurse should not expect that the levothyroxine will be started at a high dose and tapered down as needed.

    B. INCORRECT: The nurse should not expect that the client's dosage will remain the same throughout treatment.

    C. INCORRECT: The nurse should not expect that the client's dosage will be adjusted daily based on blood levels.

    D. **CORRECT:** The nurse should expect that levothyroxine will be started at a low dose and gradually increased over several weeks. This is especially important in older adult clients to prevent toxicity.

    Ⓝ NCLEX® Connection: Pharmacological Therapies, Medication Administration

4. A. INCORRECT: Bilirubin can be present in the urine with liver or biliary disorders, but is not monitored during somatropin therapy.

    B. INCORRECT: Protein can be present in the urine during stress, infection, or glomerular disorders, but is not monitored during somatropin therapy.

    C. INCORRECT: Potassium is not expected to be present in a urine specimen.

    D. **CORRECT:** A large amount of calcium can be present in the urine of a client who takes somatropin. This puts the client at risk for renal calculi.

    Ⓝ NCLEX® Connection: Pharmacological Therapies, Adverse Effects/Contraindications/ Side Effects/Interactions

5. A. INCORRECT: Edema and hypervolemia, rather than hypovolemia, are adverse effects of vasopressin.

   B. INCORRECT: Calcium imbalance is not an adverse effect of vasopressin.

   C. INCORRECT: Glucose imbalance is not an adverse effect of vasopressin.

   D. **CORRECT:** Cardiac effects, such as hypertension and angina pectoris, are serious adverse effects of vasopressin for which the nurse should monitor.

   Ⓝ NCLEX® Connection: Pharmacological Therapies, Adverse Effects/Contraindications/ Side Effects/Interactions

6. A. **CORRECT:** Acute adrenal insufficiency (adrenal crisis) is the greatest risk to a client who has Addison's disease, is taking a glucocorticoid, and is undergoing surgery. To prevent acute adrenal insufficiency, supplemental doses are administered during times of increased stress.

   B. INCORRECT: Instruction on coughing and deep breathing is important, but is not the nurse's priority for this client.

   C. INCORRECT: Obtaining additional data from the client about past medical history is important, but is not the nurse's priority for this client.

   D. INCORRECT: Inserting an indwelling urinary catheter is important, but is not the nurse's priority for this client.

   Ⓝ NCLEX® Connection: Pharmacological Therapies, Adverse Effects/Contraindications/ Side Effects/Interactions

7. *Using the ATI Active Learning Template: Medication*

   A. Therapeutic Use

   - Levothyroxine replaces T_4 and is used as thyroid hormone replacement therapy. Replacement of T_4 also raises T_3 levels, because some T_4 is converted into T_3.

   B. Adverse Effects

   - Adverse effects are essentially the same as manifestations of hyperthyroidism: cardiac symptoms, such as hypertension and angina pectoris; insomnia; anxiety; weight loss; heat intolerance; increased body temperature; tremors; and menstrual irregularities.

   C. Nursing Interventions

   - The nurse should monitor thyroid function tests: T_3, T_4, and TSH.

   D. Client Teaching

   - Instruct the client to take levothyroxine on an empty stomach, usually 1 hr before breakfast.
   - Instruct the client that thyroid replacement therapy is usually lifelong.
   - Monitor for adverse effects that indicate that the dosage needs to be reduced.
   - Adverse effects include cardiac effects, chest pain, hypertension, and palpitations, especially in older adults.

   Ⓝ NCLEX® Connection: Pharmacological Therapies, Expected Actions/Outcomes

UNIT 11   Medications Affecting the Immune System

CHAPTERS

› Immunizations

When reviewing the chapters in this unit, keep in mind the relevant sections of the NCLEX® outline, in particular:

Client Needs: Pharmacological Therapies

› Relevant topics/tasks include:

  » Adverse Effects/Contraindications/Side Effects/Interactions

    › Identify a contraindication to the administration of a prescribed or over-the-counter medication to the client.

  » Expected Actions/Outcomes

    › Use resources to check on purposes and actions of pharmacological agents.

  » Medication Administration

    › Administer a subcutaneous, intradermal, or intramuscular medication.

chapter **36**

Overview

- Administration of a vaccine causes production of antibodies that prevent illness from a specific microbe.

- Active natural immunity develops when the body produces antibodies in response to exposure to a live pathogen. Active artificial immunity develops when an immunization is administered and the body produces antibodies in response to exposure to a killed or attenuated virus.

- Passive natural immunity occurs when antibodies are passed from the mother to the newborn/infant through the placenta and then breastfeeding. Passive artificial immunity is temporary, and occurs after antibodies in the form of immune globulins are administered to an individual who requires immediate protection against a disease after exposure has occurred.

- Immunizations can be made from killed viruses or live, attenuated, or weakened viruses.

MEDICATION CLASSIFICATION: VACCINATIONS

- Childhood Vaccinations (See www.cdc.gov for updates.)
  - ○ Diphtheria and tetanus toxoids and acellular pertussis vaccine (DTaP) – Administer doses at 2, 4, 6, and 15 to 18 months, and at 4 to 6 years.
  - ○ Tetanus and diphtheria toxoids and pertussis vaccine (Tdap) – Administer one dose at 11 to 12 years.
  - ○ Tetanus and diphtheria (Td) booster – Administer one dose every 10 years following DTaP.
  - ○ Haemophilus influenza Type B (Hib) – Administer doses at 2, 4, 6, and at 12 to 15 months.
  - ○ Rotavirus (RV) oral vaccine
    - ▪ Two formulations are available. The infant may be administered either formulation. The first dose of either form should not be initiated for infants 15 weeks or older. Maximum age for any vaccination with an RV vaccine is 8 months.
      - □ RV-5 vaccine (RotaTeq) should be administered as a three-dose series at ages 2, 4, and 6 months.
      - □ RV-1 (Rotarix) vaccine should be administered as two-dose series at 2 and 4 months.
    - ▪ All doses should be completed by age 8 months.
  - ○ Inactivated poliovirus vaccine (IPV) – Administer doses at 2, 4, and 6 to 18 months, and at 4 to 6 years.
  - ○ Measles, mumps, and rubella vaccine (MMR) – Administer doses at 12 to 15 months and at 4 to 6 years.
  - ○ Varicella vaccine – Administer one dose at 12 to 15 months and 4 to 6 years, or two doses administered 4 weeks apart if administered after age 13 years.
  - ○ Pneumococcal conjugate vaccine (PCV) – Administer doses at 2, 4, 6, and 12 to 15 months.

○ Hepatitis A – Administer two doses after age 12 months. Administer the second dose 6 to 18 months after the first.

○ Hepatitis B – Administer within 12 hr after birth with additional doses at age 1 to 2 months and 6 to 18 months.

○ Seasonal influenza vaccine

▪ Administer trivalent inactivated influenza vaccine (TIV) annually, beginning at age 6 months.

▪ Starting at age 2 years, the live, attenuated influenza vaccine (LAIV) (nasal spray) can be used. LAIV is contraindicated for children who have asthma, children age 2 to 4 years who have had wheezing during the past year, or children who have a medical condition that puts them at risk for influenza complications

▪ October through November is the ideal time, and December is acceptable.

○ Meningococcal vaccine (MCV4) – Administer one dose at age 11 to 12 years (earlier if specific risk factors are present).

○ Human papillomavirus (HPV2 or HPV4) – Administer three doses over a 6-month period for males and females 9 to 12 years of age. Administer only HPV4 (Gardasil) to males; administer either HPV4 or HPV2 (Cervarix) to females.

• Adult Vaccinations: for adults age 19 and older (See www.cdc.gov for updates.)

○ Td booster – Administer at least one dose of Tdap, and then Td every 10 years.

○ MMR – Administer one or two doses at ages 19 to 49.

○ Varicella vaccine – Two doses should be administered to adults who do not have evidence of previous infection. A second dose should be administered for adults who had only one previous dose. Pregnant women needing protection against varicella should wait until the postpartum period for vaccination.

○ Pneumococcal polysaccharide vaccine (PPV) – Vaccinate adults who are immunocompromised, have a chronic disease, smoke cigarettes, or live in a long-term care facility. CDC guidelines should be followed for revaccination. If a client is not previously vaccinated or has no evidence of disease then one dose should be administered at age 65.

○ Hepatitis A – Administer two doses 6 to 12 months apart for high-risk individuals.

○ Hepatitis B – Administer three doses for high-risk individuals. There must be at least 4 weeks between doses one and two, and at least 8 weeks between doses two and three.

○ Seasonal Influenza Vaccine

▪ One dose annually is recommended for all adults.

▪ Note that LAIV, administered as a nasal spray, is only indicated for adults under age 50 who are not pregnant or immunocompromised.

○ MCV4 – Students entering college and living in college dormitories if not previously immunized. Meningococcal polysaccharide vaccine (MPSV4) is recommended for adults older than 56 years. Revaccination may be recommended after 5 years for adults at high risk for infection.

○ HPV2 or HPV4 – Three doses are recommended for females up to age 26 who were not vaccinated as children. If not vaccinated as children, HPV4 is recommended for males age 19 to 21, and for males 22 to 26 who have a high risk for human papilloma virus.

○ Herpes zoster vaccine – A one-time dose is recommended for all adults over age 60 years.

Purpose

- Expected Pharmacological Action
  - Immunizations produce antibodies that provide active immunity. Immunizations can take months to have an effect but confer long-lasting protection against infectious diseases.
- Therapeutic Uses
  - Eradication of infectious diseases (polio, smallpox)
  - Prevention of childhood and adult infectious diseases and their complications (measles, diphtheria, mumps, rubella, tetanus, *H. influenza*)

Complications, Contraindications, and Precautions

- Anaphylactic reaction to a vaccine is a contraindication for further doses of that vaccine.
- Anaphylactic reaction to a vaccine or to any of its components, including egg protein, is a contraindication to use of subsequent vaccines containing that substance.
- Moderate or severe illnesses with or without fever are contraindications. The common cold and other minor illnesses are not contraindications.
- Contraindications to vaccinations require the provider to analyze data and weigh the risks that come with immunizing or not immunizing.
- Immunocompromised individuals are defined by the CDC as those with hematologic or solid tumors, congenital immunodeficiency, or on long-term immunosuppressive therapy, including corticosteroids.

IMMUNIZATIONS	
ADVERSE EFFECTS	CONTRAINDICATIONS/PRECAUTIONS
DTaP	
› Local reaction at injection site › Fever and irritability › Crying that cannot be consoled, lasting up to 3 hours › Seizures › Rare: acute encephalopathy	› An occurrence of encephalopathy 7 days after the administration of the DTaP immunization › Seizures within 3 days of vaccination › History of uncontrollable crying or temperature of 40.5° C (105° F) or higher that occurs within 48 hr of vaccination
Haemophilus influenza type b conjugate vaccine	
› Mild local reactions, low-grade fever › Fever (temperature greater than 38.5° C [101.3° F]), vomiting, crying can occur	› Children less than 6 weeks of age
Rotavirus vaccine	
› Irritability › Mild, temporary nausea/vomiting	› Infants who have severe combined immunodeficiency (SCID) › Use caution in infants who are immunocompromised from HIV infection or medication administration, or who have chronic GI disorders.

IMMUNIZATIONS	
ADVERSE EFFECTS	CONTRAINDICATIONS/PRECAUTIONS
IPV	
› Local reaction at injection site › Rare: vaccine-associated paralytic poliomyelitis	› Pregnancy (unless the woman is at high risk for contracting polio, in which case the immunization may be prescribed during pregnancy) › Confirmed allergy to streptomycin, neomycin, or polymyxin B
MMR	
› Local reaction at injection site › Rash, fever, swollen glands › Possibility of joint pain lasting for days to weeks › Risk for anaphylaxis and thrombocytopenia	› Pregnancy or the possibility of pregnancy within 4 weeks › Clients who are immunocompromised (with HIV infection or from medication administration) › Recent transfusion with blood products › History of thrombocytopenia › If tuberculosis skin test (TST) and MMR are both needed but not administered on same day, delay TST for 4 to 6 weeks after MMR
Varicella vaccine	
› Varicella-like rash, local or generalized (such as vesicles on the body)	› Pregnancy or the possibility of pregnancy within 4 weeks › Pregnant women should avoid close proximity to children recently vaccinated › Cancers of the blood and lymphatic system › Allergy to gelatin and neomycin › Clients who are immunocompromised (with HIV infection or from medication administration) › Recent transfusion with blood products
PCV and PPV	
› Mild local reactions, fever › No serious adverse effects	› Safety during pregnancy has not been established.
Hepatitis A and B vaccines	
› Local reaction at injection site, mild fever › Anaphylaxis	› Hep A: pregnancy may be a contraindication › Hep B: allergy to baker's yeast
Seasonal influenza vaccine	
› Inactivated: mild local reaction, fever › Live attenuated: headache, cough, fever › Rare: risk for Guillain-Barré syndrome manifested by ascending paralysis, beginning with weakness of lower extremities and progressing to difficulty breathing	› LAIV, administered as nasal spray, is contraindicated for adults over 50 years; children under 2 years; and adults and children who are immunocompromised, have a chronic disease, or are receiving certain antiviral medications. Pregnant women should not receive the live vaccine. › History of Guillain-Barré syndrome

| IMMUNIZATIONS | |
ADVERSE EFFECTS	CONTRAINDICATIONS/PRECAUTIONS
MCV4	
› Mild local reaction › Rare: risk of allergic response	› Severe allergic reaction to a previous dose
HPV2 or HPV4 vaccine	
› Mild local reaction and fever › Fainting shortly after receiving vaccination	› Pregnancy › Allergy to baker's yeast
Herpes Zoster	
› Mild local reaction at injection site	› Clients who are immunocompromised (with HIV infection or from medication administration)

Interactions

- None significant

Nursing Administration

- For infants and children

  - Obtain parental consent for children.

  - Note the date, route, and site of vaccination on the child's immunization record at the time of immunization.

  - Administer IM vaccinations in the vastus lateralis muscle in infants and young children, and in the deltoid muscle for older children and adolescents.

  - Administer subcutaneous injections in the outer aspect of the upper arm or anterolateral thigh.

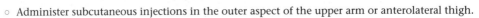
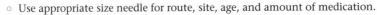

  - Use appropriate size needle for route, site, age, and amount of medication.

  - Use strategies to minimize discomfort.

  - Provide for distraction.

  - Administer oral vaccines early in clinic visit before injections and painful or potentially distressing procedures.

  - Do not allow the child to delay the procedure.

  - Encourage the parent to use comforting measures such as cuddling and pacifiers during procedure, and measures such as application of cool compresses to injection site or gentle movement of the involved extremity after the procedure.

  - Provide praise afterward.

  - Apply a colorful bandage if appropriate.

- ○ Instruct parents to avoid administration of aspirin to children to treat fever or local reaction because of the risk of the development of Reye's syndrome
- ○ Instruct parents to premedicate infants and children with nonopioid analgesic/antipyretic prior to immunizations and for the following 24 hr. Use acetaminophen for infants 2 to 6 months. Parents may administer ibuprofen starting at 6 months of age.
- ○ Instruct parents to apply topical anesthetic prior to the injection.
- For adults
  - ○ Administer subcutaneous vaccinations in the outer aspect of the upper arm or anterolateral thigh.
  - ○ Administer IM vaccinations into the deltoid muscle.
- For clients of all ages
  - ○ Have emergency medications and equipment on standby in case the client experiences an allergic response, such as anaphylaxis.
  - ○ Follow storage and reconstitution directions. If reconstituted, use within 30 min.
  - ○ Provide written vaccine information sheets and review the content with parents or clients.
  - ○ Instruct parents and clients to observe for complications and to notify the provider if side effects occur.
  - ○ Document administration of vaccines including date, route and site of vaccination; type, manufacturer, lot number, and expiration of vaccine; name; address; and signature.

Nursing Evaluation of Medication Effectiveness

- Depending on therapeutic intent, effectiveness can be evidenced by:
  - ○ Improvement of local reaction to vaccination with absence of pain, fever, and swelling at the site of injection.
  - ○ Development of immunity.

APPLICATION EXERCISES

1. A nurse is caring for several clients who came to the clinic for a seasonal influenza vaccination. Which of the following clients could receive the vaccine via nasal spray rather than an injection?

    A. A 1-year-old with no health problems

    B. A 17-year-old who has a hypersensitivity to penicillin

    C. A 25-year-old who is pregnant

    D. A 52-year-old who takes a multivitamin supplement

2. A nurse is reinforcing teaching to a group of parents about immunizations. Which of the following vaccines should the nurse tell the parents is administered to children younger than 1 year of age and not to older children or adults?

    A. Pneumococcal vaccine

    B. Meningococcal vaccine

    C. Varicella vaccine

    D. Rotavirus vaccine

3. A nurse is administering RV, DTaP, Hib, PCV, and IPV vaccinations to a 4-month-old infant in an outpatient facility. Which of the following actions should the nurse plan to take? (Select all that apply.)

    _____ A. Administer any oral vaccine before giving injectable vaccine.

    _____ B. Administer subcutaneous injections in the anterolateral thigh.

    _____ C. Administer IM injections in the deltoid muscle.

    _____ D. Administer infant a pacifier during vaccine injections.

    _____ E. Instruct parents to administer aspirin prior to the vaccination to prevent inflammation.

4. A 12-month-old child just received her first measles, mumps, and rubella (MMR) vaccine. For which of the following possible reactions to this vaccine should the nurse teach the parents to monitor? (Select all that apply.)

    _____ A. Rash

    _____ B. Redness and discomfort at injection site

    _____ C. Bruising on multiple areas of body

    _____ D. Fainting

    _____ E. Inconsolable crying

5. A nurse is caring for a group of clients who are not protected against varicella. Which of the following clients should receive a varicella vaccination at this time?

    A. 24-year-old woman in the third trimester of pregnancy

    B. 3-year-old child who has Wilms' tumor and is receiving chemotherapy

    C. 2-month-old infant who has no health problems

    D. 32-year-old man who has essential hypertension

6. A nurse is planning to administer human papilloma virus (HPV) vaccine (Gardasil) to an 11-year-old female in an outpatient facility. Use the ATI Active Learning Template: Medication to complete this item to include the following:

    A. Therapeutic Use: Identify the therapeutic use for the HPV vaccine in this client.

    B. Adverse Effects: Identify two the client should watch for.

    C. Nursing Interventions: Describe contraindications to receiving HPV vaccine.

    D. Client Education: Describe two teaching points the client who receives a first dose of HPV vaccine.

APPLICATION EXERCISES KEY

1. A. INCORRECT: Children under 2 years of age are not eligible to receive the live, attenuated influenza vaccine (LAIV). The 1-year-old should instead receive inactivated seasonal influenza vaccine by injection.

    B. **CORRECT:** A 17-year-old can be vaccinated for influenza with the LAIV via nasal spray. A hypersensitivity to penicillin is not a contraindication for an influenza vaccination.

    C. INCORRECT: The LAIV is contraindicated during pregnancy. Instead, this client should receive the inactivated influenza vaccine via injection.

    D. INCORRECT: Clients over age 50 are not eligible for the LAIV. Instead, this client should receive the inactivated influenza vaccine via injection.

    Ⓝ NCLEX® Connection: Health Promotion and Maintenance, Health Promotion/Disease Prevention

2. A. INCORRECT: Pneumococcal vaccine (PPV) is recommended for adults who have certain health risks.

    B. INCORRECT: Meningococcal vaccine is recommended for adults and children.

    C. INCORRECT: Varicella vaccine is recommended for adults and children.

    D. **CORRECT:** Rotavirus vaccine is administered only to infants less than 8 months of age.

    Ⓝ NCLEX® Connection: Health Promotion and Maintenance, Health Promotion/Disease Prevention

3. A. **CORRECT:** In order to ensure that the full dose of an oral vaccine, such as that for rotavirus (RV), is completely ingested by the infant, administer the oral vaccine before any potentially upsetting or painful injections or procedures.

    B. **CORRECT:** Subcutaneous vaccinations may be administered in either the anterolateral thigh or the outer aspect of the upper arm to infants and children.

    C. INCORRECT: The deltoid muscle is not fully developed in infants and generally should not be used for IM injections until the child begins to walk. The nurse should use the vastus lateralis muscle for vaccinations in the infant.

    D. INCORRECT: Giving the infant a pacifier during injections is a comfort measure that the nurse should encourage.

    E. **CORRECT:** Aspirin should not be used for infants or young children due to the potential for Reye's syndrome. Acetaminophen may be used prior to immunizations and for 24 hr afterward for infants age 2 to 6 months. Older infants and children may be administered ibuprofen.

    Ⓝ NCLEX® Connection: Health Promotion and Maintenance, Health Promotion/Disease Prevention

4. A. **CORRECT:** A rash, fever, and swollen glands can develop in children 1 to 2 weeks following MMR vaccination.

    B. **CORRECT:** Local irritation at the injection site can occur following MMR vaccination.

    C. **CORRECT:** Temporary thrombocytopenia, causing bruising or hemorrhage, can occur occasionally following MMR vaccination.

    D. INCORRECT: Fainting is an adverse reaction that can occur with HPV vaccination.

    E. INCORRECT: Inconsolable crying can occur in some infants following acellular pertussis (DTaP) vaccination.

    Ⓝ NCLEX® Connection: Health Promotion and Maintenance, Health Promotion/Disease Prevention

5. A. INCORRECT: A woman in the third trimester of pregnancy should wait until the postpartum period for varicella vaccination. This is a live vaccine that is not safe for pregnant women.

    B. INCORRECT: Immunocompromised clients and those with cancer who are receiving chemotherapy generally should not be vaccinated for varicella.

    C. INCORRECT: A 2-month-old infant is too young to receive varicella vaccine, which usually is started at age 12 to 15 months.

    D. **CORRECT:** A 32-year-old man who has essential hypertension and did not receive two doses of varicella vaccine earlier in life should be vaccinated. Essential hypertension is not a contraindication for this vaccine.

    Ⓝ NCLEX® Connection: Health Promotion and Maintenance, Health Promotion/Disease Prevention

6. *Using the ATI Active Learning Template: Medication*
    A. Therapeutic Use
       • HPV vaccine (Gardasil) prevents infection from four types of HPV. It can prevent cervical, vaginal, and vulvar cancer; genital warts; and precancerous lesions caused by HPV types 6, 11, 16, and 18. Because HPV vaccine can only prevent, rather than treat, infection from HPV, it is recommended that males and females between the ages of 11 and 12 years receive the vaccine. It can be administered to children as young as 9 and to young adults up to 26 years of age.
    B. Adverse Effects
       • HPV vaccine can cause localized redness and swelling at the injection site. It has caused fainting in some children who receive the vaccine. In rare cases, it can cause Guillain-Barré syndrome.
    C. Nursing Interventions
       • Contraindications to receiving HPV include a true allergy to yeast and pregnancy.
    D. Client Education
       • Instruct client and family about the possible adverse effects, and tell them that the common adverse effects are mild and temporary. Tell the client and family that three doses of the vaccine are administered within 6 months. The second dose is administered 2 months after the first dose, and the third dose is administered 6 months after the first dose.

    Ⓝ NCLEX® Connection: Health Promotion and Maintenance, Health Promotion/Disease Prevention

UNIT 12   Medications for Infection

CHAPTERS

› Principles of Antimicrobial Therapy
› Antibiotics Affecting the Bacterial Cell Wall
› Antibiotics Affecting Protein Synthesis
› Urinary Tract Infections
› Mycobacterial, Fungal, and Parasitic Infections
› Viral Infections, HIV, and AIDS

NCLEX® CONNECTIONS

When reviewing the chapters in this unit, keep in mind the relevant sections of the NCLEX® outline, in particular:

Client Needs: Pharmacological and Parenteral Therapies

› Relevant topics/tasks include:

» Adverse Effects/Contraindications/Side Effects/Interactions

› Identify symptoms/evidence of an allergic reaction.

» Medication Administration

› Evaluate the appropriateness/accuracy of a medication order for the client per institution policy, including reconciling orders.

» Parenteral/Intravenous Therapy

› Evaluate the client's response to intermittent parenteral fluid therapy.

Overview

- Antimicrobial therapy (often termed "antibiotic therapy") is the use of medications to treat infections caused by bacteria, viruses, and fungi.
- Antimicrobials (natural or synthetic) must use selective toxicity to kill or otherwise control microbes without destroying host cells. Methods of actions include the following.
  - Destroying the cell wall that is present in bacteria but not in mammals
  - Inhibiting the conversion of an enzyme unique for a particular bacteria's survival
  - Impairing protein synthesis in the bacteria ribosomes, which never are identical to mammalian cells
- New antimicrobials must be continually created due to changes in DNA of micro-organisms, called conjugation, which produces resistance to multiple existing drugs.
- Suprainfection is a type of resistance caused when normal flora are killed by use of an antibiotic, thus favoring the emergence of a new infection that is difficult to eliminate.
- Classifications of antimicrobial medications are based on:
  - Defining which microbes are susceptible to each medication.
    - Narrow-spectrum antibiotics – sensitive to only a few types of bacteria
    - Broad-spectrum antibiotics – sensitive to a wide variety of bacteria
  - The mechanism of action of each antibacterial medication.
    - Bactericidal medications are directly lethal to the micro-organism.
    - Bacteriostatic medications slow the growth of the micro-organism, but it is actually destroyed by the client's immune system response of phagocytic cells (macrophages, neutrophils) to eliminate the bacteria.
- Multiple factors determine which medication is selected for clinical use (antibacterial, antifungal, and antiviral medication).

Selection of Antimicrobials

- Identification of the Causative Agent
  - Laboratory testing is performed on body fluids, such as blood, urine, sputum, or wound drainage, to determine the micro-organism causing the infection.
    - Gram stain: An aspirate of the body fluid is examined under a microscope, where micro-organisms may be identified directly.
    - Culture of the fluid: The aspirate is applied to culture medium, and colonies of the micro-organism are grown over several days. A culture may be preferable to gram stain in cases in which positive identification cannot be made by the first method.
      - Culture should be obtained prior to treatment with antibiotics.
      - Fluid for culture should be carefully collected to prevent contamination and unnecessary antimicrobial treatment.

- Sensitivity of the Micro-Organism to the Antimicrobial
  - For organisms where resistance is common, a test for sensitivity of the organism to various antimicrobials is performed.
    - Disk diffusion test (also called Kirby-Bauer test) is most common. The degree of medication sensitivity is determined by the amount of bacteria-free zone on the disk.
    - Serial dilution method is a quantitative method using several test tubes with varying amounts of the antibiotic that helps determine the necessary amount of antibiotic to treat a specific infection.
      - Minimum inhibitory concentration (MIC) – the amount of antibiotic to completely inhibit bacterial growth but does not kill the bacteria.
      - Minimum bactericidal concentration (MBC) – the lowest concentration of the antibiotic that kills 99.9% of the bacteria.
      - Antibiotic dosage should be adjusted to produce the concentration equal to or greater than the MIC to kill the bacteria.
    - Gradient diffusion uses a disk and strips with varying concentrations of antibiotic. The antibiotic concentration needed is identified when the bacteria no longer grow.
- Host Factors
  - Immune System of Client
    - In a person who has an intact immune system, the antibiotic works with host defense systems to suppress organisms. Both bactericidal and bacteriostatic antibiotics may be used.
    - An immunocompromised person needs strong bactericidal antibiotics, as opposed to bacteriostatic medication.
  - Site of the Infection
    - Certain sites are difficult for antimicrobials to reach and achieve the MIC.
      - Infections in cerebral spinal fluid, where the blood-brain barrier must be crossed (meningitis).
      - Bacterial infiltration within the heart (endocarditis). Infectious micro-organisms vegetate on the thrombus developed from the injured endocardium and are then covered and concealed by a new thrombus, making it difficult for normal defense mechanisms and antibiotics to kill the bacteria.
      - Purulent abscesses anywhere within the body due to poor blood supply.
      - Surgical removal of drainage increases the effect of antimicrobials.
      - Foreign objects (pacemaker, joint prosthesis, vascular grafts, heart valves, surgical mesh) are attacked by phagocytic cells and become less able to destroy micro-organisms that colonize around the foreign object.
  - Age of the Client
    - Infants are at increased danger of antibiotic toxicity because of undeveloped kidney and liver function, causing slow excretion of the antibiotic.
    - Older adult clients can develop toxicity because of reduction in drug metabolism and excretion.
  - Pregnancy
    - Antibiotics can harm the developing fetus by crossing over to the placenta.
      - Gentamicin causes hearing loss in the infant.
      - Tetracyclines cause discoloration of the infant's developing teeth and increased chance of toxicity to the antibiotic in the mother.
    - Antimicrobials are generally avoided in mothers who are breastfeeding because of possible danger to the nursing infant.

○ Presence of a previous allergic reaction, especially with penicillin. (Clients should not receive penicillin after an allergic reaction, narrowing the antibiotic choice for those clients.)

○ Combination Therapy

- Combining more than one antimicrobial can cause additive, potentiative, or antagonistic effects.

  □ Treats severe infections

  □ Treats infections caused by more than one micro-organism

  □ Prevents resistant bacteria from causing an infection, such as tuberculosis

  □ Decreases the chance of toxicity by reducing necessary dosage

  □ Produces more effective treatment than use of only one antibiotic medication

- Combining antimicrobials can cause adverse effects.

  □ Increased resistance to antimicrobials

  □ Increased cost of therapy

  □ More adverse or toxic reactions

  □ Antagonistic effects among the various antibiotics

  □ Increased risk for a suprainfection

Prophylactic Use

- Indications for prophylactic use include prevention of

  ○ Infections for clients undergoing surgery of the gastrointestinal (GI) tract, cardiac or vascular surgery, orthopedic surgery, some gynecologic surgeries

  ○ Influenza with oseltamivir (Tamiflu)

  ○ Sexually transmitted infections following sexual exposure

- Limit prophylactic use of antimicrobials to individuals who have

  ○ Prosthetic heart valves prior to dental or other procedures because of the danger of bacterial endocarditis

  ○ Recurring urinary tract infections

Preventive Nursing Measures

- Perform hand hygiene before and after each client contact to prevent spread of infection.

- Recognize invasive procedures that increase the chance of infection (e.g., indwelling urinary catheter, IV catheter, heart catheterization).

- Encourage health measures to prevent infections by having the client maintain an up-to-date immunization status.

- Instruct clients to take the full course of antibiotics prescribed to prevent medication resistance and recurrence of infection.

- Use infection control procedures to prevent transmission of resistant micro-organisms.

  ○ Practice proper use of infection control principles, such as use of aseptic technique, isolation, and proper assignment of rooms within facilities.

- Monitor effectiveness of treatment.

  ○ Check posttreatment culture to determine whether it is negative for bacteria.

  ○ Monitor the client for clinical improvement (e.g., improved breath sounds and fever).

APPLICATION EXERCISES

1. A nurse is reviewing a plan of care for a client who has an infected wound of the arm. Which of the following actions should the nurse perform first?

    A. Administer antibiotic medication.

    B. Obtain a culture of the wound.

    C. Instruct the client on the purpose of antibiotics.

    D. Apply a dressing to the client's wound.

2. A nurse is reviewing a client's laboratory findings to identify which antibiotic the provider may prescribe to treat the client's urinary tract infection. Which of the following urine tests would provide this information?

    A. Gram stain

    B. Culture

    C. Sensitivity

    D. Specific gravity

3. A nurse is reviewing information with a newly licensed nurse on client conditions that decrease the effectiveness of antimicrobial therapy. Which of the following client conditions should the nurse include in the information? (Select all that apply.)

    _____ A. A client who has meningitis

    _____ B. A client who has a pacemaker

    _____ C. A client who has endocarditis

    _____ D. A client who has pneumonia

    _____ E. A client who has pyelonephritis

4. A nurse is caring for a group of clients who are receiving antimicrobial therapy. Which of the following clients is the priority for the nurse to monitor for manifestations of antibiotic toxicity?

    A. Adolescent client who has a sinus infection

    B. Older adult client who has prostatitis

    C. New mother who has mastitis

    D. Middle adult client who has a urinary tract infection

5. A nurse is reviewing the records of several clients. Which of the following clients should the nurse expect to be prescribed prophylactic antimicrobial therapy? (Select all that apply.)

_____ A. A client who suspects exposure to a sexually transmitted infection

_____ B. A client who is having orthopedic surgery

_____ C. A client who has a prosthetic heart valve and is scheduled for dental work

_____ D. A client who has recurrent urinary tract infections

_____ E. A client who has an upper respiratory infection

6. A nurse is helping develop a handout for newly hired nurses on ways to prevent the spread of micro-organisms. What information should the nurse include? Use the ATI Active Learning Template: Basic Concept to complete this item. Include the following:

A. Related Content: Determine one related concept.

B. Underlying Principles: Describe one related to the concept.

C. Nursing Interventions: Identify five related to the concept.

APPLICATION EXERCISES KEY

1. A. INCORRECT: Administering antibiotic medication will treat the wound infection, but this is not the first action the nurse should take.

    B. **CORRECT:** When using the urgent vs. nonurgent approach to care, the nurse's priority action is to obtain a culture of the wound before initiating antibiotic therapy. Obtaining a culture after therapy is started will cause inaccurate results.

    C. INCORRECT: Instructing the client on the purpose of antibiotics is an important part of reinforcing teaching about the need for treatment, but this is not the first action the nurse should take.

    D. INCORRECT: Applying a dressing to the wound will promote absorption of drainage and prevent the spread of infection, but this is not the first action the nurse should take.

    Ⓝ NCLEX® Connection: Pharmacological Therapies, Medication Administration

2. A. INCORRECT: A gram stain determines whether a gram-negative or gram-positive organism is causing the infection.

    B. INCORRECT: A culture determines the type of micro-organism that might be causing the infection.

    C. **CORRECT:** A sensitivity test identifies the most effective antibiotic to be used to treat a specific micro-organism.

    D. INCORRECT: A specific gravity test determines the dilution of the urine and does not provide information on the type of micro-organism or antibiotic to be used to treat the infection.

    Ⓝ NCLEX® Connection: Pharmacological Therapies, Medication Administration

3. A. **CORRECT:** The client who has meningitis can have difficulty responding to antimicrobial therapy because of the blood-brain barrier.

    B. **CORRECT:** The client who has a pacemaker can have difficulty responding to antimicrobial therapy due to colonization of micro-organisms around the pacemaker and the inability of phagocytic cells to destroy the micro-organisms.

    C. **CORRECT:** The client who has endocarditis can have difficulty responding to antimicrobial therapy because the antibiotic might be unable to penetrate the vegetative thrombus that develops on the injured endocardium.

    D. INCORRECT: A client who has pneumonia should respond effectively to antimicrobial therapy because of the vascularity of the pulmonary tissue.

    E. INCORRECT: A client who has pyelonephritis should respond to antimicrobial therapy effectively because of the vascularity of the kidney tissue and filtration system.

    Ⓝ NCLEX® Connection: Pharmacological Therapies, Adverse Effects/Contraindications/ Side Effects/Interactions

4. A. INCORRECT: An adolescent client who has a sinus infection should be able to metabolize and excrete the medication. Therefore, the client has a low risk of developing antibiotic toxicity.

    B. **CORRECT:** An older adult client has impaired drug metabolism and excretion due to age-related changes. Therefore, the nurse should identify this client as the one at greatest risk for medication toxicity.

    C. INCORRECT: A new mother who has mastitis should be able to metabolize and excrete the medication. Therefore, she has a low risk of developing antibiotic toxicity.

    D. INCORRECT: A middle adult client who has a urinary tract infection should be able to metabolize and excrete the medication. Therefore, the client has a low risk of developing antibiotic toxicity.

    Ⓝ NCLEX® Connection: Pharmacological Therapies, Adverse Effects/Contraindications/ Side Effects/Interactions

5. A. **CORRECT:** A client who suspects exposure to a sexually transmitted infection should be treated with prophylactic antimicrobial therapy to prevent an infection.

    B. **CORRECT:** A client who is having orthopedic surgery should be treated with prophylactic antimicrobial therapy to prevent an infection.

    C. **CORRECT:** A client who is having dental work and has a prosthetic heart valve should receive prophylactic antimicrobial therapy to prevent an infection.

    D. **CORRECT:** A client who has recurrent urinary tract infections should be treated with prophylactic antimicrobial therapy to prevent an infection.

    E. INCORRECT: Upper respiratory infections can be viral in origin. Resistance to antimicrobial therapy can occur when antibiotics are taken needlessly. Prophylactic antibiotics are prescribed before the infection occurs.

    Ⓝ NCLEX® Connection: Pharmacological Therapies, Expected Actions/Outcomes

6. *Using ATI Active Learning Template: Basic Concept*

    A. Related Content
    *   Preventive nursing measures

    B. Underlying Principles
    *   Controlling the spread of infection to health care professionals and clients in a health care setting

    C. Nursing Interventions
    *   Perform hand hygiene before and after each client contact.
    *   Be aware of invasive procedures that increase the chance of developing an infection.
    *   Encourage the client to maintain up-to-date immunization status.
    *   Instruct the client to take all antibiotics prescribed by the provider.
    *   Implement infection control measures: aseptic technique, isolation, proper assignment of rooms.
    *   Evaluate effectiveness of antimicrobial therapy.

    Ⓝ NCLEX® Connection: Pharmacological Therapies, Expected Actions/Outcomes

chapter **38**

Overview

- Antibiotics that affect the cell wall are bactericidal. This group of antibiotics includes penicillins, cephalosporins, carbapenems, and monobactams.

MEDICATION CLASSIFICATION: PENICILLINS

- Select Prototype Medication: penicillin G potassium (Pfizerpen) – a narrow-spectrum medication for IM or IV use
- Other Medications
  - Narrow-spectrum
    - Penicillin G benzathine (Bicillin L-A) for IM use
    - Penicillin V (Penicillin VK) for oral use
  - Broad-spectrum
    - Amoxicillin-clavulanate (Augmentin) for oral use
    - Ampicillin for oral or IV use
  - Antistaphylococcal
    - Nafcillin (Nallpen) for IM or IV use
  - Antipseudomonas
    - Ticarcillin-clavulanate (Timentin) for IV use
    - Piperacillin tazobactam (Zosyn) for IV use

Purpose

- Expected Pharmacological Action – Penicillins destroy bacteria by weakening the bacterial cell wall.
- Therapeutic Uses
  - Penicillins are the medication of choice for gram-positive cocci such as *Streptococcus pneumoniae* (pneumonia and meningitis), *Streptococcus viridans* (infectious endocarditis), and *Streptococcus pyogenes* (pharyngitis).
  - Penicillins are the medication of first choice for meningitis caused by gram–negative cocci *Neisseria meningitides*.
  - Penicillins are the medication of choice for the treatment of syphilis caused by *Spirochete treponema pallidum*.
  - Extended-spectrum penicillin (piperacillin, ticarcillin) is effective against organisms such as *Pseudomonas aeruginosa, Enterobacter species, Proteus, Bacteroides fragilis*, and *Klebsiella*.
  - Penicillins are used as prophylaxis against bacterial endocarditis in at-risk clients prior to dental and other procedures.

Complications

ADVERSE EFFECTS	NURSING INTERVENTIONS/CLIENT EDUCATION
› Allergies/anaphylaxis	› Interview clients for prior allergy. › Advise clients to wear an allergy identification bracelet. › Observe clients for 30 min following administration of parenteral penicillin.
› Renal impairment	› Monitor kidney function. › Monitor I&O.
› Hyperkalemia/dysrhythmias (high doses of penicillin G potassium) › Hypernatremia (IV ticarcillin)	› Monitor cardiac status and electrolyte levels.

Contraindications/Precautions

- Penicillins are contraindicated for clients who have a severe history of allergies to penicillin, cephalosporin, or imipenem.
- Clients who are allergic to one penicillin should be considered cross-allergic to other penicillins and at risk for a cross allergy to cephalosporin.

- Use cautiously in clients who have or are at risk for kidney dysfunction (clients who are acutely ill, older adults, or young children).

Interactions

MEDICATION/FOOD INTERACTIONS	NURSING INTERVENTIONS/CLIENT EDUCATION
› Penicillin inactivates aminoglycosides when mixed in the same IV solution.	› Do not mix penicillin and aminoglycosides in the same IV solution.
› Probenecid (Probalan) delays excretion of penicillin.	› Probenecid may be added to penicillin therapy to prolong action.

Nursing Administration

- Instruct clients that penicillin V, amoxicillin, and amoxicillin-clavulanate may be taken with meals. All others should be taken with a full glass of water 1 hr before meals or 2 hr after.
- Instruct clients to report any indications of an allergic response such as skin rash, itching, or hives.
- IM injection should be performed cautiously to avoid injection into a nerve or an artery.
- Advise clients to complete the entire course of therapy regardless of presence of symptoms.

MEDICATION CLASSIFICATION: CEPHALOSPORINS

- Select Prototype Medication: cephalexin (Keflex) – 1st generation
- Other Medications
  - 1st generation – cefazolin (Kefzol)
  - 2nd generation – cefaclor, cefotetan
  - 3rd generation – ceftriaxone (Rocephin), cefotaxime (Claforan)
  - 4th generation – cefepime (Maxipime)

Purpose

- Expected Pharmacological Action
  - Cephalosporins are beta-lactam antibiotics, similar to penicillins that destroy bacterial cell walls causing destruction of micro-organisms.
  - Cephalosporins are grouped into four generations. Each subsequent generation of cephalosporins is:
    - More likely to reach cerebrospinal fluid.
    - Less likely to be destroyed by beta-lactamase.
    - More effective against gram-negative organisms and anaerobes.
- Therapeutic Uses
  - Cephalosporins are broad-spectrum bactericidal medications with a high therapeutic index that treat urinary tract infections, postoperative infections, pelvic infections, and meningitis.

Complications

ADVERSE EFFECTS	NURSING INTERVENTIONS/CLIENT EDUCATION
› Allergic/hypersensitivity/anaphylaxis › Possible cross-sensitivity to penicillin	› If indications of allergy appear (urticaria, rash, hypotension, and/or dyspnea) stop cephalosporin immediately, and notify the provider. › Question client carefully regarding past history of allergy to a penicillin or other cephalosporin, and notify the provider if present.
› Bleeding tendencies with use of cefotetan and ceftriaxone	› Avoid use in clients who have bleeding disorders and those taking anticoagulants. › Observe for signs of bleeding. › Monitor prothrombin time and bleeding time. Abnormal levels can require discontinuation of medication. › Administer parenteral vitamin K.
› Thrombophlebitis with IV infusion	› Rotate injection sites. › Administer as a diluted intermittent infusion or, if a bolus dose is prescribed, administer slowly over 3 to 5 min and in a dilute solution.
› Pain with IM injection	› Administer IM injection deep in large muscle mass.
› Antibiotic-associated pseudomembranous colitis	› Observe for diarrhea and notify the provider. › Medication should be discontinued.

Contraindications/Precautions

- Cephalosporins should not be given to clients who have a history of severe allergic reactions to penicillins.

- Use cautiously in clients who have renal impairment or bleeding tendencies.

Interactions

MEDICATION/FOOD INTERACTIONS	NURSING INTERVENTIONS/CLIENT EDUCATION
› Disulfiram reaction (intolerance to alcohol) occurs with combined use of cefotetan, cefazolin, cefoperazone, and alcohol.	› Instruct clients not to consume alcohol while taking these cephalosporins.
› Probenecid delays renal excretion.	› Monitor I&O.

Nursing Administration

- Instruct clients to complete the prescribed course of therapy, even though symptoms can resolve before the full course of antimicrobial treatment is completed.

- Advise clients to take oral cephalosporins with food.

- Instruct clients to store oral cephalosporin suspensions in a refrigerator.

MEDICATION CLASSIFICATION: CARBAPENEMS

- Select Prototype Medication: imipenem-cilastatin (Primaxin)
- Other Medication: meropenem (Merrem IV)

Purpose

- Expected Pharmacological Action – Carbapenems are beta-lactam antibiotics that destroy bacterial cell walls, causing destruction of micro-organisms.

- Therapeutic Uses

  ○ Broad antimicrobial spectrum is effective for serious infections such as pneumonia, peritonitis, and urinary tract infections caused by gram-positive cocci, gram-negative cocci, and anaerobic bacteria.

  ○ Resistance develops when imipenem is used alone to treat *Pseudomonas aeruginosa*. A combination of antipseudomonal medications should be used to treat this micro-organism.

Complications

ADVERSE EFFECTS	NURSING INTERVENTIONS/CLIENT EDUCATION
› Allergy/hypersensitivity › Possible cross-sensitivity to penicillin or cephalosporins	› Monitor for indications of allergic reactions, such as rashes or pruritus. › Question clients carefully regarding past history of allergy to a penicillin or other cephalosporin and notify provider if present.
› Gastrointestinal symptoms (nausea, vomiting, diarrhea)	› Observe for manifestations and notify the provider if they occur. › Monitor I&O.
› Suprainfection	› Monitor for indications of colitis (diarrhea, oral thrush, or vaginal yeast infection).

Interactions

MEDICATION/FOOD INTERACTIONS	NURSING INTERVENTIONS/CLIENT EDUCATION
› Imipenem-cilastatin can reduce blood levels of valproic acid (Depakote). Breakthrough seizures are possible.	› Avoid using together. If concurrent use is unavoidable, monitor for increased seizure activity.

Contraindications/Precautions

- Imipenem-cilastatin is a Pregnancy Risk Category C medication.
- Use cautiously in clients who have renal impairment.

Nursing Administration

- Instruct clients to complete the prescribed course of antimicrobial therapy, even though manifestations can resolve before the full course is completed.

MEDICATION CLASSIFICATION: OTHER INHIBITORS

- Select Prototype Medications
  - Vancomycin (Vancocin)
  - Aztreonam (Azactam): classified as a monobactam
  - Fosfomycin (Monurol)

Purpose

- Expected Pharmacological Action – This group of antibiotics destroys bacterial cell walls, causing destruction of micro-organisms.
- Therapeutic Uses
  - They are the antimicrobials of choice for:
    - Serious infections caused by methicillin-resistant *Staphylococcus aureus*, *E. coli*, or *Staphylococcus epidermidis*.
    - Antibiotic-associated pseudomembranous colitis caused by *Clostridium difficile*.

Complications

ADVERSE EFFECTS	NURSING INTERVENTIONS/CLIENT EDUCATION
› Ototoxicity	› Monitor for indications of hearing loss. › Instruct clients to notify the provider if changes in hearing acuity develop. › Monitor vancomycin levels.
› Infusion reactions (rashes, flushing, tachycardia, and hypotension, sometimes called "red man syndrome")	› Administer vancomycin slowly over 60 min.
› IV injection site thrombophlebitis	› Rotate injection sites. › Monitor the infusion site for redness, swelling, and inflammation.
› Renal toxicity	› Monitor I&O and kidney function tests. › Monitor vancomycin trough levels.

Interactions

MEDICATION/FOOD INTERACTIONS	NURSING INTERVENTIONS/CLIENT EDUCATION
› Increased risk for ototoxicity when vancomycin is used concurrently with another medication that also produces ototoxicity (loop diuretics and aminoglycoside antibiotics).	› Monitor for hearing loss.

Contraindications/Precautions

- Contraindicated for clients who have allergy to corn/corn products or previous allergy to vancomycin.
- Use cautiously in clients who have renal impairment, hearing impairment, or older adults.

Nursing Administration

- Monitor vancomycin trough levels routinely after blood levels have reached a steady state. Peak levels may also be prescribed.
- IV dose may be adjusted based on creatinine clearance levels if renal insufficiency is present.

Nursing Evaluation of Medication Effectiveness

- Depending on therapeutic intent, effectiveness can be evidenced by:
  - Reduction of clinical manifestations such as fever, pain, inflammation, and adventitious breath sounds.
  - Resolution of infection.

APPLICATION EXERCISES

1. A nurse is caring for a client admitted with a cerebral spinal fluid (CSF) infection caused by a highly resistant gram-negative bacteria. Which of the following cephalosporin IV antibiotics should the nurse expect to be effective in treating this infection?

    A. Cefaclor

    B. Cefazolin (Kefzol)

    C. Cefepime (Maxipime)

    D. Cephalexin (Keflex)

2. A nurse in an outpatient facility is preparing to administer nafcillin (Nallpen) IM to an adult client who has an infection. Which of the following actions should the nurse plan to take? (Select all that apply.)

_____ A. Select a 25-gauge, ½-inch needle for the injection.

_____ B. Administer the medication deeply into the ventrogluteal muscle.

_____ C. Ask the client about allergy to penicillin before administering the medication.

_____ D. Monitor the client for 30 min following the injection.

_____ E. Tell the client to expect a temporary rash to occur following the injection.

3. A nurse is preparing to administer cefotaxime (Claforan) IV to a client who has a severe infection and has been receiving cefotaxime for the past week. Which of the following findings indicates a potentially serious adverse reaction to this medication and should be reported to the provider?

    A. Diaphoresis

    B. Epistaxis

    C. Diarrhea

    D. Alopecia

4. A nurse is taking a medication history for a hospitalized client who is to receive imipenem-cilastatin (Primaxin) IV. Which of the following medications taken by the client places the client at risk for medication interaction?

    A. Regular insulin (Humulin R)

    B. Furosemide (Lasix)

    C. Valproic acid (Depakote)

    D. Ferrous sulfate (Feosol)

5. A nurse is preparing to administer ceftriaxone (Rocephin) 0.5 g IM to a client in a long-term care facility. Available is ceftriaxone diluted to 350 mg/mL. How many mL should the nurse administer? (Round the answer to the nearest tenth.)

6. A nurse is assisting with care of a client who has a new prescription for vancomycin (Vancocin) IV to treat a serious wound infection. What information about this medication should the nurse reinforce with the client? Use the ATI Active Learning Template: Medication to complete this item to include the following:

A. Therapeutic Use: Identify for vancomycin in this client.

B. Adverse Effects: Identify two the client should watch for.

C. Diagnostic Tests: Describe two diagnostic tests to monitor for this client.

D. Nursing Actions: Describe two nursing actions for client taking vancomycin.

APPLICATION EXERCISES KEY

1. A. INCORRECT: Cefaclor, a second-generation cephalosporin, is unlikely to be effective against a highly resistant gram-negative bacterial infection in the CSF.

    B. INCORRECT: Cefazolin, a first-generation cephalosporin, is unlikely to be effective against a highly resistant gram-negative bacterial infection in the CSF.

    C. **CORRECT:** Cefepime, a fourth-generation cephalosporin, is more likely to be effective against this infection than earlier generationr medications. Later generation cephalosporin medications are more effective against gram-negative bacteria, more resistant to being destroyed by beta-lactamase, and more able to penetrate the CSF than early generation forms.

    D. INCORRECT: Cephalexin, a first-generation cephalosporin, is unlikely to be effective against a highly resistant gram-negative bacterial infection in the CSF.

    Ⓝ NCLEX® Connection: Pharmacological Therapies, Expected Actions/Outcomes

2. A. INCORRECT: A 25-gauge, ½-inch needle is too small and short for an IM injection of nafcillin to an adult client. Although the needle size/length should be chosen for each specific client, an example of a correctly sized IM needle for an adult would be 19- to 22-gauge and 1½ inches.

    B. **CORRECT:** It is important to administer nafcillin IM into a deep muscle mass, such as the ventrogluteal site.

    C. **CORRECT:** It is important to ask the client about allergy to penicillin or other antibiotics before administering nafcillin. In general, a documented allergy to another penicillin or to a cephalosporin is a contraindication for administering a penicillin medication.

    D. **CORRECT:** When administering a parenteral penicillin or other antibiotic, it is important to monitor the client for 30 min for an allergic reaction.

    E. INCORRECT: A rash is not an expected reaction after nafcillin administration. A rash can be a manifestation of allergy to the medication.

    Ⓝ NCLEX® Connection: Pharmacological Therapies, Medication Administration

3. A. INCORRECT: Diaphoresis is not an adverse effect of cefotaxime.

    B. INCORRECT: Epistaxis is not an adverse effect of cefotaxime.

    C. **CORRECT:** Diarrhea caused by cefotaxime and other cephalosporins should be reported to the provider. Severe diarrhea can indicate the client has developed antibiotic-associated pseudomembranous colitis, which could be life-threatening.

    D. INCORRECT: Alopecia is not an adverse effect of cefotaxime.

    Ⓝ NCLEX® Connection: Pharmacological Therapies, Adverse Effects/Contraindications/
    Side Effects/Interactions

4.   A. INCORRECT: Regular insulin, an antidiabetic medication, does not interact with imipenem-cilastatin.

      B. INCORRECT: Furosemide, a loop diuretic, does not interact with imipenem-cilastatin.

      C. **CORRECT:** Imipenem-cilastatin decreases blood levels of valproic acid, an antiseizure medication, putting the client at risk for increased seizure activity. Combination of these two medications should be avoided. If they must be taken concurrently, the nurse should monitor the client for seizures.

      D. INCORRECT: Ferrous sulfate does not interact with imipenem-cilastatin.

      (N) NCLEX® Connection: Pharmacological Therapies, Adverse Effects/Contraindications/ Side Effects/Interactions

5.   **1.4** mL

Using Ratio and Proportion		
STEP 1: *What is the unit of measurement to calculate?* mL	STEP 5: *What is the quantity of the dose available?* 1 mL	STEP 8: *Reassess to determine whether the amount to give makes sense.*
STEP 2: *What is the dose needed?* *Dose needed = Desired* 0.5 g	STEP 6: *Set up an equation and solve for X.*	If there is 350 mg/mL and the prescribed amount is 0.5 g (500 mg), it makes sense to give 1.4 mL. The nurse should administer ceftriaxone injection 1.4 mL IM.
STEP 3: *What is the dose available? Dose available = Have* 350 mg	$\dfrac{\text{Have}}{\text{Quantity}} = \dfrac{\text{Desired}}{\text{X}}$ $\dfrac{350 \text{ mg}}{1 \text{ mL}} = \dfrac{500 \text{ mg}}{\text{X mL}}$	
STEP 4: *Should the nurse convert the units of measurement?* Yes (g ≠ mg) 1 g = 1,000 mg 0.5 g = 500 mg	X = 1.4285 STEP 7: *Round if necessary.* 1.4285 = 1.4	

Using Desired Over Have		
STEP 1: *What is the unit of measurement to calculate?* mL	STEP 5: *What is the quantity of the dose available?* 1 mL	STEP 8: *Reassess to determine whether the amount to give makes sense.*
STEP 2: *What is the dose needed?* *Dose needed = Desired* 0.5 g	STEP 6: *Set up an equation and solve for X.*	If there is 350 mg/mL and the prescribed amount is 0.5 g (500 mg), it makes sense to give 1.4 mL. The nurse should administer ceftriaxone injection 1.4 mL IM.
STEP 3: *What is the dose available? Dose available = Have* 350 mg	$\dfrac{\text{Desired x Quantity}}{\text{Have}} = \text{X}$ $\dfrac{500 \text{ mg x 1 mL}}{350 \text{ mg}} = \text{X mL}$	
STEP 4: *Should the nurse convert the units of measurement?* Yes (g ≠ mg) 1 g = 1,000 mg 0.5 g = 500 mg	1.4285 = X STEP 7: *Round if necessary.* 1.4285 = 1.4	

Using Dimensional Analysis

STEP 1: *What is the unit of measurement to calculate?*
mL

STEP 2: *What quantity of the dose available?*
1 mL

STEP 3: *What is the dose available? Dose available = Have*
350 mg

STEP 4: *What is the dose needed? Dose needed = Desired*
0.5 g

STEP 5: *Should the nurse convert the units of measurement?*
Yes

$$\frac{1,000 \text{ mg}}{1 \text{ g}}$$

STEP 6: *Set up an equation of factors and solve for X.*

$$X = \frac{\text{Quantity}}{\text{Have}} \times \frac{\text{Conversion (Have)}}{\text{Conversion (Desired)}} \times \frac{\text{Desired}}{}$$

$$X \text{ mL} = \frac{1 \text{ mL}}{350 \text{ mg}} \times \frac{1,000 \text{ mg}}{1 \text{ g}} \times \frac{0.5 \text{ g}}{}$$

$$X = 1.4285$$

STEP 7: *Round if necessary.*
1.4285 = 1.4

STEP 8: *Reassess to determine whether the amount to give makes sense.*
If there is 350 mg/mL and the prescribed amount is 0.5 g (500 mg), it makes sense to give 1.4 mL. The nurse should administer ceftriaxone injection 1.4 mL IM.

(N) NCLEX® Connection: Pharmacological Therapies, Dosage Calculation

6. *Using the ATI Active Learning Template: Medication*

A. Therapeutic Use

- Vancomycin is an antibiotic that kills bacteria by disrupting their cell wall. The IV form treats serious infections caused by gram-positive bacteria, such as methicillin-resistant *Staphylococcus aureus*, *E. Coli*, or *Staphylococcus epidermidis*.

B. Adverse Effects

- Infusion reaction, sometimes called "red man syndrome," which causes a flushed face/neck, tachycardia, and hypotension
- Ototoxicity, manifested by hearing loss
- Renal toxicity manifested by acute renal failure
- Thrombophlebitis at the IV site

C. Diagnostic Tests

- Renal function tests and trough vancomycin levels in order to determine if toxicity is occurring
- Peak vancomycin levels
- WBC to determine if the infection is being successfully treated

D. Nursing Actions

- Infuse vancomycin over at least 60 min/dose to prevent an infusion reaction.
- Monitor the IV site for redness, pain, or other manifestations of thrombophlebitis.
- Monitor I&O, and notify the provider for oliguria or other indications of acute renal injury.
- Monitor the client for hearing loss.
- Ask the client about allergy to antibiotics before administering the medication. Watch for allergic manifestations during and after the infusion.

(N) NCLEX® Connection: Pharmacological Therapies, Expected Actions/Outcomes

chapter 39

Overview

- Antibiotics affecting protein synthesis can be bacteriostatic, such as tetracyclines and macrolides, or bactericidal, such as aminoglycosides.

- Uses include infections of the respiratory, gastrointestinal (GI), urinary, and reproductive tract and infections caused by rickettsia.

MEDICATION CLASSIFICATION: TETRACYCLINES

- Select Prototype Medication: tetracycline
- Other Medications: doxycycline (Vibramycin), minocycline (Minocin), demeclocycline

Purpose

- Expected Pharmacological Action
  - Tetracyclines are broad-spectrum antibiotics that inhibit micro-organism growth by preventing protein synthesis (bacteriostatic).
- Therapeutic Uses
  - Administered topically and orally to treat acne vulgaris and topically for periodontal disease
  - Used as first-line medication for
    - Rickettsial infections, such as typhus fever or Rocky Mountain spotted fever
    - Infections of the urethra or cervix caused by *Chlamydia trachomatis*
    - Brucellosis
    - Pneumonia caused by *Mycoplasma pneumonia*
    - Lyme disease
    - Anthrax
    - GI infections caused by *Helicobacter pylori*

Complications

ADVERSE EFFECTS	NURSING INTERVENTIONS/CLIENT EDUCATION
› GI discomfort (cramping, nausea, vomiting, diarrhea, and esophageal ulceration)	› Monitor for nausea, vomiting, and diarrhea. › Monitor the client's I&O. › Doxycycline and minocycline may be taken with meals. › Avoid taking at bedtime to reduce esophageal ulceration.
› Yellow/brown tooth discoloration and/or hypoplasia of tooth enamel	› Avoid administration to children younger than 8 years of age and to pregnant women.
› Hepatotoxicity (lethargy, jaundice)	› Avoid administration of high daily doses IV.
› Photosensitivity (exaggerated sunburn)	› Advise clients to take precautions when in the sun, such as wearing protective clothing and using sunscreen.
› Suprainfection of the bowel – antibiotic-associated pseudomembranous colitis (diarrhea, yeast infections of the mouth, pharynx, vagina, and bowels)	› Instruct clients to notify the provider if diarrhea occurs.
› Dizziness, lightheadedness, with minocycline	› Instruct clients to report these findings if they occur and to take care with ambulation.

Contraindications/Precautions

- Tetracyclines are Pregnancy Risk Category D medications.
- Use of tetracycline during pregnancy after the fourth month can cause staining of the deciduous teeth, but will not have a permanent effect on permanent teeth. In general, tetracyclines should not be given to women who are pregnant or to young children.
- Use cautiously in clients who have liver and kidney disease. Doxycycline and minocycline may be used in clients who have kidney disease.

Interactions

MEDICATION/FOOD INTERACTIONS	NURSING INTERVENTIONS/CLIENT EDUCATION
› Interaction with milk products, calcium or iron supplements, laxatives containing magnesium such as magnesium hydroxide (Milk of Magnesia), and antacids causes formation of nonabsorbable chelates, thus reducing the absorption of tetracycline.	› Tetracycline should be taken on an empty stomach with a full glass of water. › Minocycline may be taken with meals. › Administer tetracyclines at least 1 hr before and 2 hr after taking food and supplements containing calcium and magnesium.
› Tetracycline decreases the efficacy of oral contraceptives.	› Advise client to use an alternative form of birth control.
› Both minocycline and doxycycline increase the risk of digoxin toxicity.	› Monitor digoxin level carefully if taking concurrently.

Nursing Administration

- Instruct clients to take tetracyclines on an empty stomach with a full glass of water. Minocycline may be taken with food.

- Taking any of the tetracyclines just before lying down increases the chance of esophageal ulceration and should be avoided.

- Instruct clients to maintain a 2-hr interval between ingestion of chelating agents and medications.

- Instruct clients to complete the prescribed course of antimicrobial therapy, even though manifestations can resolve before the full course is completed.

Nursing Evaluation of Medication Effectiveness

- Depending on therapeutic intent, effectiveness can be evidenced by the following.
  - A decrease in the clinical manifestations of infection, such as clear breath sounds
  - Resolution of yeast infections of the mouth, vagina, and bowels
  - Resolution of acne vulgaris facial lesions

MEDICATION CLASSIFICATION: MACROLIDES

- Select Prototype Medication: erythromycin
- Other medication: azithromycin (Zithromax)

Purpose

- Expected Pharmacological Action
  - Erythromycin slows the growth of micro-organisms by inhibiting protein synthesis (bacteriostatic) but can be bactericidal if given for susceptible bacteria at high enough doses.

- Therapeutic Uses
  - Used to treat infections in clients who have a penicillin allergy, such as for prophylaxis against rheumatic fever and bacterial endocarditis
  - Used for clients who have Legionnaires' disease, whooping cough (pertussis), and acute diphtheria (eliminates the carrier state of diphtheria)
  - Used for chlamydia infections (urethritis and cervicitis; pneumonia caused by *Mycoplasma pneumoniae*; respiratory tract infections caused by *Streptococcus pneumoniae* and group A *Streptococcus pyogenes*)

Complications

ADVERSE EFFECTS	NURSING INTERVENTIONS/CLIENT EDUCATION
› GI discomfort (nausea, vomiting, epigastric pain)	› Administer erythromycin with meals. › Observe for GI manifestations and notify the provider.
› Prolonged QT interval causing dysrhythmias and possible sudden cardiac death	› Use in clients who have prolonged QT intervals is not recommended. › Avoid concurrent use with medications that affect hepatic drug metabolizing enzymes.
› Ototoxicity with high-dose therapy	› Monitor for hearing loss, vertigo, and ringing in ear. Notify provider if these occur.

Contraindications/Precautions

- Contraindicated in clients who have pre-existing liver disease, or in clients who have existing QT prolongation.

Interactions

MEDICATION/FOOD INTERACTIONS	NURSING INTERVENTIONS/CLIENT EDUCATION
› Erythromycin inhibits metabolism of antihistamines, theophylline, carbamazepine, warfarin, and digoxin, which can lead to toxicity of these medications.	› To minimize toxicity, avoid using erythromycin with these medications if possible. If they must be used concurrently, monitor carefully for toxicity.
› Verapamil, diltiazem, HIV protease inhibitors, antifungal medications, and nefazodone inhibit hepatic drug-metabolizing enzymes, which can lead to erythromycin toxicity, causing a tachydysrhythmia and possible cardiac arrest.	› Concurrent use is not recommended.

Nursing Administration

- Administer oral preparation on an empty stomach (1 hr before meals or 2 hr after) with a full glass of water, unless GI upset occurs.
- Azithromycin may be administered with food.
- The IV form of erythromycin is used only for severe infections or when a client cannot take oral doses.
- Instruct clients to complete the prescribed course of antimicrobial therapy, even though manifestations can resolve before the full course is completed.
- Carefully monitor the PT/INR of clients who take warfarin concurrently with erythromycin.
- Monitor liver function tests for therapy lasting more than 1 to 2 weeks.

Nursing Evaluation of Medication Effectiveness

- Depending on therapeutic intent, effectiveness can be evidenced by a decrease in the clinical manifestations of infection (clear lung sounds; improvement of sore throat, cough, and urinary tract symptoms; and resolution of bacterial endocarditis with negative blood cultures).

MEDICATION CLASSIFICATION: AMINOGLYCOSIDES

- Select Prototype Medication: gentamicin
- Other Medications
  - Amikacin
  - Tobramycin
  - Neomycin
  - Streptomycin
  - Paromomycin (oral)

Purpose

- Expected Pharmacological Action
  - Aminoglycosides are bactericidal antibiotics that destroy micro-organisms by disrupting protein synthesis.
- Therapeutic Uses
  - Aminoglycosides are the medication of choice against *aerobic gram-negative bacilli,* such as *Escherichia coli, Klebsiella pneumoniae, Proteus mirabilis,* and *Pseudomonas aeruginosa.*
  - Paromomycin (oral aminoglycoside) is used for intestinal amebiasis and tapeworm infections.
  - Oral neomycin is often used prior to surgery of the GI tract to suppress normal flora, and topically to treat infections of the eye, ear, and skin.
  - Streptomycin is used, along with other medications, to treat active tuberculosis and to treat a variety of other serious infections caused by gram-positive, gram-negative, or acid-fast bacteria.

Complications

ADVERSE EFFECTS	NURSING INTERVENTIONS/CLIENT EDUCATION
› Ototoxicity – cochlear damage (hearing loss) and vestibular damage (loss of balance)	› Monitor for tinnitus (ringing in the ears), headache, hearing loss, nausea, dizziness, and vertigo. › Instruct clients to notify the provider if tinnitus, hearing loss, or headaches occur. › Stop aminoglycoside if manifestations occur. Do baseline audiometric studies (hearing test).
› Nephrotoxicity related to high total cumulative dose resulting in acute tubular necrosis (proteinuria, casts in the urine, dilute urine, elevated BUN, creatinine levels)	› Monitor I&O, BUN, and creatinine levels. › Report hematuria or cloudy urine.
› Intensified neuromuscular blockade resulting in respiratory depression or muscle weakness	› Closely monitor use in clients who have myasthenia gravis, clients taking skeletal muscle relaxants, and clients receiving general anesthetics.
› Hypersensitivity (rash, pruritus, paresthesia of hands and feet, and urticaria)	› Monitor for allergic effects.
Streptomycin	
› Neurologic disorder (peripheral neuritis, optic nerve dysfunction, tingling/numbness of the hands and feet)	› Instruct clients to promptly report any manifestations to the provider.

Contraindications/Precautions

- Use cautiously in clients who have kidney impairment, pre-existing hearing loss, or myasthenia gravis.
- Use cautiously in clients taking ethacrynic acid (increases risk for ototoxicity), amphotericin B, cephalosporins, vancomycin (increases risk for nephrotoxicity), and neuromuscular blocking agents such as tubocurarine.
- Clients who have kidney impairment should receive reduced doses of aminoglycosides.

Interactions

MEDICATION/FOOD INTERACTIONS	NURSING INTERVENTIONS/CLIENT EDUCATION
› Penicillins inactivate aminoglycosides when mixed in the same IV solution.	› Do not mix aminoglycosides and penicillins in the same IV solution.
› When administered concurrently with other ototoxic medications (such as loop diuretics), the risk for ototoxicity greatly increases.	› Monitor frequently for hearing loss with concurrent medication use.

Nursing Administration

- Most aminoglycosides (such as gentamicin and amikacin) are administered only by IM or IV routes. Some others (such as neomycin) can be administered either orally or topically.
- Measure aminoglycoside levels based on dosing schedules.
  - Once-a-day dosing: only trough level needs to be measured.
  - Divided doses
    - Peak – 30 min after administration of aminoglycoside intramuscularly or 30 min after an IV infusion has finished
    - Trough – right before the next dose

Nursing Evaluation of Medication Effectiveness

- Depending on therapeutic intent, effectiveness can be evidenced by a decrease in clinical manifestations of infection (clear lung sounds, improvement of urinary tract effects, wound healing).

APPLICATION EXERCISES

1. A nurse is reinforcing teaching with a client prescribed tetracycline to treat a GI infection caused by *Helicobacter pylori*. Which of the following client statements indicates understanding of the teaching?

    A. "I will take this medication with a full glass of milk."

    B. "I will let my doctor know if I start having diarrhea."

    C. "I can stop taking this medication when I feel completely well."

    D. "I can take this medication just before bedtime."

2. A nurse is administering gentamicin by IV infusion at 0900. The gentamicin will take 1 hr to infuse. When should the nurse plan for a peak serum level of gentamicin to be drawn?

    A. 1000

    B. 1030

    C. 1100

    D. 1130

3. A nurse is caring for a client who is starting a course of gentamicin IV for a serious respiratory infection. For which of the following adverse effects should the nurse monitor? (Select all that apply.)

    _____ A. Drowsiness

    _____ B. Hematuria

    _____ C. Muscle weakness

    _____ D. Difficulty swallowing

    _____ E. Vertigo

4. A nurse is caring for a client who has subacute bacterial endocarditis and is being treated with several antibiotics, including IM streptomycin. The nurse should monitor this client for which of the following adverse effects of streptomycin?

    A. Extremity paresthesias

    B. Urinary retention

    C. Severe constipation

    D. Complex partial seizures

5. A nurse is caring for a client who is being prepared for extensive colorectal surgery. Which of the following oral antibiotics should the nurse expect to be prescribed for this client in order to suppress normal flora in the GI tract?

    A. Amikacin

    B. Gentamicin

    C. Neomycin

    D. Erythromycin

6. A nurse in an outpatient facility is reinforcing teaching about oral erythromycin with a client who has pneumonia. What should the nurse reinforce with the client about this medication? Use the ATI Active Learning Template: Medication to complete this item to include the following:

    A. Therapeutic Use: Describe the therapeutic use for erythromycin in this client.

    B. Adverse Effects: Identify two adverse effects the client should watch for.

    C. Diagnostic Tests: Describe two diagnostic tests to monitor for clients taking erythromycin.

    D. Nursing Interventions: Describe two nursing actions for clients taking erythromycin.

APPLICATION EXERCISES KEY

1. A. INCORRECT: Tetracycline can form a nonabsorbable chelate when taken with dairy products. It should be taken with water on an empty stomach.

    B. **CORRECT:** Diarrhea can indicate that the client is developing a suprainfection, which can be very serious. The client should notify the provider if diarrhea occurs.

    C. INCORRECT: The client should be advised to take the full prescription of tetracycline and not to stop the medication if he begins to feel well.

    D. INCORRECT: Taking tetracycline in the morning will help prevent esophageal ulceration, which can occur if taken just before lying down at night.

    N NCLEX® Connection: Pharmacological Therapies, Adverse Effects/Contraindications/ Side Effects/Interactions

2. A. INCORRECT: The infusion should be completed at 1000, but that is not the time for the peak serum level to be drawn.

    B. **CORRECT:** The peak serum level should be drawn at 1030, 30 min after the 1-hr IV infusion is complete. The trough level should be drawn just before the infusion is started.

    C. INCORRECT: It would not be correct to draw the peak serum level 1 hr following the end of the IV infusion.

    D. INCORRECT: It would not be correct to draw the peak serum level 1.5 hr following the end of the IV infusion.

    N NCLEX® Connection: Pharmacological Therapies, Medication Administration

3. A. INCORRECT: Drowsiness is not an adverse effect of gentamicin.

    B. **CORRECT:** Hematuria is an indication of acute kidney toxicity caused by gentamicin.

    C. **CORRECT:** Muscle weakness and respiratory depression can occur in clients taking gentamicin as a result of neuromuscular blockade.

    D. INCORRECT: Difficulty swallowing does not occur as an adverse effect of gentamicin.

    E. **CORRECT:** Vertigo, ataxia, and hearing loss are indications of ototoxicity that can occur in clients taking gentamicin.

    N NCLEX® Connection: Pharmacological Therapies, Adverse Effects/Contraindications/ Side Effects/Interactions

4.   A.   **CORRECT:** Paresthesias of the hands and feet can occur in clients taking streptomycin. Streptomycin has many other severe adverse effects, and is usually used to treat infections either in combination with other antibiotics or to treat severe infections where other antibiotics failed.

     B.   INCORRECT: Streptomycin causes nephrotoxicity rather than urinary retention.

     C.   INCORRECT: Streptomycin does not cause severe constipation.

     D.   INCORRECT: Streptomycin does not cause complex partial seizures.

     Ⓝ   NCLEX® Connection: Pharmacological Therapies, Adverse Effects/Contraindications/ Side Effects/Interactions

5.   A.   INCORRECT: Amikacin, an aminoglycoside antibiotic, is not used preoperatively for bowel surgery, and is only available for IM or IV use.

     B.   INCORRECT: Gentamicin, an aminoglycoside antibiotic, is not used preoperatively to suppress normal flora in the GI tract. It is not available as an oral medication, but can be administered IM, IV, and intrathecally.

     C.   **CORRECT:** Neomycin, an aminoglycoside antibiotic, is administered orally prior to GI surgery in order to rid the bowel of normal flora.

     D.   INCORRECT: Erythromycin, a broad-spectrum antibiotic, can be administered orally or parenterally, but is not used to suppress normal flora preoperatively.

     Ⓝ   NCLEX® Connection: Pharmacological Therapies, Expected Actions/Outcomes

6. *Using the ATI Active Learning Template: Medication*

A. Therapeutic Use

- Erythromycin inhibits protein synthesis in the cells of susceptible micro-organisms, usually gram-positive bacteria. Erythromycin can be either bacteriostatic or bactericidal, depending on the organism and on the medication dosage. It is sometimes used to treat infections in clients who are allergic to penicillin.

B. Adverse Effects

- The most common adverse effects of erythromycin are GI effects, including abdominal pain, nausea, vomiting, and diarrhea. Hepatotoxicity with abdominal pain, anorexia, fatigue, and possibly jaundice can occur after 1 to 2 weeks of erythromycin therapy. Erythromycin can cause a prolonged QT interval on ECG, which can lead to potentially fatal tachydysrhythmias. Ototoxicity can occur if erythromycin is given in high doses, especially for prolonged periods.

C. Diagnostic Tests

- Monitor liver function tests for clients who take erythromycin over a period of several weeks. If the client is concurrently taking warfarin or digoxin with erythromycin, carefully monitor PT/INR or digoxin levels. Monitor WBC for effectiveness of erythromycin treatment (decrease to normal levels).

D. Nursing Interventions

- Instruct the client to take erythromycin on an empty stomach, 1 hr before or 2 hr after meals, and with a full glass of water. Some forms of erythromycin may be taken with meals if GI distress occurs, so check the prescribing reference before reinforcing teaching with the client.

- Remind the client of adverse effects to watch for, and to call the provider for severe GI distress, manifestations of liver toxicity, and ototoxicity.

- Advise client that the medication should be taken as prescribed and not stopped if the client is feeling better.

(N) NCLEX® Connection: Pharmacological Therapies, Expected Actions/Outcomes

chapter **40**

Overview

- Sulfonamides, trimethoprim, and urinary antiseptics are medications used to treat urinary tract infections.

- Other medications used include penicillins, aminoglycosides, cephalosporins, and fluoroquinolones.

- Medications are used to treat active infections and prophylaxis of recurrent infections for susceptible individuals.

- Regimens with these medications may be a single-dose, a short course of 3 days, or the traditional course of 7 days.

MEDICATION CLASSIFICATION: SULFONAMIDES AND TRIMETHOPRIM

- Select Prototype Medications
  - Sulfamethoxazole-trimethoprim (SMZ-TMP, Bactrim, Septra)
  - Sulfadiazine
  - Trimethoprim

Purpose

- Expected Pharmacological Action
  - Sulfonamides and trimethoprim inhibit bacterial growth by preventing the synthesis of folic acid. Folic acid is essential for the production of DNA, RNA, and proteins.
- Therapeutic Uses
  - SMZ-TMP is used to treat urinary tract infections.
    - Causative agents include *Escherichia coli*, *klebsiella*, proteus, enterobacter, and *Neisseria gonorrhoeae*.
    - Other infections include otitis media, bronchitis, shigellosis, and *Pneumocystis jiroveci* pneumonia.

Complications

ADVERSE EFFECTS/ MEDICATION INTERACTIONS	NURSING INTERVENTIONS/CLIENT EDUCATION
› Hypersensitivity, including Stevens-Johnson syndrome	› Do not administer SMZ-TMP to client who has allergies to » Sulfonamides (sulfa) » Thiazide diuretics (hydrochlorothiazide [Microzide]) » Sulfonylurea-type oral hypoglycemics (tolbutamide) » Loop diuretics (furosemide [Lasix]) › Stop SMZ-TMP at the first indication of hypersensitivity, such as rash.
› Blood dyscrasias (hemolytic anemia, agranulocytosis, leukopenia, thrombocytopenia, aplastic anemia)	› Draw baseline and periodic CBC levels to detect any hematologic disorders. › Observe for bleeding episodes, sore throat, or pallor. › If the above symptoms occur, instruct the client to notify the provider.
› Crystalluria (crystalline aggregates in the kidneys, ureters, and bladder causing irritation and obstruction that leads to acute kidney injury)	› Maintain adequate oral fluid intake. › Instruct the client to drink 2 to 3 L/day. › Monitor for urine output of at least 1,200 mL each day.
› Kernicterus (jaundice, increased bilirubin levels, which is neurotoxic to infants)	› Avoid administering SMZ-TMP during the first trimester to prevent birth defects of the fetus. › Avoid administering SMZ-TMP to women who are pregnant near term or breastfeeding, and infants younger than 2 months (risk of kernicterus).
› Photosensitivity	› Advise the client to avoid prolonged exposure to sunlight, use sunscreen, and wear appropriate protective clothing.
› Sulfonamides can increase the effects of warfarin (Coumadin), phenytoin (Dilantin), sulfonylurea oral hypoglycemics, and tolbutamide.	› Reduced dosages of these medications can be required during SMZ-TMP therapy. › Monitor laboratory levels (prothrombin time and INR, phenytoin levels, and blood glucose levels).

Contraindications/Precautions

- SMZ-TMP is contraindicated in clients who have folate deficiency (increases risk of megaloblastic anemia).

- Use cautiously in clients who have renal dysfunction. Reduced dosage of SMZ-TMP is recommended.

 • Administer with caution in adults older than age 65 years who take angiotensin-converting enzyme (ACE) inhibitors or angiotensin II receptor blockers (ARB) because of risk for hyperkalemia.

Nursing Considerations

- Instruct clients to take SMZ-TMP on an empty stomach with a full glass of water.

- Instruct clients to complete the prescribed course of antimicrobial therapy, even though manifestations can resolve before the full course is completed.

Nursing Evaluation of Medication Effectiveness

- Depending on therapeutic intent, effectiveness can be evidenced by improvement of infection symptoms, such as improvement of urinary tract manifestations (decreased frequency, burning, and pain during urination) and negative urine cultures.

MEDICATION CLASSIFICATION: URINARY TRACT ANTISEPTICS

- Select Prototype Medication: nitrofurantoin (Furadantin) and nitrofurantoin macrocrystals (Macrodantin, Macrobid)
- Other Medications: methenamine (Hiprex, Urex)

Purpose

- Expected Pharmacological Action

  ○ Nitrofurantoin is a broad-spectrum urinary antiseptic with bacteriostatic and bactericidal action. Bacterial injury occurs by damaging DNA.

- Therapeutic Uses

  ○ Acute urinary tract infections

  ○ Prophylaxis for recurrent lower urinary tract infections

Complications

ADVERSE EFFECTS/ MEDICATION INTERACTIONS	NURSING INTERVENTIONS/CLIENT EDUCATION
› Gastrointestinal (GI) discomfort (anorexia, nausea, vomiting, and diarrhea)	› Administer nitrofurantoin with milk or meals. › Reduce dosage, and use macrocrystalline tablet to reduce GI discomfort.
› Hypersensitivity reactions with severe pulmonary manifestations (dyspnea, cough, chest pain, fever, chills, and alveolar infiltrations)	› Advise the client to stop medication and call provider if this occurs. › Pulmonary manifestations should subside within several days after nitrofurantoin is discontinued. › Advise the client not to receive nitrofurantoin agents again.
› Blood dyscrasias (agranulocytosis, leukopenia, thrombocytopenia, megaloblastic anemia, and hepatotoxicity)	› Do baseline CBC, and perform periodic blood tests to include liver function tests. › Monitor for easy bruising and epistaxis (nose bleeding). › Notify provider if manifestations occur.
› Peripheral neuropathy (numbness, tingling of the hands and feet, muscle weakness)	› Instruct the client to notify provider if these findings occur. › Avoid chronic use of nitrofurantoin; it is not recommended for clients who have kidney failure.
› Headache, drowsiness, dizziness	› Instruct the client to notify provider if these findings occur.

Contraindications/Precautions

- Nitrofurantoin is contraindicated in clients who have renal dysfunction and creatinine clearance less than 40 mL/min. Impaired renal function will increase the risk of medication toxicity because of inability to excrete nitrofurantoin.

Nursing Considerations

- Inform clients that urine will have a brownish discoloration.
- Encourage clients to administer with food if GI manifestations occur.
- Instruct clients to complete the prescribed course of antimicrobial therapy, even though manifestations can resolve before the full course is completed.
- Remind clients to avoid crushing tablets because of the possibility of tooth staining.
- Instruct clients to prevent pregnancy while taking nitrofurantoin (can cause infant birth defects).

Nursing Evaluation of Medication Effectiveness

- Depending on therapeutic intent, effectiveness may be evidenced by the following.
  - Improvement of infection symptoms, such as improvement of urinary tract symptoms (decreased frequency, burning, and pain during urination) and negative urine cultures
  - Resolution of GI disturbances, which can include anorexia, diarrhea, nausea, and vomiting

MEDICATION CLASSIFICATION: FLUOROQUINOLONES

- Select Prototype Medication: ciprofloxacin (Cipro)
- Other Medications: ofloxacin, moxifloxacin (Avelox), levofloxacin (Levaquin), norfloxacin (Noroxin)

Purpose

- Expected Pharmacological Action
  - Fluoroquinolones are bactericidal as a result of inhibition of the enzyme necessary for DNA replication.
- Therapeutic Uses
  - Broad-spectrum antimicrobials used for a wide variety of micro-organisms, such as aerobic gram-negative bacteria, gram-positive bacteria, *klebsiella*, and *E. coli*
  - Alternative to parenteral antibiotics for clients who have severe infections
  - Urinary, respiratory, and GI tract infections; infections of bones, joints, skin, and soft tissues
  - Medication of choice for prevention of anthrax in clients who have inhaled anthrax spore

Complications

ADVERSE EFFECTS/ MEDICATION INTERACTIONS	NURSING INTERVENTIONS/CLIENT EDUCATION
› GI discomfort (nausea, vomiting, diarrhea)	› Administer medications accordingly.
› Achilles tendon rupture	› Instruct the client to observe for clinical manifestations of pain, swelling, and redness at Achilles tendon site, and to notify the provider if they occur.
	› Ciprofloxacin should be discontinued. The client should not exercise until inflammation subsides.
› Suprainfection (thrush, vaginal yeast infection)	› Instruct the client to observe for clinical manifestations of yeast infection (cottage cheese/curd-like lesions on the mouth and genital area) and to notify the provider if they occur.
› Phototoxicity (severe sunburn) when exposed to direct and indirect sunlight, and sunlamps even when sunscreen is applied	› Instruct the client to avoid sun exposure and to wear protective clothing and sunscreen at all times.
	› Discontinue immediately (ciprofloxacin and other fluoroquinolones) if phototoxicity occurs.

Contraindications/Precautions

- Ciprofloxacin should not be administered to children younger than 18 years of age (due to risk of Achilles tendon rupture), unless the child is being treated for *E. coli* infections of urinary tract or inhalational anthrax. (Ciprofloxacin is the only fluoroquinolone approved for children.)

- Ciprofloxacin is contraindicated in clients who have myasthenia gravis.

- Ciprofloxacin increases the risk for developing *Clostridium difficile* infection by decreasing normal intestinal bacteria.

- Ciprofloxacin and several other fluoroquinolone medications can effect the CNS (dizziness, headache, restlessness, confusion). Use with caution in older adults and those who have cardiovascular disorders.

Interactions

MEDICATION/FOOD INTERACTIONS	NURSING INTERVENTIONS/CLIENT EDUCATION
› Cationic compounds (aluminum-magnesium antacids, iron salts, sucralfate, milk and dairy products) decrease absorption of ciprofloxacin.	› Administer cationic compounds 6 hr before or 2 hr after ciprofloxacin.
› Plasma levels of theophylline (Theolair) can increase with concurrent use of ciprofloxacin.	› Monitor levels, and adjust dosage accordingly.
› Plasma levels of warfarin (Coumadin) can increase with concurrent use of ciprofloxacin.	› Monitor prothrombin time and INR, and adjust the dosage of warfarin accordingly.

Nursing Considerations

- Ciprofloxacin is available in oral and intravenous forms.
  - Discontinue other IV infusions or use another IV site when administering IV ciprofloxacin.
- Decrease doses of ciprofloxacin in clients who have renal dysfunction.
- Intravenous ciprofloxacin should be administered in a dilute solution slowly over 60 min in a large vein.
- For inhalation anthrax infection, ciprofloxacin is administered every 12 hr for 60 days.
- Instruct clients to complete the prescribed course of antimicrobial therapy, even though symptoms may resolve before the full course is completed.

Nursing Evaluation of Medication Effectiveness

- Depending on therapeutic intent, effectiveness can be evidenced by the following.
  - Improvement of infection symptoms (improvement of urinary tract symptoms [decreased frequency, burning, and pain during urination], negative urine cultures)
  - No evidence of suprainfection, such as absence of cottage cheese or curd-like lesions in the mouth and genital areas

MEDICATION CLASSIFICATION: URINARY TRACT ANALGESIC

- Select Prototype Medication: phenazopyridine (Pyridiate, Pyridium, Urogesic)

Purpose

- Expected Pharmacological Action
  - The medication is an azo dye that functions as a local anesthetic on the mucosa of the urinary tract.
- Therapeutic Uses
  - Relieve manifestations of burning on urination, pain, frequency, and urgency.
- Nursing Considerations
  - Contraindicated for a client who has acute kidney injury or chronic kidney disease.
  - Medication changes urine to an orange/red color.
  - Instruct the client that the urine might stain clothes.
  - Administer with or after meals to prevent mild GI discomfort.

APPLICATION EXERCISES

1. A nurse is reviewing a client's medication history and notes an allergy to sulfonamides. Which of the following medications are contraindicated due to this allergy? (Select all that apply.)

_____ A. Hydrochlorothiazide (Microzide)

_____ B. Metoprolol (Lopressor)

_____ C. Acetaminophen (Tylenol)

_____ D. Tolbutamide

_____ E. Furosemide (Lasix)

2. A nurse is assisting with discharge planning for a female client who has a new prescription for sulfamethoxazole-trimethoprim (Septra). Which of the following information should the nurse include in the teaching?

A. May take if pregnant.

B. Drink 1 L of water each day.

C. Take the medication on an empty stomach.

D. Discontinue medication when symptoms subside.

3. A nurse is reinforcing teaching with a client who has a new prescription for nitrofurantoin (Furadantin). Which of the following information should the nurse include in the teaching? (Select all that apply.)

_____ A. Observe for bruising on the skin.

_____ B. Take the medication with milk or meals.

_____ C. Expect brownish discoloration of urine.

_____ D. Crush the medication if difficult to swallow.

_____ E. Expect headaches and drowsiness.

4. A nurse is reinforcing teaching about ciprofloxacin (Cipro) with a female client who has a severe urinary tract infection. Which of the following information about adverse reactions should the nurse include in the teaching? (Select all that apply.)

_____ A. Observe for pain and swelling of the Achilles tendon.

_____ B. Monitor for a vaginal yeast infection.

_____ C. Check for excessive nighttime perspiration.

_____ D. Inspect the mouth for cottage cheese-like lesions.

_____ E. Take medication with a dairy product.

5. A nurse is planning to administer ciprofloxacin (Cipro) IV to a client who has cystitis. Which of the following is an appropriate action by the nurse?

    A. Administer a concentrated solution.

    B. Infuse medication over 60 min.

    C. Piggyback the solution onto existing IV medication tubing.

    D. Choose a small peripheral vein for administration.

6. A client who has a urinary tract infection is to receive phenazopyridine (Pyridium). What therapeutic uses and nursing considerations should the nurse review? Use the ATI Active Learning Template: Medication to complete this item to include the following:

    A. Expected Pharmacological Action

    B. Therapeutic Uses: Describe four.

    C. Nursing Interventions/Client Education: Include three teaching points.

APPLICATION EXERCISES KEY

1. A. **CORRECT:** Hydrochlorothiazide is contraindicated with sulfonamides, which can lead to hypersensitivity, including Stevens-Johnson syndrome.

    B. INCORRECT: Metoprolol is not contraindicated with an allergy to sulfonamides.

    C. INCORRECT: Acetaminophen is not contraindicated with an allergy to sulfonamides.

    D. **CORRECT:** Tolbutamide is a sulfonamide-type hypoglycemic medication and is contraindicated with sulfonamides, which can lead to hypersensitivity, including Stevens-Johnson syndrome.

    E. **CORRECT:** Furosemide is a sulfonamide-type diuretic medication and is contraindicated with sulfonamides, which can lead to hypersensitivity, including Stevens-Johnson syndrome.

    Ⓝ NCLEX® Connection: Pharmacological Therapies, Adverse Effects/Contraindications/ Side Effects/Interactions

2. A. INCORRECT: Sulfamethoxazole-trimethoprim is not recommended during pregnancy because it can cause birth defects and fetal kernicterus.

    B. INCORRECT: Sulfamethoxazole-trimethoprim should be taken with at least 2 to 3 L/day of water to prevent crystalluria, which results in kidney damage.

    C. **CORRECT:** The nurse should instruct the client to take sulfamethoxazole-trimethoprim on an empty stomach with a full glass of water for maximum absorption of the medication.

    D. INCORRECT: Sulfamethoxazole-trimethoprim should be taken until the prescription is completed to prevent a rebound infection.

    Ⓝ NCLEX® Connection: Pharmacological Therapies, Medication Administration

3. A. **CORRECT:** Bruising may indicate a blood dyscrasia, and the client should notify the provider if this occurs.

    B. **CORRECT:** Taking the medication with milk or meals will decrease gastrointestinal discomfort related to nausea, vomiting, anorexia, and diarrhea.

    C. **CORRECT:** A brownish discoloration of urine is a common adverse effect when taking nitrofurantoin.

    D. INCORRECT: Crushing the medication will cause staining of the teeth and is not recommended.

    E. INCORRECT: Headaches and drowsiness are not to be expected and are adverse effects of nitrofurantoin. The client should report the symptoms immediately to the provider.

    Ⓝ NCLEX® Connection: Pharmacological Therapies, Adverse Effects/Contraindications/ Side Effects/Interactions

4. A. **CORRECT:** Pain and swelling of the Achilles tendon indicate an adverse effect of ciprofloxacin and should be reported to the provider.

    B. **CORRECT:** A vaginal yeast infection is an overgrowth of *Candida albicans*, which commonly occurs when taking ciprofloxacin.

    C. INCORRECT: Alteration in perspiration is not an adverse effect of this medication.

    D. **CORRECT:** Cottage cheese-like lesions in the mouth indicates an overgrowth of *Candida albicans*, a common adverse effect when taking ciprofloxacin.

    E. INCORRECT: Milk and other dairy products contain calcium ions that reduce the effect of ciprofloxacin. The medication should be taken 6 hr before or 2 hr after ingesting dairy products.

    Ⓝ NCLEX® Connection: Pharmacological Therapies, Adverse Effects/Contraindications/ Side Effects/Interactions

5. A. INCORRECT: Ciprofloxacin should be administered in a dilute solution to minimize irritation of the vein.

    B. **CORRECT:** Ciprofloxacin should be administered IV over 60 min to minimize irritation of the vein.

    C. INCORRECT: Ciprofloxacin should not be administered with other IV medication. A new IV site should be started as needed.

    D. INCORRECT: Ciprofloxacin should be administered using a large vein to minimize the risk of phlebitis.

    Ⓝ NCLEX® Connection: Pharmacological Therapies, Medication Administration

6. *Using the ATI Active Learning Template: Medication*

    A. Expected Pharmacological Action
       • Phenazopyridine is an azo dye, which acts as a local anesthetic on the mucosa of the urinary tract. It is not an antibiotic.

    B. Therapeutic Uses
       • Relieves manifestations of burning, urgency, pain, and frequency upon urination

    C. Nursing Interventions/Client Education
       • Instruct client that urine will turn orange/red in color.
       • Urine can stain clothing.
       • Take the medication with or after meals to prevent mild gastrointestinal discomfort.
       • Frequently prescribed in addition to an antibiotic.

    Ⓝ NCLEX® Connection: Pharmacological Therapies, Expected Actions/Outcomes

chapter 41

Overview

- *Mycobacterium tuberculosis* is a slow-growing pathogen that necessitates long-term treatment. Long-term treatment increases the risk for toxicity, poor client adherence, and development of medication-resistant strains. Treatment for tuberculosis requires the use of at least two medications to which the pathogen is susceptible.

- Metronidazole (Flagyl) is the medication of choice for parasitic infections.

- Antifungal medications belong to a variety of chemical families and are used to treat systemic and superficial mycoses.

MEDICATION CLASSIFICATION: ANTIMYCOBACTERIAL (ANTITUBERCULOSIS)

- Select Prototype Medication: isoniazid (Laniazid)

- Other Medications

  - Pyrazinamide

  - Ethambutol (Myambutol) bacteriostatic only to *M. tuberculosis*

  - Rifapentine (Priftin)

Purpose

- Expected Pharmacological Action

  - This medication is highly specific for mycobacteria. Isoniazid inhibits growth of mycobacteria by preventing synthesis of mycolic acid in the cell wall.

- Therapeutic Uses

  - Indicated for active and latent tuberculosis

    - Latent: Isoniazid only – 6 to 9 months, or isoniazid with rifapentine once weekly for 3 months (rifapentine is contraindicated in children under age 12, clients who have HIV, and pregnant women).

    - Active: Several antimycobacterial medications must be used to treat a client who has active tuberculosis in order to decrease medication resistance. Multiple medication therapy includes isoniazid, for a minimum of 6 months.

    - The initial phase (induction phase) focuses on eliminating the active tubercle bacilli, which will result in noninfectious sputum. The second phase (continuation phase) works toward eliminating any other pathogens in the body. Length of treatment varies and may be as short as 6 months for medication-sensitive tuberculosis (2 months for the initial phase and 4 months for the continuation phase) or as long as 24 months for medication-resistant infections.

Complications

ADVERSE EFFECTS	NURSING INTERVENTIONS/CLIENT EDUCATION
› Peripheral neuropathy (tingling, numbness, burning, and pain resulting from deficiency of pyridoxine, vitamin B_6)	› Instruct clients to observe for manifestations and notify the provider if they occur. › Administer 50 to 200 mg vitamin B_6 daily.
› Hepatotoxicity (anorexia, malaise, fatigue, nausea, and yellowish discoloration of skin and eyes)	› Instruct clients to observe for manifestations and notify the provider if they occur. › Monitor liver function tests. › Instruct clients to avoid consumption of alcohol. › Medication might need to be discontinued if liver function test results are elevated.
› Hyperglycemia and decreased glucose control in clients who have diabetes mellitus	› Monitor blood glucose. › Clients who have diabetes mellitus can require additional antidiabetic medication.

Contraindications/Precautions

- Isoniazid is contraindicated for clients who have liver disease.
- Use cautiously in older clients, and those who have diabetes mellitus or alcohol use disorder.

Interactions

MEDICATION/FOOD INTERACTIONS	NURSING INTERVENTIONS/CLIENT EDUCATION
› Isoniazid inhibits metabolism of phenytoin, leading to buildup of medication and toxicity. Ataxia and incoordination can indicate toxicity.	› Monitor levels of phenytoin. Dosage of phenytoin might need to be adjusted based on phenytoin levels.
› Concurrent use of alcohol, rifampin, and pyrazinamide increases the risk for hepatotoxicity.	› Instruct clients to avoid alcohol consumption. › Monitor liver function.

Nursing Administration

- Usually administered orally. When given IM, ensure that the solution is free of crystals and inject deeply into a large muscle.
- For active tuberculosis, direct observation therapy (DOT) is used to ensure adherence.
- Advise clients to take isoniazid 1 hr before meals or 2 hr after. If gastric discomfort occurs, the client can take isoniazid with meals.
- Instruct clients to complete the prescribed course of antimicrobial therapy, even though manifestations might resolve before the full course is completed.

MEDICATION CLASSIFICATION: ANTIMYCOBACTERIAL (ANTITUBERCULOSIS)

- Select Prototype Medication: rifampin (Rifadin)

Purpose

- Expected Pharmacological Action
  - Rifampin is bactericidal as a result of inhibition of protein synthesis
- Therapeutic Uses
  - Rifampin is a broad-spectrum antibiotic effective for gram-positive and gram-negative bacteria, *M. tuberculosis*, and *M. leprae*.
  - Rifampin is given in combination with at least one other antituberculosis medication to help prevent antibiotic resistance.

Complications

ADVERSE EFFECTS	NURSING INTERVENTIONS/CLIENT EDUCATION
› Discoloration of body fluids	› Inform clients of expected orange color of urine, saliva, sweat, and tears.
› Hepatotoxicity (jaundice, anorexia, and fatigue)	› Monitor liver function. › Inform clients regarding manifestations of anorexia, fatigue, and malaise, and instruct them to notify the provider if they occur. › Instruct clients to avoid alcohol.
› Mild GI discomfort associated with anorexia, nausea, and abdominal discomfort	› Abdominal discomfort is mild and usually does not require intervention.

Contraindications/Precautions

- Use cautiously in clients who have liver dysfunction.

Interactions

MEDICATION/FOOD INTERACTIONS	NURSING INTERVENTIONS/CLIENT EDUCATION
› Rifampin accelerates metabolism of warfarin (Coumadin), oral contraceptives, protease inhibitors, and NNRTIs (medications for HIV), resulting in diminished effectiveness.	› Increased dosages of HIV medications can be necessary. › Monitor PT and INR. › Clients might need to use alternative form of birth control.
› Concurrent use with isoniazid and pyrazinamide increases risk of hepatotoxicity.	› Instruct clients to avoid alcohol consumption. › Monitor liver function.

Nursing Administration

- Administer orally or by IV route.
- Administer oral rifampin 1 hr before or 2 hr after meals. Absorption is decreased if given with food.

Nursing Evaluation of Medication Effectiveness

- Depending on therapeutic intent, effectiveness can be evidenced by:
  - Improvement of tuberculosis manifestations, such as clear breath sounds, no night sweats, increased appetite, and no afternoon rises of temperature.
  - Three negative sputum cultures for tuberculosis, usually taking 3 to 6 months to achieve.

MEDICATION CLASSIFICATION: ANTIPROTOZOALS

- Select Prototype Medication: metronidazole (Flagyl)

Purpose

- Expected Pharmacological Action
  - Metronidazole is a broad-spectrum antimicrobial with bactericidal activity against anaerobic micro-organisms.
- Therapeutic Uses
  - Treatment of protozoal infections (intestinal amebiasis, giardiasis, trichomoniasis) and obligate anaerobic bacteria (*Bacteroides fragilis*, antibiotic-induced *Clostridium difficile*, *Gardnerella vaginalis*)
  - Prophylaxis for clients who will have surgical procedures and are high-risk for anaerobic infection (vaginal, abdominal, colorectal surgery)
  - Treatment of *H. pylori* in combination with tetracycline and bismuth salicylate in clients who have peptic ulcer disease

Complications

ADVERSE EFFECTS	NURSING INTERVENTIONS/CLIENT EDUCATION
› GI discomfort (nausea, vomiting, dry mouth, and metallic taste)	› Advise clients to observe for effects and to notify the provider.
› Darkening of urine	› Advise clients that this is a harmless effect of metronidazole.
› CNS manifestations (numbness of extremities, ataxia, and seizures)	› Advise clients to notify the provider if manifestations occur.
	› Stop metronidazole.

Contraindications/Precautions

- Contraindicated in active CNS disorders, blood dyscrasias, and during lactation. Contraindicated in the first trimester of pregnancy in clients who have trichomoniasis.
- Use cautiously in clients who have renal, cardiac, or seizure disorders and in older adults.

Interactions

MEDICATION/FOOD INTERACTIONS	NURSING INTERVENTIONS/CLIENT EDUCATION
› Alcohol causes a disulfiram-like reaction.	› Advise clients to avoid alcohol consumption.
› Metronidazole inhibits inactivation of warfarin.	› Monitor prothrombin time and INR, and adjust warfarin dosage accordingly.

Nursing Administration

- Administer by oral or IV route.
- Instruct clients to complete the prescribed course of antimicrobial therapy, even though manifestations might resolve before the full course is completed.

Nursing Evaluation of Medication Effectiveness

- Depending on therapeutic intent, effectiveness can be evidenced by improvement of manifestations (resolution of bloody mucoid diarrhea, formed stools, negative stool results for amoeba and *Giardia*, decrease or absence of watery vaginal/urethral discharge, negative blood cultures for anaerobic organisms in the CNS, blood, bones and joints, and soft tissues).

MEDICATION CLASSIFICATION: ANTIFUNGALS

- Select Prototype Medications
  - Amphotericin B (Amphotec), a polyene antibiotic for systemic mycoses
  - Ketoconazole, an azole for treating both superficial and systemic mycoses
- Other Medications
  - Flucytosine (Ancobon)
  - Nystatin (Nystop)
  - Miconazole (Monistat)
  - Clotrimazole (Lotrimin)
  - Terbinafine (Lamisil)
  - Fluconazole (Diflucan)
  - Griseofulvin (Grifulvin)

Purpose

- Expected Pharmacological Action

  ○ Amphotericin B is an antifungal agent that acts on fungal cell membranes to cause cell death. Depending on concentration, these agents can be fungistatic (slows growth on the fungus) or fungicidal (destroys the fungus).

- Therapeutic Uses

  ○ Antifungals are the treatment of choice for systemic fungal infection (*Candidiasis, Aspergillosis, Cryptococcosis, Mucormycosis*) and nonopportunistic mycoses, (*Blastomycosis, Histoplasmosis, Coccidioidomycosis*).

  ○ Some antifungals treat superficial fungal infections: dermatophytic infections (tinea pedis [ringworm of the foot], tinea cruris [ringworm of the groin]); candida infections of the skin and mucous membranes; and fungal infections of the nails (*Onychomycosis*).

Complications

ADVERSE EFFECTS	NURSING INTERVENTIONS/CLIENT EDUCATION
Amphotericin B	
› Infusion reactions (fever, chills, rigors, and headache) 1 to 3 hr after initiation	› A test dose of 1 mg amphotericin B, infused slowly IV, may be prescribed to monitor client reaction. › Pretreat with diphenhydramine and acetaminophen. › Meperidine (Demerol) or dantrolene may be given for rigors.
› Thrombophlebitis	› Observe infusion sites for indications of erythema, swelling, and pain. › Rotate injection sites. › Administer in a large vein and administer heparin before infusing amphotericin B.
› Nephrotoxicity	› Obtain baseline kidney function (BUN and creatinine) and do weekly kidney function tests. › Monitor I&O. › Infuse 1 L saline on the day of amphotericin B infusion.
› Hypokalemia	› Monitor electrolyte levels, especially potassium. › Administer potassium supplements accordingly.
› Bone marrow suppression	› Obtain baseline CBC and hematocrit, and monitor weekly.
Ketoconazole	
› Hepatotoxicity (anorexia, nausea, vomiting, jaundice, dark urine, and clay-colored stools)	› Obtain baseline liver function studies, and monitor liver function monthly. › If manifestations occur, notify provider and discontinue medication.

› Effects on sex hormones
  » In males, gynecomastia (enlargement of breast), decreased libido, erectile dysfunction
  » In females, irregular menstrual flow
	› Advise clients to observe for these effects and to notify the provider.

Contraindications/Precautions

- Amphotericin B should be used with caution in clients who have suppressed bone marrow, renal dysfunction, or anemia.

Interactions

MEDICATION/FOOD INTERACTIONS	NURSING INTERVENTIONS/CLIENT EDUCATION
› Aminoglycosides (gentamicin, streptomycin, cyclosporine) have additive nephrotoxic risk when used concurrently with antifungal medications.	› Avoid use of these antimicrobials when clients are taking amphotericin B due to additive nephrotoxicity risk.
› Antifungal effects of flucytosine are potentiated with concurrent use of amphotericin B. › Fluconazole is Pregnancy Risk Category C in low dose and Category D in high dose; contraindicated during lactation.	› Potentiating the effects of flucytosine allows for a reduction in amphotericin B dosages.
› Azole antibiotics increase levels of multiple medications, including digoxin, warfarin, and sulfonylurea antidiabetic medications.	› If concurrent administration is necessary, carefully monitor for toxicity.

Nursing Administration

- Amphotericin B is highly toxic and should be reserved for severe life-threatening fungal infections.
- Amphotericin B should be infused slowly over 2 to 4 hr by the IV route, because oral preparation is poorly absorbed in the GI tract. Observe solutions for precipitation and discard if precipitates are present. Renal damage can be lessened with administration of 1 L saline solution on the day of amphotericin B infusion.
- Instruct clients to complete the prescribed course of antimicrobial therapy, even though manifestations might resolve before the full course is completed.
- Antifungals for topical use to treat superficial vulvovaginal candidiasis may be applied as vaginal suppository or cream.

Nursing Evaluation of Medication Effectiveness

- Depending on therapeutic intent, effectiveness can be evidenced by:
  - Improvement of findings of systemic fungal infections, such as clear breath sounds and negative chest x-rays.
  - Improvement of findings of superficial infections, such as clear mucus membranes, clear nails, and intact skin.

APPLICATION EXERCISES

1. A nurse is caring for a client who has diabetes mellitus and pulmonary tuberculosis and has a new prescription for isoniazid (Laniazid). Which of the following supplements should the nurse expect to administer to prevent an adverse effect of isoniazid?

    A. Ascorbic acid

    B. Pyridoxine

    C. Folic acid

    D. Cyanocobalamin

2. A nurse is infusing IV amphotericin B for a client who has a severe fungal infection. The nurse starts the infusion at 0800. When should the nurse begin to monitor the client for indications of an infusion reaction?

    A. 0805

    B. 0830

    C. 0900

    D. 1200

3. A nurse is administering IV amphotericin B to a client who has a systemic fungal infection. The nurse should monitor which of the following laboratory values? (Select all that apply.)

    _____ A. Blood glucose

    _____ B. Serum amylase

    _____ C. Serum potassium

    _____ D. Hematocrit

    _____ E. Serum creatinine

4. A nurse is reinforcing teaching with a client who is beginning a course of metronidazole (Flagyl) to treat an infection. The nurse should instruct the client to stop taking metronidazole and notify the provider if which of the following adverse effects occur?

    A. Metallic taste

    B. Nausea

    C. Ataxia

    D. Dark-colored urine

5. A nurse is reinforcing teaching with a client who has active tuberculosis about his treatment regimen. The client asks why he must take four different medications. Which of the following replies by the nurse is appropriate? "Taking multiple antituberculosis medications

    A. decreases the chance for a severe allergic reaction to any of the medications."

    B. reduces the chance that the TB bacteria will become resistant to the medications."

    C. minimizes the chance of adverse effects caused by any of the medications."

    D. lessens the chance that you will have a positive tuberculin test indefinitely."

6. A nurse in an outpatient facility is reinforcing teaching with a client who has latent tuberculosis (TB) and is about to begin taking isoniazid (Laniazid) twice weekly for 6 months. What should the nurse teach the client about this medication? Use the ATI Active Learning Template: Medication to complete this item to include the following:

    A. Therapeutic Use: Describe the therapeutic use for isoniazid in this client.

    B. Adverse Effects: List two adverse effects the client should watch for.

    C. Diagnostic Tests: Describe one to monitor for clients taking isoniazid.

    D. Nursing Actions: Describe two for clients taking isoniazid.

APPLICATION EXERCISES KEY

1. A. INCORRECT: Ascorbic acid (vitamin C) is not administered to prevent an adverse effect of isoniazid.

   B. **CORRECT:** Pyridoxine (vitamin B₆) is frequently prescribed along with isoniazid to prevent peripheral neuropathy for clients who have increased risk factors, such as diabetes mellitus or alcohol use disorder.

   C. INCORRECT: Folic acid is not administered to prevent an adverse effect of isoniazid.

   D. INCORRECT: Cyanocobalamin (vitamin B₁₂) is not administered to prevent an adverse effect of isoniazid.

   Ⓝ NCLEX® Connection: Pharmacological Therapies, Adverse Effects/Contraindications/ Side Effects/Interactions

2. A. INCORRECT: The nurse does not yet need to monitor the client for an infusion reaction 5 min following the start of the infusion.

   B. INCORRECT: The nurse does not need to monitor the client for an infusion reaction 30 min following the start of the infusion.

   C. **CORRECT:** Infusion reactions to amphotericin B can begin 1 to 3 hr after the infusion begins. The nurse should start monitoring for a reaction at 0900.

   D. INCORRECT: The nurse should not start to monitor for an infusion reaction 4 hr after the beginning of the infusion.

   Ⓝ NCLEX® Connection: Pharmacological Therapies, Adverse Effects/Contraindications/ Side Effects/Interactions

3. A. INCORRECT: Amphotericin B does not affect blood glucose levels.

   B. INCORRECT: Amphotericin B does not cause pancreatitis. Monitoring serum amylase is unnecessary.

   C. **CORRECT:** Hypokalemia is a serious adverse effect of amphotericin B. The nurse should monitor serum potassium values for hypokalemia.

   D. **CORRECT:** Amphotericin B can cause bone marrow suppression. Hematocrit and platelet count should be monitored periodically.

   E. **CORRECT:** Amphotericin B can cause nephrotoxicity. Kidney function (with serum creatinine, BUN, creatinine clearance) should be monitored.

   Ⓝ NCLEX® Connection: Pharmacological Therapies, Adverse Effects/Contraindications/ Side Effects/Interactions

4.   A. INCORRECT: A metallic taste in the mouth is an adverse effect of metronidazole, but it is not necessary to stop the medication and notify the provider.

     B. INCORRECT: Nausea is an adverse effect of metronidazole, but it is not necessary to stop taking the medication. The client should notify the provider of GI manifestations.

     C. **CORRECT:** Ataxia, tremors, paresthesias of the extremities, and seizures are manifestations of CNS toxicity. The client should stop taking the medication and notify the provider if any of these effects occur.

     D. INCORRECT: Dark-colored urine is a harmless effect, and it is not necessary to stop taking the medication the notify the provider.

     Ⓝ NCLEX® Connection: Pharmacological Therapies, Adverse Effects/Contraindications/ Side Effects/Interactions

5.   A. INCORRECT: Taking several antituberculosis medications concurrently does not decrease the chance of an allergic reaction to any of the individual medications.

     B. **CORRECT:** If the client took only one medication to treat active tuberculosis, resistance to the medication would occur quickly. Taking three or four different medications decreases the possibility of resistance.

     C. INCORRECT: Taking several antituberculosis medications concurrently does not minimize the chance of adverse effects to any of the medications. Risk for liver toxicity increases when more than one medication that causes liver toxicity is taken, such as isoniazid (Laniazid), rifampin (Rifadin), and pyrazinamide.

     D. INCORRECT: Taking several antituberculosis medications concurrently does not change the fact that the client will have a positive tuberculin test indefinitely.

     Ⓝ NCLEX® Connection: Pharmacological Therapies, Expected Actions/Outcomes

6. *Using the ATI Active Learning Template: Medication*

A. Therapeutic Use

- A client who has latent tuberculosis has been infected by *Mycobacterium tuberculosis* and can be at risk for (but has not yet developed) active tuberculosis. Certain clients who have latent tuberculosis, such as those who are immunocompromised or who have recently immigrated to the U.S. from a country where active TB is common, can require treatment with isoniazid, with or without rifapentine (Priftin), in order to prevent the onset of active TB. The client who has latent TB has a positive tuberculin test but a negative sputum culture and negative chest x-ray for TB. The client cannot infect others with tuberculosis unless the infection becomes active.

B. Adverse Effects

- Paresthesias in the extremities caused by vitamin B_6 deficiency

- Hepatotoxicity

C. Diagnostic Tests

- The client who starts isoniazid should have baseline liver function testing and be tested periodically throughout treatment.

D. Nursing Actions

- Instruct the client to watch for paresthesias, and to take pyridoxine (vitamin B_6) daily to reverse the effect if they occur.

- Reinforce teaching with the client about indications of hepatitis (anorexia, fatigue, nausea, jaundice) and that the provider should be notified if these occur.

- Remind the client that isoniazid must be taken as prescribed and should not be stopped until the entire course of treatment is completed.

- The client with latent tuberculosis does not feel ill, and the nurse should be sure that the client understands why it is important to continue with treatment.

Ⓝ NCLEX® Connection: Pharmacological Therapies, Expected Actions/Outcomes

chapter 42

Overview

- Most antiviral medications act by altering viral reproduction. Antiviral medications are only effective during viral replication. Therefore, they are ineffective when the virus is dormant.

- The human immunodeficiency virus (HIV) is a retrovirus. A retrovirus must attach to a host cell in order to replicate. RNA is changed into DNA using the enzyme reverse transcriptase.

- Antiretroviral agents are used to treat HIV infections. These medications do not cure HIV infection and do not decrease the risk of passing HIV infection to others.

  - Antiretroviral agents may act by preventing the virus from entering the cells (fusion/entry inhibitors and CCR5 antagonists). Others act by inhibiting enzymes needed for HIV replication (nucleoside reverse transcriptase inhibitors [NRTIs], nonnucleoside reverse transcriptase inhibitors [NNRTIs], protease inhibitors [PIs], and an integrase inhibitor [INSTI]).

  - Highly active antiretroviral therapy (HAART) involves using three to four HIV medications in combination with other antiretroviral medications to reduce medication resistance, adverse effects, and dosages.

  - HAART is an aggressive treatment method using three or more different medications to reduce the amount of virus and increase CD4 counts.

  - In addition to HAART, clients who have HIV infection take additional medications to treat adverse effects of antiretrovirals and to treat or prevent secondary infections, such as pneumocystis pneumonia.

  - Skipping doses or taking decreased dosages of antiretroviral medications causes medication resistance and possible treatment failure.

MEDICATION CLASSIFICATION: ANTIVIRALS

- Select Prototype Medications
  - Acyclovir (Zovirax): oral, topical, and IV
  - Ganciclovir (Cytovene): oral, IV
- Other Medications
  - Interferon alfa-2b (Intron A)
  - Lamivudine (Epivir)
  - Oseltamivir (Tamiflu)
  - Ribavirin (Rebetol)
  - Amantadine
  - Boceprevir (Victrelis)
  - Telaprevir (Incivek)

Purpose

- Expected Pharmacological Action – Acyclovir and ganciclovir prevent the reproduction of viral DNA and thus interrupts cell replication.

- Therapeutic Uses

  - Acyclovir is used to treat herpes simplex and varicella-zoster viruses

  - Ganciclovir is used for treatment and prevention of cytomegalovirus (CMV). Prevention therapy using ganciclovir is given for clients who have HIV/AIDS, organ transplants, and other immunocompromised states.

  - Interferon alfa-2b and lamivudine are used to treat hepatitis B and C.

  - Oseltamivir is used to treat influenza A and B.

  - Ribavirin is used to treat respiratory syncytial virus and influenza.

  - Boceprevir and telaprevir are protease inhibitors used to treat hepatitis C virus (HCV).

Complications

ADVERSE EFFECTS	NURSING INTERVENTIONS/CLIENT EDUCATION
Acyclovir	
› Phlebitis and inflammation at the site of infusion	› Rotate IV injection sites. › Monitor IV sites for swelling and redness.
› Nephrotoxicity	› Administer acyclovir infusion slowly over 1 hr. › Ensure adequate hydration during infusion and 2 hr after to minimize nephrotoxicity by administering IV fluids and increasing oral fluid intake as prescribed.
› Mild discomfort associated with oral therapy (nausea, headache, diarrhea)	› Observe for manifestations and notify the provider.
Ganciclovir	
› Suppressed bone marrow, including leukocytes and thrombocytes	› Obtain baseline CBC and platelet count. › Administer granulocyte colony-stimulating factors. › Monitor WBC, absolute neutrophil, and platelet counts frequently during treatment.
› Fever, headache, nausea, diarrhea	› Advise client to report these findings.
› Teratogenic and embryotoxic; suppresses sperm production.	› Warn female clients to prevent pregnancy. › Warn male clients about possible sterility.

Contraindications/Precautions

- Acyclovir should be used cautiously in clients who have renal impairment or dehydration, and clients taking nephrotoxic medications.

- Ganciclovir is contraindicated in pregnancy and in clients who have a neutrophil count less than 500/mm^3 or platelet counts less than 25,000/mm^3; and should be used cautiously in infants younger than 3 months, older adults, and clients who have dehydration, renal insufficiency, or malignant disorders.

Interactions

MEDICATION/FOOD INTERACTIONS	NURSING INTERVENTIONS/CLIENT EDUCATION
Acyclovir	
› Probenecid can decrease elimination of acyclovir.	› Monitor for medication toxicity.
› Concurrent use of zidovudine may cause drowsiness.	› Use with caution.
Ganciclovir	
› Cytotoxic medications can cause increased toxicity.	› Use together with caution.

Nursing Administration

- Acyclovir
    - For topical administration, advise clients to put on rubber gloves to avoid transfer of virus to other areas of the body.
    - Administer IV infusion slowly over 1 hr or longer.
    - Inform clients to expect symptom relief but not cure.
    - Instruct clients to wash affected area with soap and water three to four times/day and to keep the lesions dry after washing.

    - Advise clients to refrain from sexual contact while lesions are present.
    - Clients who have healed herpetic lesions should continue to use condoms to prevent transmission of the virus.
- Ganciclovir
    - Administer IV infusion slowly, with an infusion pump, over at least 1 hr.
    - Administer oral medication with food and encourage extra fluid intake during therapy.
    - Administer intraocular for CMV retinitis.
    - Avoid getting ganciclovir solution or powder on skin. Wash well if contact occurs.
- Instruct clients to complete the prescribed course of antimicrobial therapy, even though manifestations might resolve before the full course is completed.

Nursing Evaluation of Medication Effectiveness

- Depending on therapeutic intent, effectiveness can be evidenced by improvement of findings, such as healed genital lesions, decreased inflammation and pain, and improvement in vision.

MEDICATION CLASSIFICATION: ANTIRETROVIRALS – FUSION/ENTRY INHIBITORS

- Select Prototype Medication: enfuvirtide (Fuzeon) subcutaneous

Purpose

- Expected Pharmacological Action – decreases and limits the spread of HIV by blocking HIV from attaching to and entering CD4 T cell
- Therapeutic Use – treatment of HIV that is unresponsive to other antiretrovirals

Complications

ADVERSE EFFECTS	NURSING INTERVENTIONS/CLIENT EDUCATION
› Localized reaction at injection site.	› Rotate injection sites. Monitor for swelling and redness.
› Bacterial pneumonia	› Auscultate breath sounds prior to start of therapy. Monitor for signs of pneumonia, such as fever, cough, or shortness of breath.
› Systemic reaction (fever, chills, rash, hypotension)	› Monitor for medication reaction. Discontinue and notify the provider.

Contraindications/Precautions

- Enfuvirtide is contraindicated in clients who have medication hypersensitivity.
- This medication is Pregnancy Risk Category B.

Interactions

- None significant

Nursing Administration

- Enfuvirtide is only administered subcutaneously. Rotate injection sites and avoid previous skin reaction areas.
- Monitor for bacterial pneumonia.
- Monitor for systemic hypersensitivity reaction.
- Instruct client to take exactly as prescribed to minimize development of resistance.

Nursing Evaluation of Medication Effectiveness

- Depending on therapeutic intent, effectiveness can be evidenced by a reduction of symptoms and absence of opportunistic infection.

MEDICATION CLASSIFICATION: ANTIRETROVIRALS – CCR5 ANTAGONISTS

- Select Prototype Medication: maraviroc (Selzentry)

Purpose

- Expected Pharmacological Action – prevents HIV from entering lymphocytes by binding to CCR5 on cell membranes
- Route of Administration – oral
- Therapeutic Use – treats HIV infection in conjunction with other antiretroviral medications

Complications

ADVERSE EFFECTS	NURSING INTERVENTIONS/CLIENT EDUCATION
› Cough and upper respiratory tract infections	› Instruct client to report respiratory findings.
› CNS effects, such as dizziness, paresthesias	› Advise client to move carefully from lying or sitting to standing and prevent injury caused by dizziness.
› Hepatotoxicity (jaundice, right upper quadrant pain, nausea) often preceded by allergic reaction (hives, rash)	› Advise client to stop maraviroc and notify provider for these findings.

Contraindications/Precautions

- Contraindicated as the first medication to treat clients who have newly diagnosed HIV infection and also contraindicated with existing liver disease or during lactation.
- Use caution in clients who have existing cardiovascular disorders and in older adults.
- Pregnancy Risk Category B.

Interactions

MEDICATION/FOOD INTERACTIONS	NURSING INTERVENTIONS/CLIENT EDUCATION
› Most protease inhibitors raise maraviroc levels.	› Maraviroc dosage may need to be reduced.
› Rifampin, efavirenz, phenytoin, some other anticonvulsants, and St. John's wort decrease maraviroc levels.	› Maraviroc levels may need to be increased.

Nursing Administration

- Administer orally in conjunction with other antiretroviral medications.
- Monitor liver function tests, blood pressure, and CBC at baseline and periodically during treatment.

Nursing Evaluation of Medication Effectiveness

- Decrease in manifestations of HIV infection and remaining free from opportunistic infections

MEDICATION CLASSIFICATION: ANTIRETROVIRALS – NRTIs

- Select Prototype Medication: zidovudine (Retrovir)
- Other Medications
  - Didanosine (Videx)
  - Stavudine (Zerit)
  - Lamivudine (Epivir)
  - Abacavir (Ziagen)
- Combination Medications: fixed medication dosages in one tablet or capsule
  - Abacavir, lamivudine, zidovudine (Trizivir)
  - Abacavir, lamivudine (Epzicom)
  - Lamivudine, zidovudine (Combivir)

Purpose

- Expected Pharmacological Action – reduces HIV symptoms by inhibiting DNA synthesis and thus viral replication
- Therapeutic Use – first-line antiretrovirals to treat HIV infection
- Route of Administration – oral, IV

Complications

ADVERSE EFFECTS	NURSING INTERVENTIONS/CLIENT EDUCATION
› Zidovudine can cause suppressed bone marrow, resulting in anemia, agranulocytosis (neutropenia), and thrombocytopenia	› Monitor CBC and platelets. Instruct the client to monitor for bleeding, easy bruising, sore throat, and fatigue.
› Lactic acidosis	› Monitor for indications of lactic acidosis, such as hyperventilation, nausea, and abdominal pain. Pregnancy increases the risk of lactic acidosis.
› Nausea, vomiting, diarrhea	› Take medication with food to reduce gastric irritation. Monitor fluids and electrolytes.
› Hepatomegaly/fatty liver	› Monitor liver enzymes.

Contraindications/Precautions

- These medications are Pregnancy Risk Category C. Pregnancy increases risk for lactic acidosis, liver enlargement, and fatty liver.
- These medications are contraindicated in clients who have medication hypersensitivity.
- Use with caution in clients who have liver disease and bone marrow suppression.

Interactions

MEDICATION/FOOD INTERACTIONS	NURSING INTERVENTIONS/CLIENT EDUCATION
› Probenecid, valproic acid, and methadone can increase zidovudine.	› Reduce dosage. Monitor for medication toxicity.
› Ganciclovir or medications that decrease bone marrow production can further suppress bone marrow.	› Use together with caution.
› Rifampin and ritonavir can reduce zidovudine levels.	› Adjust dosage if needed.
› Phenytoin can alter both medication levels.	› Monitor medication levels.

Nursing Administration

- Monitor for bone marrow suppression. Obtain baseline CBC and platelets at the start of therapy and monitor periodically as needed.
- Anemia may be treated with epoetin alfa or transfusions.
- Neutropenia may be treated with colony-stimulating factors.
- Remind the client to take exactly as prescribed to minimize development of medication resistance.

Nursing Evaluation of Medication Effectiveness

- Depending on therapeutic intent, effectiveness can be evidenced by a reduction of symptoms and absence of opportunistic infection.

MEDICATION CLASSIFICATION: ANTIRETROVIRALS – NNRTIs

- Select Prototype Medications
  - Delavirdine (Rescriptor)
  - Efavirenz (Sustiva)
- Other Medications
  - Nevirapine (Viramune)
  - Etravirine (Intelence)

Purpose

- Expected Pharmacological Action – NNRTIs act directly on reverse transcriptase to stop HIV replication.
- Therapeutic Uses
  - Primary HIV-1 infection
  - Often used in combination with other antiretroviral agents to prevent medication resistance
- Route of administration – oral

Complications

ADVERSE EFFECTS	NURSING INTERVENTIONS/CLIENT EDUCATION
› Rash, which can become serious and lead to Stevens-Johnson syndrome	› Monitor for rash. Treat with diphenhydramine, if prescribed. › Notify the provider for fever or blistering.
› Flulike symptoms, headache, fatigue	› Monitor for adverse reactions. › Encourage rest and adequate oral fluid intake.
› CNS manifestations: dizziness, drowsiness, insomnia, nightmares (especially efavirenz)	› Advise client that these findings should decrease after first few weeks of therapy. › Client should not drive or operate machinery until effects are known.

Contraindications/Precautions

- Efavirenz is Pregnancy Risk Category D, including the first trimester. Delavirdine is Pregnancy Risk Category C.

- These medications are contraindicated in clients who have medication hypersensitivity.

- Use with caution in clients who have liver disease.

Interactions

MEDICATION/FOOD INTERACTIONS	NURSING INTERVENTIONS/CLIENT EDUCATION
› Antacids can decrease absorption of delavirdine.	› Allow 1 hr between medications.
› NNRTIs can increase effects of benzodiazepines, antihistamines, calcium channel blockers, ergot alkaloids, quinidine, warfarin, and others.	› Monitor for medication toxicity.
› Rifampin and phenytoin can cause decrease in levels of delavirdine.	› Do not use together.
› Didanosine can reduce both medications' absorption.	› Allow 1 hr between medications.
› NNRTIs can cause increase in sildenafil level.	› Monitor for hypotension and changes in vision. Use together with caution.

Nursing Administration

- Advise client to take exactly as prescribed and not skip doses to minimize development of resistance.

- Monitor for rash.

- Efavirenz should be taken at bedtime on an empty stomach to minimize adverse CNS effects.

- Advise client to take NNRTIs exactly as prescribed to minimize medication resistance.

Nursing Evaluation of Medication Effectiveness

- Depending on therapeutic intent, effectiveness can be evidenced by a reduction of symptoms and absence of any opportunistic infection.

MEDICATION CLASSIFICATION: ANTIRETROVIRALS – PROTEASE INHIBITORS

- Select Prototype Medication: ritonavir (Norvir)
- Other Medications
  - Saquinavir (Invirase)
  - Indinavir (Crixivan)
  - Fosamprenavir (Lexiva)
  - Nelfinavir (Viracept)
  - Lopinavir/ritonavir combination (Kaletra)

Purpose

- Expected Pharmacological Action – Protease inhibitors act against HIV-1 and HIV-2 to alter and inactivate the virus by inhibiting enzymes needed for HIV replication.
- Therapeutic Uses
  - Used to treat HIV infections.
  - Ritonavir is usually given with other PIs to increase their effect.
- Route of administration – oral

Complications

ADVERSE EFFECTS	NURSING INTERVENTIONS/CLIENT EDUCATION
› Bone loss/osteoporosis	› Advise client to eat a diet high in calcium and vitamin D. › Severe bone loss is treated with medications such as raloxifene and alendronate.
› Diabetes mellitus/ hyperglycemia	› Monitor serum glucose. Adjust diet and administer antidiabetic medications as prescribed. Advise clients to monitor for increased thirst and urine output.
› Hypersensitivity reaction	› Monitor for rash. Notify the provider if rash develops.
› Nausea and vomiting	› Take medication with food to reduce GI effects and increase absorption.
› Elevated serum lipids	› Monitor for hyperlipidemia. Adjust diet.
› Thrombocytopenia, leukopenia	› Monitor CBC. Monitor for indications of infection (fever, sore throat). Monitor for bleeding (blood in stool, bruising).

Contraindications/Precautions

- Protease inhibitors are Pregnancy Risk Category B medications.
- Use with caution in clients who have liver disease.
- Contraindicated with many other medications. Advise the client to notify the provider before taking any new medications.

Interactions

MEDICATION/FOOD INTERACTIONS	NURSING INTERVENTIONS/CLIENT EDUCATION
› All protease inhibitors (especially ritonavir) cause multiple medications (e.g., quinidine) to raise to toxic levels.	› Check any new medication with list of medications that must be avoided in clients taking protease inhibitors.
› Ritonavir can increase medication levels of sildenafil, tadalafil, and vardenafil.	› Use with caution. Dosages may need to be reduced.
› Ritonavir decreases levels of ethynyl estradiol in oral contraceptives.	› Instruct clients to use an alternative form of birth control.
› Phenobarbital, phenytoin, carbamazepine, and St. John's wort significantly reduce the level of protease inhibitors.	› Avoid concurrent use or adjust dosages.

Nursing Administration

- Instruct clients to report all other medications, including over-the-counter and herbal medications, to the provider.

- Except for indinavir (Crixivan), protease inhibitors should be given with food to increase absorption.

- Give concurrently with another antiretroviral to reduce risk of medication resistance.

Nursing Evaluation of Medication Effectiveness

- Depending on therapeutic intent, effectiveness can be evidenced reduction of HIV manifestations and absence of opportunistic infections.

MEDICATION CLASSIFICATION: ANTIRETROVIRALS – INTEGRASE INHIBITORS (INSTIs)

- Select Prototype Medication: raltegravir (Isentress)

Purpose

- Expected Pharmacological Action – interferes with the enzyme integrase to prevent HIV replication within the cell

- Therapeutic Use – a first-line treatment for HIV when combined with two to three other antiretroviral medications

- Route of administration – oral

Complications

ADVERSE EFFECTS	NURSING INTERVENTIONS/CLIENT EDUCATION
› Headache and difficulty sleeping	› Advise client to notify provider if these findings occur.
› Skin rash, which can indicate Stevens-Johnson syndrome or other serious disorder such as allergy	› Notify provider if rash or other skin manifestations occur.
› Liver injury (anorexia, nausea, right upper quadrant pain, jaundice)	› Monitor liver function tests. › Notify provider for indications of liver injury.

Contraindications/Precautions

- Contraindicated during lactation.
- Pregnancy Risk Category C.
- Use cautiously in clients younger than 16 years, older adult clients, or clients who have existing liver disorders.

Interactions

MEDICATION/FOOD INTERACTIONS	NURSING INTERVENTIONS/CLIENT EDUCATION
› Raltegravir may be decreased with concurrent use of rifampin or the combination tipranavir/ritonavir.	› Raltegravir dosage can need to be increased.

Nursing Administration

- Raltegravir may be taken with or without food.
- Monitor baseline and periodic liver function tests and CBC.
- Instruct client to take exactly as prescribed without skipping doses to prevent medication resistance.

Nursing Evaluation of Medication Effectiveness

- Depending on therapeutic intent, effectiveness can be evidenced by reduction of HIV manifestations and absence of opportunistic infections.

APPLICATION EXERCISES

1. A nurse is caring for a client who has a new diagnosis of HIV infection and is beginning combination oral NRTIs (abacavir, lamivudine, and zidovudine [Trizivir]). The client asks how medications work to treat HIV. Which of the following responses by the nurse is appropriate?

   A. "These medications block HIV entry into cells."

   B. "These medications weaken the cell wall of the HIV virus."

   C. "These medications inhibit enzymes to prevent HIV replication."

   D. "These medications prevent protein synthesis within the HIV cell."

2. A nurse is reinforcing teaching with a client about preventing medication resistance while taking highly active antiretroviral therapy (HAART) for HIV infection. Which of the following instructions should the nurse include about resistance?

   A. Taking low dosages of antiretroviral medication minimizes resistance.

   B. Taking one antiretroviral medication at a time minimizes resistance.

   C. Taking medication at the same times daily without skipping doses minimizes resistance.

   D. Changing the medication regimen when adverse effects occur minimizes resistance.

3. A nurse is caring for a client who takes several antiretroviral medications, including the NRTI zidovudine (Retrovir), to treat HIV infection. For which of the following adverse effects of zidovudine should the nurse monitor? (Select all that apply.)

   _____ A. Fatigue

   _____ B. Visual disturbances

   _____ C. Ataxia

   _____ D. Hyperventilation

   _____ E. Vomiting

4. A nurse is caring for a client who is taking ritonavir (Norvir), a protease inhibitor, to treat HIV infection. For which of the following abnormalities in laboratory values should the nurse monitor?

   A. Increased TSH and T_4 levels

   B. Decreased ALT and AST levels

   C. Hypoglycemia

   D. Hyperlipidemia

5. A nurse is caring for a client who is starting enfuvirtide (Fuzeon) to treat HIV infection. For which of the adverse reactions should the nurse monitor? (Select all that apply.)

_____ A. Stools or emesis for bleeding

_____ B. Breath sounds for pneumonia

_____ C. Level of consciousness for cerebral edema

_____ D. Injection site for erythema

_____ E. Blood pressure for hypersensitivity reaction

6. A nurse is administering IV acyclovir (Zovirax) to a client who has varicella and is immunocompromised. Which of the following nursing actions is appropriate?

A. Administer a test dose of 0.1 mg acyclovir before starting the regular infusion.

B. Decrease fluid intake during and for 2 hr following acyclovir infusion to prevent fluid overload.

C. Administer acyclovir infusion over at least 1 hr.

D. Monitor for a severe infusion reaction within 15 min after acyclovir infusion is started.

7. A nurse is caring for a client who is immunocompromised and is receiving ganciclovir IV twice daily to prevent cytomegalovirus (CMV). What instructions should the nurse reinforce with the client about this medication? Use the ATI Active Learning Template: Medication to complete this item to include the following:

A. Therapeutic Use: Identify for ganciclovir in this client.

B. Adverse Effects: Identify two.

C. Diagnostic Tests: Describe two the nurse should monitor.

D. Nursing Interventions: Describe two nursing actions for clients taking ganciclovir.

APPLICATION EXERCISES KEY

1.   A. INCORRECT: The fusion/entry inhibitor enfuvirtide (Fuzeon) and the CCR5 antagonist maraviroc (Selzentry) are newer antiretroviral medications that work by blocking HIV entry into cells.

   B. INCORRECT: Some bactericidal antibiotics, such as penicillin, work by weakening the cell walls of bacteria.

   C. **CORRECT:** The NRTI antiretroviral medications work by inhibiting the enzyme reverse transcriptase and preventing HIV replication.

   D. INCORRECT: Some antibiotics, such as the aminoglycosides, kill bacteria by preventing protein synthesis within the cell.

   (N) NCLEX® Connection: Pharmacological Therapies, Expected Actions/Outcomes

2.   A. INCORRECT: Taking low dosages of the medication may cause medication resistance.

   B. INCORRECT: Taking a combination of antiretroviral medications helps prevent resistance to each medication. Resistance occurs quickly if only one medication is taken.

   C. **CORRECT:** Skipping even a few doses of antiretroviral medication can promote medication resistance, which can cause treatment failure. The nurse should emphasize the importance of taking each dose of medication exactly as prescribed.

   D. INCORRECT: Changing the medication regimen when adverse effects occur can promote medication resistance.

   (N) NCLEX® Connection: Pharmacological Therapies, Medication Administration

3.   A. **CORRECT:** Fatigue is a manifestation of anemia that can occur in clients taking zidovudine. Neutropenia can also occur, causing a high risk for infection.

   B. INCORRECT: Visual disturbances are not an expected adverse effect of zidovudine.

   C. INCORRECT: Ataxia is not an expected adverse effect of zidovudine.

   D. **CORRECT:** Hyperventilation is a finding that can occur if the client develops lactic acidosis, a serious adverse effect of zidovudine.

   E. **CORRECT:** Vomiting and other GI effects can occur in the client who takes zidovudine.

   (N) NCLEX® Connection: Pharmacological Therapies, Adverse Effects/Contraindications/ Side Effects/Interactions

4. A. INCORRECT: Increased TSH and T4 levels indicate hyperthyroidism, which is not an adverse effect of ritonavir.

    B. INCORRECT: An increase, rather than a decrease, in liver function tests, including AST and ALT levels, can occur as an adverse effect of ritonavir. Serum transaminase also can be elevated, indicating liver injury.

    C. INCORRECT: Hyperglycemia indicating a possible onset or worsening of diabetes mellitus, rather than hypoglycemia, can occur as an adverse effect of ritonavir.

    D. **CORRECT:** Hyperlipidemia with increased cholesterol and triglyceride levels can occur as an adverse effect of ritonavir.

    Ⓝ NCLEX® Connection: Pharmacological Therapies, Adverse Effects/Contraindications/ Side Effects/Interactions

5. A. INCORRECT: Bleeding is not an adverse effect of enfuvirtide.

    B. **CORRECT:** Bacterial pneumonia with fever, cough, and difficulty breathing are manifestations of an adverse reaction to enfuvirtide. The nurse should evaluate breath sounds regularly.

    C. INCORRECT: Cerebral edema is not an adverse reaction to enfuvirtide.

    D. **CORRECT:** Enfuvirtide is administered subcutaneously, and injection-site reactions such as pain, redness, itching, and bruising are common.

    E. **CORRECT:** A systemic allergic reaction can occur when taking enfuvirtide. Manifestations of hypersensitivity include rash, hypotension, fever, and chills.

    Ⓝ NCLEX® Connection: Pharmacological Therapies, Adverse Effects/Contraindications/ Side Effects/Interactions

6. A. INCORRECT: A test dose of acyclovir is not necessary. Acyclovir does not cause frequent severe allergic reactions.

    B. INCORRECT: It is important to increase, rather than decrease, fluid intake during and for 2 hr following acyclovir infusing in order to prevent nephrotoxicity.

    C. **CORRECT:** It is important o administer IV acyclovir slowing, over at least 1 hr, in order to prevent nephrotoxicity.

    D. INCORRECT: A severe infusion reaction is not an expected effect during acyclovir infusion.

    Ⓝ NCLEX® Connection: Pharmacological Therapies, Medication Administration

7. *Using the ATI Active Learning Template: Medication*

A. Therapeutic Use
- Ganciclovir prevents reproduction of viral DNA and thus prevents viral cell replication. Its only use is to prevent or treat cytomegalovirus in clients who are immunocompromised.

B. Adverse Effects
- Minor discomforts, such as fever, headache, and nausea
- Suppresses the bone marrow, causing a decrease in WBCs, especially granulocytes
- Causes thrombocytopenia frequently
  ○ Client should report any discomforts and be sure to report new onset of fatigue, easy bruising, or sore throat.

C. Diagnostic Tests
- Client blood counts, especially WBC, absolute neutrophil count, and thrombocyte count
  ○ The nurse should expect ganciclovir therapy to be interrupted for an absolute neutrophil count of less than 500/mm³ or a thrombocyte count of less than 25,000/mm³.

D. Nursing Interventions
- Monitor blood counts.
- Prepare to administer granulocyte colony-stimulating factors for a low absolute neutrophil count.
- Monitor I&O and encourage the client to increase fluid intake.
- Avoid direct contact with the powder from oral ganciclovir or the IV solution and wash well if contact occurs.

(N) NCLEX® Connection: Pharmacological Therapies, Expected Actions/Outcomes

Berman, A. J., & Snyder S. (2012). *Fundamentals of nursing: Concepts, process, and practice* (9th ed.). Upper Saddle River, NJ: Prentice-Hall.

Dudek, S. G. (2010). *Nutrition essentials for nursing practice* (6th ed.). Philadelphia: Lippincott Williams & Wilkins.

Ford, S. M., & Roach, S. S. (2013). *Roach's introductory clinical pharmacology* (10th ed.). Philadelphia: Lippincott Williams & Wilkins.

Grodner, M., Roth, S. L., & Walkingshaw, B. C. (2012). *Nutrition Foundations and clinical applications of nutrition: A nursing approach* (5th ed.). St. Louis, MO: Mosby.

Ignatavicius, D. D., & Workman, M. L. (2013). *Medical-surgical nursing* (7th ed.). St. Louis, MO: Saunders.

Lehne, R. A. (2013). *Pharmacology for nursing care* (8th ed.). St. Louis: Saunders.

Lilley, L. L., Harrington, S., & Snyder, J. S. (2014). *Pharmacology and the nursing process* (7th Ed.). St. Louis, MO: Mosby.

Lowdermilk, D. L., Perry, S. E., Cahsion, M. C., & Aldean, K. R. (2012). *Maternity & women's health care* (10th ed.). St. Louis, MO: Mosby.

Potter, P. A., Perry, A. G., Stockert, P., & Hall, A. (2013). *Fundamentals of nursing* (8th ed.). St. Louis, MO: Mosby.

Smeltzer, S. C., Bare, B. G., Hinkle, J. L., & Cheever, K. H. (2010). *Brunner and Suddarth's textbook of medical-surgical nursing* (12th ed.). Philadelphia: Lippincott Williams & Wilkins.

Touhy, T. A., & Jett, K. F. (2012) *Ebersole & Hess' toward healthy aging: Human needs and nursing response* (8th ed.). St. Lois, MO: Mosby.

Wilson, B. A., Shannon, M. T., & Shields, K. M. (2013). *Pearson nurse's drug guide 2013*. Upper Saddle River, NJ: Prentice Hall.

CONTENT _____ REVIEW MODULE CHAPTER _____

TOPIC DESCRIPTOR_____

Related Content (e.g. delegation, levels of prevention, advance directives)	Underlying Principles	Nursing Interventions › Who? › When? › Why? › How?

Appendix

CONTENT _____ REVIEW MODULE CHAPTER _____

TOPIC DESCRIPTOR_____

DESCRIPTION OF PROCEDURE:

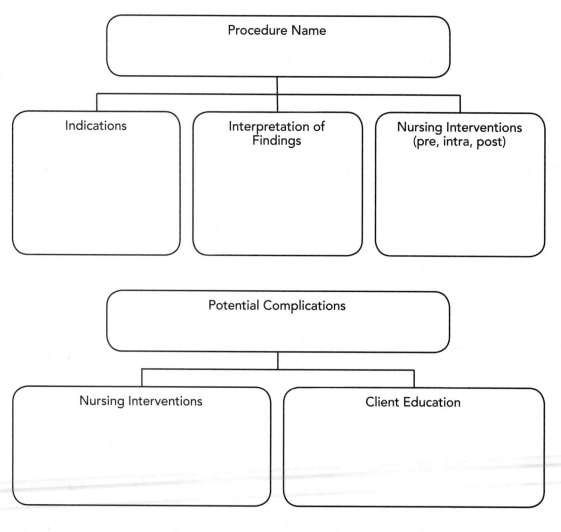

Procedure Name

Indications

Interpretation of Findings

Nursing Interventions (pre, intra, post)

Potential Complications

Nursing Interventions

Client Education

CONTENT _____   REVIEW MODULE CHAPTER _____

TOPIC DESCRIPTOR_____

| Alteration in Health (Diagnosis) | Client Problem Related to Alteration in Health | Pathophysiology Related to Client Problem |

Safety Considerations

Assessment

- Past Medical History
- Medications
- Risk Factors
- Laboratory Data
- Objective and Subjective Data
- Diagnostic Procedures/ Surgical Interventions

Teamwork and Collaboration

- Discharge Planning
- Interprofessional Care
- Coordination of Client Care

Nursing Interventions (Evidence-Based)

Client Education

Outcomes/Evaluations

Appendix

CONTENT _____ REVIEW MODULE CHAPTER _____

TOPIC DESCRIPTOR_____

```
┌─────────────────────────────────────┐
│         Developmental Stage          │
│                                      │
└─────────────────────────────────────┘
```

Physical Development	Cognitive Development	Age-Appropriate Activities

```
┌─────────────────────────────────────┐
│           Health Promotion           │
│                                      │
└─────────────────────────────────────┘
```

Immunizations	Health Screening	Nutrition	Injury Prevention

CONTENT _____ REVIEW MODULE CHAPTER _____

TOPIC DESCRIPTOR_____

MEDICATION _____

EXPECTED PHARMALOGICAL ACTION:

Therapeutic Uses

Adverse Effects

Nursing Interventions

Contraindications

Client Education

Medication/Food Interactions

Medication Administration

Evaluation of Medication Effectiveness

Appendix

CONTENT _____ REVIEW MODULE CHAPTER _____

TOPIC DESCRIPTOR _____

DESCRIPTION OF SKILL:

```
                          ┌─────────────────────────────┐
                          │      Procedure Name          │
                          │                              │
                          └─────────────────────────────┘
                                       │
         ┌─────────────────────────────┼─────────────────────────────┐
┌─────────────────┐        ┌─────────────────────┐        ┌─────────────────────┐
│   Indications   │        │ Nursing Interventions│        │ Outcomes/Evaluations│
│                 │        │  (pre, intra, post)  │        │                     │
│                 │        │                      │        │                     │
│                 │        │                      │        │                     │
│                 │        │                      │        │                     │
└─────────────────┘        └─────────────────────┘        └─────────────────────┘


                          ┌─────────────────────────────┐
                          │   Potential Complications    │
                          │                              │
                          └─────────────────────────────┘
                                       │
              ┌────────────────────────┴────────────────────────┐
┌───────────────────────────┐              ┌───────────────────────────┐
│   Nursing Interventions    │              │     Client Education       │
│                            │              │                            │
│                            │              │                            │
│                            │              │                            │
└───────────────────────────┘              └───────────────────────────┘
```

CONTENT _____ REVIEW MODULE CHAPTER _____

TOPIC DESCRIPTOR_____

DESCRIPTION OF PROCEDURE:

```
                        ┌─────────────────────────────┐
                        │      Procedure Name          │
                        └─────────────────────────────┘
```

Indications	Nursing Interventions (pre, intra, post)	Outcomes/Evaluations

```
                        ┌─────────────────────────────┐
                        │   Potential Complications    │
                        └─────────────────────────────┘
```

Nursing Interventions	Client Education